A GUIDE TO
ORAL COMMUNICATION
IN VETERINARY MEDICINE

A GUIDE TO ORAL COMMUNICATION IN VETERINARY MEDICINE

Ryane E. Englar, DVM, DABVP (Canine and Feline Practice)

Associate Professor
University of Arizona College of Veterinary Medicine
Oro Valley, AZ

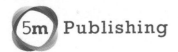 Publishing

First published 2020

Copyright © Ryane E. Englar 2020

Published by
5M Publishing Ltd,
Benchmark House,
8 Smithy Wood Drive,
Sheffield, S35 1QN, UK
Tel: +44 (0) 1234 81 81 80
www.5mpublishing.com

A Catalogue record for this book is available from the British Library

ISBN 9781789180954

Book layout by Toynbee Editorial Services Ltd, Great Easton, UK

Printed by Replika Press Pvt Ltd, India

Photos by the author unless otherwise indicated

Contents

Contents   v
About the Author   xv
Preface   xvii
Dedication   xxi
Acknowledgments   xxv
About the companion website   xxxi
List of Acronyms   xxxiii

PART I   CLINICAL COMMUNICATION AS AN INTEGRAL PART OF THE VETERINARY PROFESSION   1

CHAPTER 1   WHAT DO OUR CLIENTS UNDERSTAND? THE EVOLUTION OF THE DOCTOR–PATIENT RELATIONSHIP, PATIENT AUTONOMY, AND HEALTH LITERACY   3

    1.1 The Development of Medical Paternalism   4
    1.2 The Limitations of Medical Paternalism   6
    1.3 The Evolution of Relationship–Centered Care   7
    1.4 The Modernization of Medicine Drives Relationship–Centered Care   8
    1.5 The Concept of Health Literacy   10
    1.6 How Do Health Literacy and Relationship–Centered Care Apply to Veterinary Medicine?   15

CHAPTER 2   HOW CAN WE HELP OUR CLIENTS TO UNDERSTAND? THE EMERGENCE OF CLINICAL COMMUNICATION AS A TEACHABLE SCIENCE   27

    2.1 Connectivity and the Provider–Patient Relationship   28
    2.2 Past Assumptions about Relationship-Centered Care   29
    2.3 Challenging Past Assumptions   29
    2.4 The Kalamazoo Consensus Statement and Relationship-Centered Care   31
    2.5 The Changing Face of Medical Education   32

2.6 The Changing Face of Veterinary Education 33

2.7 Communication as a Teachable Skill 36

2.8 Present-Day Challenges Associated with Teaching
Communication 39

2.9 The Future of Communication Training in Veterinary Curricula 42

CHAPTER 3 **HOW CAN WE STRUCTURE THE CONSULTATION FROM THE VANTAGE POINT OF CLINICAL COMMUNICATION? THE CALGARY–CAMBRIDGE GUIDE AS A BLUEPRINT FOR A COLLABORATIVE CONSULTATION** **49**

3.1 The Shift from Medical Paternalism to Relationship-Centered Care 49

3.2 Relationship-Centered Care in Veterinary Medicine 50

3.3 The Development of Consultation Models 50

3.4 The Calgary–Cambridge Model 53

3.5 The Revised Calgary–Cambridge Model for Veterinary Patients 57

3.6 Limitations of Consultation Models 58

PART II **DEFINING ORAL COMMUNICATION SKILLS AS THEY RELATE TO THE VETERINARY CONSULTATION** **65**

CHAPTER 4 **FIRST IMPRESSIONS** **67**

4.1 Our Journey through Healthcare as Consumers 67

4.2 The Veterinary Client's Experience 69

4.3 Starting the Client's Journey off on the Right Foot 69

4.4 Prep Work May Seem Silly, But ... 70

4.5 Greeting the Client: What the Veterinary Team Can Learn from
Human Healthcare 71

4.6 Greeting the Veterinary Client: Finding Common Ground 74

4.7 Attending to the Client's Comfort 78

4.8 Acknowledging and Attending to the Patient 80

CHAPTER 5 **DEFINING ENTRY-LEVEL COMMUNICATION SKILLS: REFLECTIVE LISTENING** **85**

5.1 Introduction to Reflective Listening 86

5.2 Clinical Conversations, Defined 87

5.3 Why Should Healthcare Providers Listen? 87

5.4 Why Is Effective Listening such a Difficult Task? 88

5.5 Active or Reflective Listening, Defined 89

5.6 Active Listening Requires Preparation 90

5.7 Active Listening in Veterinary Practice 91

5.8 Examples of Active Listening Statements in Veterinary Consultations 92

CHAPTER 6 **DEFINING ENTRY-LEVEL COMMUNICATION SKILLS:
EMPATHY** **98**

6.1 Cognitive Empathy 98
6.2 Missed Opportunities for Empathetic Displays in Healthcare 99
6.3 Emotional Empathy 103
6.4 The Impact of Empathy on Case Outcomes 103
6.5 Empathy versus Sympathy 104
6.6 The Human–Animal Bond Creates Opportunities for Empathy
in Veterinary Practice 105
6.7 The Dangers of Making Assumptions about Client Emotions 106
6.8 When Might Clients Become Emotional? 106
6.9 The Challenges Associated with Empathetic Displays in
Clinical Practice 107
6.10 Displaying Empathy through Actions in Clinical Practice 109
6.11 Displaying Empathy through Words in Clinical Practice 109
6.12 The Potential Dangers of Empathy in Clinical Practice: the
Client's Perspective 111
6.13 The Potential Dangers of Empathy in Clinical Practice: the
Clinician's Perspective 111
6.14 The Decline of Empathy? 113

CHAPTER 7 **DEFINING ENTRY-LEVEL COMMUNICATION SKILLS:
NONVERBAL CUES** **121**

7.1 The History of Nonverbal Cues in Clinical Conversations 123
7.2 The Importance of Nonverbal Cues in Clinical Conversations 124
7.3 What Contributes to Accuracy in Judgment Making Based
upon Fleeting Observations? 124
7.4 What Are Nonverbal Cues? 125
7.5 Kinesics 125
7.6 Proxemics 135
7.7 Paralanguage 138
7.8 Autonomic Shifts 140
7.9 Revisiting the Impact of Nonverbal Cues on Clinical
Conversations 141
7.10 When Words and Nonverbal Cues Do Not Align: How to
Handle Mixed Messages 142
7.11 Nonverbal Skills Development 143

CHAPTER 8   DEFINING ENTRY-LEVEL COMMUNICATION SKILLS:
OPEN-ENDED QUESTIONS AND STATEMENTS   149

8.1 The Comprehensive Patient History   149
8.2 Why is it Critical to Elicit the Patient's Concerns? The Human
     Medical Perspective   152
8.3 Why is it Critical to Elicit the Client's Concerns? The Veterinary
     Perspective   152
8.4 Noncompliance in Healthcare   153
8.5 The Art of Listening and the Dangers of Interrupting during History
     Taking   153
8.6 The Art of History Taking: Introducing Two Styles of Questioning 155
8.7 Closed-Ended Questions, Defined   156
8.8 The Open-Ended Question or Statement   159
8.9 Is there a Place for Both Open- and Closed-Ended Questions? 163
8.10 Client Preferences for Open-Ended Questions Based upon
     Species   164

CHAPTER 9   DEFINING SUPPLEMENTAL COMMUNICATION SKILLS:
REDUCING MEDICAL JARGON   169

9.1 Defining Medical Jargon   170
9.2 The Limitations of Medical Jargon: the Provider's Perspective 170
9.3 The Limitations of Medical Jargon: the Patient's Perspective 173
9.4 Easy-to-Understand Language Implies Transparency   178
9.5 Implications for the Veterinary Medical Profession   179
9.6 Strategies for Overcoming the Use of Medical Jargon   181

CHAPTER 10 ENHANCING RELATIONSHIP-CENTERED CARE THROUGH
PARTNERSHIP   190

10.1 The Shift towards Partnership   191
10.2 Are Veterinary Clients Experts?   192
10.3 Setting the Stage for Relationship-Centered Care   193
10.4 Establishing Partnership with the Client   194

CHAPTER 11 ELICITING THE CLIENT'S PERSPECTIVE TO ENHANCE RELATIONSHIP-
CENTERED CARE   202

11.1 Phrases that Effectively Elicit the Client's Perspective 203
11.2 Softening These Phrases   204
11.3 What Happens When We Do Not Use This Skill   205
11.4 Revisiting the Same Scenario and Eliciting the Client's Perspective 205

11.5 Eliciting the Client's Perspective Also Helps Clients Open Up about Treatment Preferences   206

CHAPTER 12 ASKING PERMISSION TO ENHANCE RELATIONSHIP-CENTERED CARE   **211**

12.1 Incorporating Permission Statements into Clinical Scenarios   213
12.2 What if the Client Doesn't Say "Yes"?   214
12.3 Alternative Phrasing of "May I?"   215
12.4 Other Clinical Scenarios that Benefit from Asking Permission   216
12.5 The Clinical Importance of Asking for Permission among Dog and Cat Owners   221

CHAPTER 13 ENHANCING RELATIONSHIP-CENTERED CARE BY ASSESSING THE CLIENT'S KNOWLEDGE   **224**

13.1 What Happens When We Do Not Assess the Client's Knowledge?   227
13.2 Revisiting the Same Scenario to Assess our Client's Knowledge   228
13.3 Other Reasons to Assess our Client's Knowledge   229
13.4 Assessing Knowledge Is Respectful   230

CHAPTER 14 MAPPING OUT THE CLINICAL CONSULTATION: SIGNPOSTING   **232**

14.1 Defining the Consultation Map   234
14.2 Using Signposting to Outline Differentials   236
14.3 Using Signposting to Discuss Treatment Plans   236
14.4 Using Signposting to Rein in a Chatty Client   237
14.5 Using Signposting to Preface Actions, Such as Reviewing the Medical Record   238
14.6 Using Mapping Statements as Caution Signs, So-Called "Warning Shots"   240

CHAPTER 15 COMMUNICATION SKILLS THAT FACILITATE CLIENT COMPREHENSION: SUMMARIZING AND CHECKING IN WITH THE CLIENT   **245**

15.1 Summarizing   247
15.2 Internal Summaries, Defined   248
15.3 End-of-Consultation Summaries   252
15.4 "Chunk and Check"   257

CHAPTER 16 COMMUNICATION SKILLS THAT FACILITATE COMPLIANCE: CONTRACTING FOR NEXT STEPS 261

16.1 Defining "Contracting for Next Steps" 263
16.2 Examples of Contracting for Next Steps in Clinical Practice 265
16.3 Contracting for Next Steps Tells the Client What to Expect 267
16.4 Contracting for Next Steps Reinforces Our Role in Patient Care 268
16.5 Modifying How Contracting for Next Steps Is Phrased 268
16.6 Be Prepared for the Client to Say "No" to the Initial Plan 269

CHAPTER 17 AGENDA-SETTING AND THE FINAL "CHECK-IN" 271

17.1 The Value of Agenda-Setting 273
17.2 The Final Check-In as a Relationship Builder 276
17.3 Pairing the Final Check-In with Appropriate Nonverbal Cues 276
17.4 What If the Client Does Not Stop Talking? 278

CHAPTER 18 DEFINING TWO NEW SKILLS THAT COMPANION-ANIMAL CLIENTS VALUE: COMPASSIONATE TRANSPARENCY AND UNCONDITIONAL POSITIVE REGARD 282

18.1 What Is Transparency in Healthcare? 285
18.2 Barriers to Transparency in Healthcare 286
18.3 Transparency in Veterinary Medicine through Words 287
18.4 Transparency in Veterinary Medicine through Actions 288
18.5 Veterinary Clinical Scenarios that Involve Transparency 288
18.6 Example of a Situation that Would Have Benefited from Transparency 289
18.7 Unconditional Positive Regard in Healthcare 290
18.8 Unconditional Positive Regard in Veterinary Medicine 291
18.9 Veterinary Clinical Scenarios that Involve Unconditional Positive Regard 292

PART III APPLYING COMMUNICATION SKILLS TO EVERYDAY CONVERSATIONS IN CLINICAL PRACTICE 297

CHAPTER 19 USING COMMUNICATION SKILLS TO INITIATE THE CONSULTATION 299

19.1 Preparing for the Visit 300
19.2 Developing Rapport 303
19.3 Identifying the Presenting Complaint 303

CHAPTER 20 USING COMMUNICATION SKILLS TO GATHER DATA: HISTORY TAKING   311

    20.1 Taking a Complete History at a Wellness Appointment   313
    20.2 Taking a Complete History at a Sick Visit   318

CHAPTER 21 USING COMMUNICATION SKILLS TO GATHER DATA: EXPLAINING AND PLANNING   325

    21.1 Explaining Physical Examination Findings in an Apparently Healthy Patient   327
    21.2 Explaining Physical Examination Findings in an Ill Patient   331
    21.3 Forward Planning   335
    21.4 Planning Next Steps in an Apparently Healthy Patient   336
    21.5 Planning Next Steps in an Ill Patient   341

PART IV TESTING YOUR UNDERSTANDING OF ORAL COMMUNICATION SKILLS IN VETERINARY MEDICINE   347

CHAPTER 22 END-OF-CHAPTER READING COMPREHENSION QUESTIONS   359

CHAPTER 23 WORKBOOK-STYLE EXERCISES   359

    Exercise 23.1 – Defining Communication Skills I   359
    Exercise 23.2 – Defining Communication Skills II   360
    Exercise 23.3 – Examples of Communication Skills in Use I   361
    Exercise 23.4 – Examples of Communication Skills in Use II   362
    Exercise 23.5 – Open- vs Closed-Ended Questions I   363
    Exercise 23.6 – Open- vs Closed-Ended Questions II   364
    Exercise 23.7 – Converting Closed-Ended Questions into Open-Ended Questions   365
    Exercise 23.8 – Converting Open-Ended Questions into Closed-Ended Questions   366
    Exercise 23.9 – Reflective Listening I   367
    Exercise 23.10 – Reflective Listening II   368
    Exercise 23.11 – Empathy I   370
    Exercise 23.12 – Empathy II   372
    Exercise 23.13 – Nonverbal Cues   374
    Exercise 23.14 – Barriers to Communication   374
    Exercise 23.15 – Reducing Barriers to Communication   375
    Exercise 23.16 – Body Language and Communication I   375

Exercise 23.17 – Body Language and Communication II · 376
Exercise 23.18 – Medical Jargon I · 377
Exercise 23.19 – Medical Jargon II · 378
Exercise 23.20 – Medical Jargon III · 379
Exercise 23.21 – Medical Jargon IV · 380
Exercise 23.22 – Medical Jargon V · 381
Exercise 23.23 – Medical Jargon VI · 382
Exercise 23.24 – Partnership · 383
Exercise 23.25 – Eliciting the Client's Perspective · 384
Exercise 23.26 – Assessing the Client's Knowledge · 385
Exercise 23.27 – Signposting I · 386
Exercise 23.28 – Signposting II · 386
Exercise 23.29 – Signposting and Transparency · 387
Exercise 23.30 – Putting It All Together · 388

CHAPTER 24 ANSWER KEY TO WORKBOOK-STYLE EXERCISES · 390

CHAPTER 25 CLINICAL VIGNETTES FOR ROLE PLAY · 409

Scenario 25.1: Greeting the Client at a Wellness Visit I · 410
Scenario 25.2: Greeting the Client at a Wellness Visit II · 410
Scenario 25.3: Greeting the Returning Client I · 410
Scenario 25.4: Greeting the Returning Client II · 411
Scenario 25.5: Taking a Clinical History at the Wellness Visit – Feline · 411
Scenario 25.6: Taking a Clinical History at the Wellness Visit – Canine · 412
Scenario 25.7: Taking a Clinical History at a Sick Visit – Feline I · 413
Scenario 25.8: Taking a Clinical History at a Sick Visit – Feline II · 414
Scenario 25.9: Taking a Clinical History at a Sick Visit – Canine I · 415
Scenario 25.10: Taking a Clinical History at a Sick Visit – Canine II · 416
Scenario 25.11: Explaining Physical Examination Findings – Feline I · 418
Scenario 25.12: Explaining Physical Examination Findings – Feline II · 419
Scenario 25.13: Explaining Physical Examination Findings – Canine I · 420
Scenario 25.14: Explaining Physical Examination Findings – Canine II · 422
Scenario 25.15: Explaining Radiographs I · 423
Scenario 25.16: Explaining Radiographs II · 424
Scenario 25.17: Explaining Radiographs III · 425

Scenario 25.18: Explaining Radiographs IV   427
Scenario 25.19: Explaining Bloodwork I   428
Scenario 25.20: Explaining Bloodwork II   429

Index   433

About the Author

Ryane E. Englar, DVM, DABVP (Canine and Feline Practice) graduated from Cornell University College of Veterinary Medicine in 2008. She practiced as an associate veterinarian in companion animal practice before transitioning into the educational realm as an advocate for pre-clinical training in primary care. She began her debut in academia as a Clinical Instructor of the Community Practice Service at Cornell University's Hospital for Animals. She then transitioned into the role of Assistant Professor as founding faculty at Midwestern University College of Veterinary Medicine. While at Midwestern University, she had the opportunity to work with the inaugural Class of 2018, the Class of 2019, and the Class of 2020. While training these remarkable young professionals, Dr. Englar became a Diplomat of the American Board of Veterinary Practitioners (ABVP; Canine and Feline Practice). She relocated to Kansas State University in May 2017 to design and debut the Clinical Skills curriculum. She is currently on faculty at the University of Arizona College of Veterinary Medicine. Her research areas of interest include clinical communication and educational outcomes.

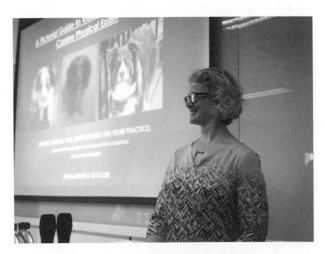

Dr. Englar is passionate about advancing education for generalists by thinking outside of the box to develop new course materials for the hands-on learner. This labor of love

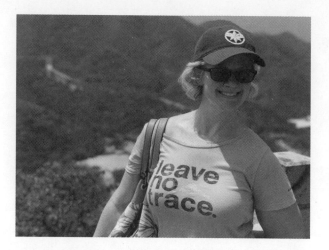

is preceded by three texts that collectively provide students and clinicians alike with functional, relatable, and practice-friendly tools for success:

- *Performing the Small Animal Physical Examination* (John Wiley & Sons, Inc., 2017)
- *Writing Skills for Veterinarians* (5M Publishing, Ltd., 2019)
- *Common Clinical Presentations in Dogs and Cats* (John Wiley & Sons, Inc., 2019)

Dr. Englar's students fuel her desire to create. They inspire her to develop the tools that they need to succeed in clinical practice. If the goal of educators, as they are tasked by the accrediting bodies, is to create "Day One", so-called "Practice-Ready" veterinarians, then this text and her others complement the mission.

When she is not teaching or advancing primary care, she trains in the art of ballroom dancing and competes nationally with her instructor, Lowell E. Fox.

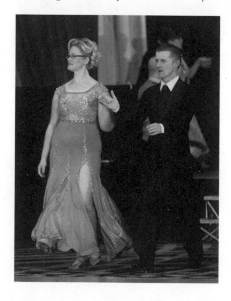

Preface

People are curious about our profession. It is why conversations about who we are and what we do follow us wherever we go: on buses or planes, boats or trains, whether travel is national or abroad. Our seatmates seem compelled to ask about our professional lives.

Animal Planet enthusiasts want to know if everything they see on television is real. They ask if there are really dog cardiologists and cat eye doctors, and if it's true that hip replacements can be performed on alpacas.

Fans of *Gray's Anatomy* and *The Good Doctor* often ask how we stomach the blood and gore of emergency medicine, trauma, and surgery. They are inspired, yet intimidated that veterinarians can wear so many hats to be so many things for so many people.

Those who are aware that mental health issues plague our community often inquire about our physical and emotional wellbeing. They ask how we find balance between bringing our patients into this world and taking them out of it. They thank us for our service. They ask us what we need.

Others do not recognize that rain precedes rainbows, and ask only what it is like to play with kittens and puppies all day. I used to cringe, but now I see it as a learning opportunity to provide a more accurate frame of reference for the professional identity that we wear on our sleeves, right alongside our hearts.

From this rather eclectic mix of questions, typically one theme emerges. Non-veterinary acquaintances often ask what propelled me to become a veterinarian. Their quest to understand me and my career aspirations often ends with a variation of this sentiment:

"Why didn't you become a human doctor?" they ask. "Don't you like people?"

The answer is shockingly simple, yet it often surprises my audience: "Yes. Yes, I like people."

It is not at all what they were expecting to hear.

In truth, to be a successful veterinarian, you have to like, care about, and respect people. Your patients are attached to owners. Your owners will come to your door with past life experiences, personalities, and perspective.

You will never have the opportunity to get to know, medically manage, operate on, treat, or cure animals unless the person who is tethered to the other end of the leash or travel carrier seeks out you and your services.

Veterinary education emphasizes how to treat animal patients – and rightly so. You cannot be a proficient clinician unless you understand the animal body, in health and disease. You cannot be a competent surgeon unless you commit your mind and muscle memory to learning anatomic landmarks, instrument ties, and gentle tissue handling skills.

Yet, in reality, you cannot take any of these actions without client consent. In the poker game of life, your clients hold the cards. They determine whether to play (commit to care), hold (consider care), or fold them (decline care altogether). In the absence of financial constraints, how you treat your patients' people determines the level of care that you and your team can provide.

Client communication is essential both to the delivery of high quality medicine and to the success of veterinary practice. Today's clients come armed with knowledge and questions. They have access to information at their fingertips that their parents and their grandparents never had. They have formulated their own opinions and ideas. They have insight and intuition.

We may be the expert in the consultation room about medicine, but they are the experts about their pets. Nothing can be accomplished in terms of healthcare unless we take active measures to deconstruct this artificial divide.

We should not fear that our client is perhaps our best resource. Our role as educator is antiquated only if we let it be, that is, if we expect to be the "sage on the stage" and assume that our client has nothing to offer us.

Quite the contrary, our client holds the key to patient outcomes. Much of whether a patient's health status improves depends upon client compliance and adherence to our recommendations. There must be client "buy-in." We lose both "buy-in" and our credibility the moment we fail to see common ground (the wellbeing of the pet) and fail to engage the client in shared decision making.

The era of relationship-centered care has only just begun. It is not going away. The fact that pet care is in many ways client-driven challenges us as professionals to partner with "pet parents" to effect change. Our ability to manage patients' healthcare rides on our willingness to listen and communicate, both of which are teachable skills.

Communication drives relationships and connectivity. It builds client loyalty and encourages client retention. It creates a safe and supportive environment for client interactions with the veterinary team. A client who feels respected is more likely to exhibit transparency with information-sharing, or ask questions about treatment options.

When there is dialogue, there is hope for mutual understanding.

Dialogue may not always lead to agreement or perfect outcomes, but it forges a bond that communicates, "I am here, and I am listening. Help me to help you help your loved one."

Communication drives action as much as it drives relationships. Communication is how we accomplish all that we do. Patient care is only as effective as we can convey its value, through words and non-verbal cues.

Communication is therefore not just an art or "soft science." Communication is not something you are either born with or without. Communication is not just a nicety or an added bonus.

Communication is an evidence-based discipline that our clients depend upon in order for them to have what they need to make educated decisions.

For that reason, communication is a job requirement as much as the capacity for clinical acumen, hand-eye coordination, and surgical prowess.

It behooves us to learn how to be better speakers so that, at the end of the day, we can be better people to other people who have called upon us. What they need is precisely what we can give, but only if we can effectively communicate our desire to help them experience, sustain, and nurture companionship.

Our clients do what they do, not in spite of this bond, but because of it, each day, every day, all so that they might come to know the love of a dog or the love of a cat.

That love and humanity speaks to us, as veterinarians.

It's our responsibility to learn how to speak back.

Dedication

I live and dream in photographs. I work best when I am surrounded by them. I smile when I look at the faces of those who mean so much, and they smile back at me. I treasure them all as snapshots in time, moments that I never want to forget, as if I ever could. I hold onto my photographs as tightly I hold onto hope. They remind me of good times, happy times, peaceful times, and younger times.

Yet, does time ever really stand still? Can a single photograph ever stop the clock between what once was, what is, and what will be? Every yesterday and every past relationship collectively set the stage for who we are today, just as every today prepares tomorrow's you for the path that lies ahead.

Albert Einstein was once quoted as saying:

> The distinction between the past, present, and future is only a stubbornly persistent illusion.

He was right. Past, present, and future blend into one another in the same way that a stream meets a river that meets the sea.

In the timeline of life, the past, present, and future create a perfect path for the imperfect journey: they are so intimately associated that they forever bind us to one another, to places and faces, to connections that, once made, will always be. People may move on. Geography may change. Relationships may end.

At the end of the day, we are a product of every experience, every memory, every bond, and every life that came before us, just as we in turn become the foundation for the lives that follow ours. In that way, the circle of life becomes the circle of meaning. Time reminds me that nothing is permanent and nothing is forever. Rather, experiences, people, and places are fluid. They can change. They can evolve.

Change can be scary at times. But change is what keeps us alive. It is what keeps our heart beating and our lungs breathing. It keeps us yearning for the next chapter. It keeps us honest and humble.

Change makes all things possible. Dreams. Goals. Aspirations.

And just like that, in the blink of an eye, days pass. So, too, do weeks, months, and years until one day we see the Bigger Picture. Like a climber who stands tall at the mountain's summit, seeing the world through a whole new lens for the very first time, we realize what and who this life is all about, what and who we live for.

We are forever shaped – and changed – by those with whom we surround ourselves. In the spirit of coming to that realization, it is only fitting that I dedicate this text to key faces from my past, present, and future – not because they are distinct entities, but because their memories co-exist in the moment that is the here and now, where they thrive inside of me.

In honor of the Past, I dedicate this text to my beloved maternal grandmother, Doris Buchanan

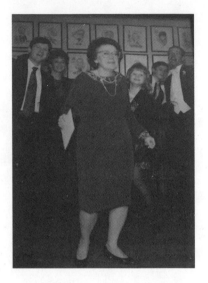

Grandma was one of my favorite cheerleaders in life. She saw in me what I hoped to convey to the world, at my very best: my passion for medicine, my commitment to science, and my perseverance to power through the obstacles to get to the Other Side. She called me her "shining star" because she saw potential in me, long before I chased after the very same opportunities that would one day chase after me.

Thank you, Grandma, for being among the first to transform my world, my present and future, by teaching me to replace the question, "Can I?" with the statement, "Yes, I can."

In honor of the Present, I dedicate this text to my parents, Jill and Richard Englar

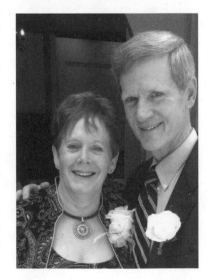

My mom is the most selfless person that I know. For as long as I can remember, she has put the needs of others before her own. Whether through her work as a licensed and certified social worker in Hospice or her concurrent career as a parent for life, she has taught me the importance of responsibility, establishing ties, engaging in dialogue, making connections, building bridges, and giving back to the community. Mom has also been the gold standard communicator for my entire life. As a child, I didn't always have the words to speak my mind. I was quiet and introverted. I thought more than I spoke. Yet Mom was always there to encourage and nurture. She gave me the time and space to develop into my own person, one that I wanted her to be proud of. As I have matured, I have come to see that Mom's strength of character comes from the power to wield words in a positive way and to deliver them responsibly, with good intent. More than that, she is a trailblazer, forever reminding me to be unafraid of the path less taken.

Thank you, Mom, for everything. It was from you that I learned to be me.

My dad is an educator whose love of teaching inspires me. As a department chair for social studies, he has also painted a realistic picture of effective leadership, and defined it in a way that I respected from the start. He showed me by example that it was possible to lead with a gentle nature rather than an iron fist. His perspective on office infrastructure, management, and business relations has been invaluable as I transition through various roles and phases in academia. As I age, I would like to think that I take after him in the classroom, both in terms of energy level and creativity in terms of thinking outside the box.

Thank you, Dad, for your work outside of the classroom, too. I appreciate you standing in as my second set of eyes to review each and every textbook draft before it goes to print, no matter what length. Somehow, you always manage to make deadline and catch that one mistake that would have gnawed at me for a lifetime.

In honor of the Future, I dedicate this text to my one and only niece, Beatrix Rae Englar-Green

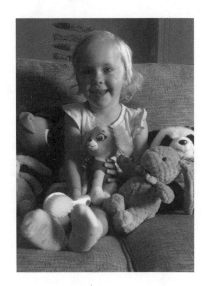

At the time that this text goes to print, Bea is the ripe age of three years young. Technology allows me to visit with her more frequently, from afar, and with every phone call, I see her developing into a beautiful person. There is no other smile like hers – and no other laugh, too. She is a burst of energy, and a ray of sunshine. She is a bold investigator with an active mind, amazing hand-eye coordination, and a refreshing sense of genuineness that is so often lost in adulthood. I see that spark in her eye, and it makes me happy. Happy to see her so full of life and living life as it was intended: joyful and free, exuberant and fun.

Bea represents the future that we all hope for, for our little ones. A future filled with opportunity, where she can flourish in any activity she sets her mind to, in a world where she can truly do anything and be anyone.

Thank you, Bea, for bringing out the kid in all of us, and for reminding me that it's okay to finally live a little, to have a laugh, and have some fun.

Acknowledgments

As youth, we are heavily influenced by what and who others think we should be. Adulthood may lessen the hold that others have over us, yet those we care for as we mature continue to shape our identity and sense of self-worth.

If someone you greatly esteem tells you that you are capable, then you are apt to believe it. If, on the other hand, someone tells you that you cannot do "X" or achieve "Y," then you reach the proverbial fork in the road, where you can go one of two ways. Either you are driven into action to prove him wrong, or you allow yourself to be crushed by the weight of another's failure to believe in you.

I wish I could say that I was the bold and daring adventurer who marched to the beat of my own drum and didn't care what other people thought. But the truth is that I was far less adventurous then, as I am now, and those were the days long before I channeled my inner Katniss Everdeen. The truth is I held onto every word that others spoke of me. Reflecting back upon those days, it strikes me as how fortuitous, how blessed I was to be surrounded by goodness and warmth, those who wished to buoy me up rather than pull me down.

Outside of my nuclear family, who has always loved and accepted me, I have always looked up to educators. Maybe it was because my father was a teacher and his colleagues became family. Maybe it's because I was a bookworm. For as long as I can remember, knowledge has always fascinated me. Others may have dreamed of power or status or some fantasied superhero trait. But in my imaginary world, I did not need a cape to fly from Point A to Point B. I just needed to think myself there.

As a child, my imagination was my greatest skill. I dreamed dreams into goals and goals into action plans. When I said at age five that I would be a veterinarian, I truly meant it with every fiber of my being. I was convinced that I could will it into reality. My professional conviction wasn't just a phase, spoken by a stubborn, strong-willed child. It was a reflection of what I had heard all along, beginning at home and continuing into the classroom: *You can do and be anything.*

Lady Bird Johnson once said it best: "Children are likely to live up to what you believe of them." Others believed that I could, and so I did.

During my formative years, I was blessed with great mentors. They may have been paid to teach me a subject, which each did, masterfully, in his own way. But more important than book learning were the lessons that each one taught me about life. At this time, I would like to acknowledge five teachers who have been invaluable to my evolution as a person and individual, scientist and doctor.

On paper, Mr. Dean Curtis taught me junior high math and science

In actuality, his life lesson to me was not to stifle imagination and to follow your dreams, even if yours are different than most.

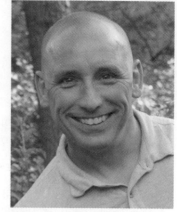

> I used to think great teachers inspire you. Now I think I had it wrong. Good teachers inspire you; great teachers show you how to inspire yourself every day of your life. They don't show you their magic. They show you how to make magic of your own. ~ Alfred Doblin

At that time, there were no interactive teaching videos and the internet was only a fraction then of what it is today. Learning about cells *on paper* did not interest me. I did not understand ribosomes or mitochondria unless they were tangible concepts that I could grasp in my own two hands. So, I asked him if I could create a three-dimensional model of a cell. Whereas most people would have looked at the kid that I was then and said, "Why?" with disdain or disbelief, he said "Why not?"

That same imagination served me well at recess. While most of my classmates were in the courtyard playing dodgeball, I was busy mapping the trajectory of boomerangs. Little did I know then that the boomerang of my childhood would later become an analogy for life. Mr. Curtis once said something to the effect of that no matter where you go in life, no matter how high, no matter how far, what matters is that you return, to your roots, to who and what you know.

On paper, Mr. Joseph Harris taught me high school inorganic chemistry

In actuality, he gave meaning to the Kreb's cycle. He made learning about carbon chains fun. He also inspired me to consider how functional groups of medicinal compounds were the key to their pharmacodynamic and pharmacokinetic effects.

> Great teachers engineer learning experiences that put students in the driver's seat and then get out of the way. ~ Ben Johnson

This foundation in clinical science prompted my interest, years later, in drug solubility, mechanism of action, route of administration, metabolism and elimination, all of which helped me to steer patient care towards solutions that would be most effective based upon chemical reactions.

On paper, Dr. Bruce Currie taught me AN SCI 100 (Domestic Animal Biology) during my first semester of undergraduate study at Cornell University, within the College of Agriculture and Life Sciences (CALS)

In actuality, he inspired new ways of thinking.

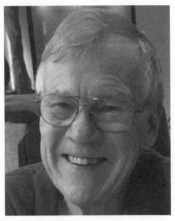

> The best teachers are those who show you where to look, but don't tell you what to see. ~ Alexandra K. Trenfor

As part of our coursework, we managed Ezra's Farm, an on-campus, student-run barnyard, to immerse ourselves in animal husbandry. We got out of the opportunity what we put into it. Dr. Currie provided the experience of a lifetime for citified students like me, who had never bottle-fed calves or stood knee-deep in pigsties. During those early morning shifts, I learned how to make connections between the basic and clinical sciences. I never again looked at an animal in quite the same way. Before Ezra's Farm, my vision was superficial: when I saw a cow, I saw a cow. I couldn't relate its movement to its structure. Ezra's Farm taught me how to translate structure into function in a way that would benefit my patients for years to come.

On paper, Dr. Abraham Bezuidenhout taught me Block 1 (The Animal Body) during my first semester of graduate study at Cornell University College of Veterinary Medicine

In actuality, he blended rigor, proficiency in patient care, compassion for humanity, and zest for life.

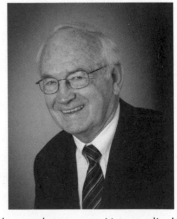

> Ideal teachers are those who use themselves as bridges over which they invite their students to cross, then having facilitated their crossing, joyfully collapse, encouraging them to create bridges of their own. ~ Nikos Kazantzakis

Dr. B pushed me harder than ever before. Initially, he was intimidating, and he did not hold back. He said what he wanted to, when he wanted to, in perfectly constructed, direct and formal statements. When he called upon you in class or in laboratory, you were expected to know the answer. You studied extra hard in his class because you had to. But you also studied extra hard because, at the end of the day, you did not want to let him down.

Dr. B's greatness as an instructor was that he gave you the blueprint to build wings, but he expected you to create them, for yourself, if you wanted to fly. Answers were not dispensed with ease and convenience. Lessons were earned. At the beginning, I thought he was just making things harder for us. I didn't know then what I do now. He ignited our potential. He gave us a shoulder to lean on and a stepstool to take that first leap in the right direction. But it was up to us to rise to the challenge, complete the climb, reach unforeseen heights, and stretch ourselves beyond our wildest dreams. Dreams were all well and good, but dreams didn't earn titles, accomplishments, or accolades. Hard work and sweat did.

On paper, Lowell E. Fox continues to teach me the art of American Smooth, International Standard, American Rhythm, and Latin dance

But were it not for his love of science and evidence-based medicine, I do not know if I could have excelled at either.

> A great teacher never stops being a student. ~ Jeffrey Benjamin

Lowell's mind is always in motion. I see the wheels turning in his mind every time he circles the dance floor. Just as he steps deliberately, with posture and poise, his mind is sharp with purpose. It sifts through details that sharpen his understanding of those who he trains.

Lowell studies his students in the same way that we study dance: methodically. He learns what each of us needs in order to succeed. He was the first to link dance to veterinary medicine in a way that made sense to me. He connected leg crawls in dance to grasshoppers, and pivots to marine life. He talked to me about microglia and compared walking actions to diabetic neuropathy. He lit a fire in me about dance because he made it relatable. The science fact of the day became a staple of our lessons. He also wasn't afraid to learn from me.

Lowell learned how I measured success, in dance and in life. He redefined for me that success is not always about the perfect outcome. It's about learning how to channel fear of the unknown into directed and deliberate action. It is about recognizing that sometimes what we think are dead ends are really just new beginnings, and that even light can come from dark. Even to this day, Lowell reminds me to push myself to reach new limits – and to break through them.

All five of these teachers influenced who I am today. In return, I do what I can to pay it forward.

I do not know what my teaching legacy will be.

I do hope that what my students glean from me is to live life fully, without regret, so that they are never haunted by "What If?" So that, instead, they can say they tried to live and they lived to try.

If they try, they may or may not succeed. But if they never try, then they will never know how it all was supposed to turn out.

About the companion website

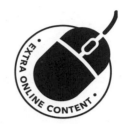

Please visit the companion website to this book at this link:

https://www.5mbooks.com/communication-videos

The website gives access to 19 supplementary videos, which are signalled with the extra online content icon at relevant points in the text. These short videos capture different communication skills that can be effectively interwoven throughout the consultation, and incorporate good and bad points of practice. As such, they are ideal training materials for young vets and vets new to practising in the UK and USA. They are also a great refresher for established vets who may want to brush up on skills that can round out their communication style.

The videos have been produced in partnership with the US-China Center for Animal Health at Kansas State University. Ryane Englar, DVM, DABVP (Canine and Feline Practice) presents each episode. Dr. Englar is the author of *Writing Skills for Veterinarians* published by 5m Publishing, as well as the forthcoming book, *The Veterinary Workbook of Small Animal Clinical Cases*.

The following subjects are covered:

- Greeting Your Client
- Reflective Listening
- Empathy
- Nonverbal Cues
- Taking a Patient History
- Open-Ended Questions
- Closed-Ended Questions
- Avoiding Medical Jargon
- Offering Partnership
- Eliciting the Client's Perspective
- Asking Permission
- Assessing the Client's Knowledge
- Mapping Out the Consultation
- Sectioning the Conversation into Bite-Size Chunks
- Contracting for the Next Steps
- Final Check-In
- Compassionate Transparency
- Unconditional Positive Regard
- Summarizing

Acronyms

AAHA	American Animal Hospital Association
ACGME	Accreditation Council for Graduate Medical Education
AKI	acute kidney injury
BUN	blood urea nitrogen
CCG	Calgary–Cambridge Guide
CDC	Centers for Disease Control and Prevention
CE	continuing education
CHF	congestive heart failure
CKD	chronic kidney disease
CPA	cardiopulmonary arrest
CPR	cardiopulmonary resuscitation
CT	computed tomography
CVO	College of Veterinarians of Ontario
DKA	diabetic ketoacidosis
EMRs	electronic medical records
FeLV	feline leukemia
FIV	feline immunodeficiency virus
HW	heartworm
HWD	heartworm disease
ICCVM	International Conference on Communication in Veterinary Medicine
IHC	Institute for Healthcare Communication
IRIS	International Renal Interest Society
MRI	magnetic resonance imaging
NAVMEC	North American Veterinary Medical Education Consortium
OSCE	objective structured clinical examination
OVC	Ontario Veterinary College
OVH	ovariohysterectomy
RCVS	Royal College of Veterinary Surgeons
RT	radiation therapy
RVC	Royal Veterinary College
SCs	standardized clients
SOPs	standard operating procedures
SPs	standardized patients
URI	upper respiratory infection
USG	urine specific gravity
UTO	urinary tract obstruction

Part I

Clinical Communication as an Integral Part of the Veterinary Profession

Chapter 1

What Do Our Clients Understand?

The Evolution of the Doctor–Patient Relationship, Patient Autonomy, and Health Literacy

The physician–patient relationship was conceptualized in the writings of Hippocrates, who was credited with authoring the Oath that to this day continues to be recited, in modified form, at commencement ceremonies for graduating doctors of innumerable disciplines.(1)

This Oath has undergone multiple transformations, yet the Oath in its original state set the stage for a tradition of paternalism in the practice of medicine.(2)

> I swear by Apollo Physician and Asclepius and Hygieia and Panaceia and all the gods and goddesses, making them my witnesses, that I will fulfill according to my ability and judgment this oath and this covenant:
>
> To hold him who has taught me this art as equal to my parents and to live my life in partnership with him, and if he is in need of money to give him a share of mine, and to regard his offspring as equal to my brothers in male lineage and to teach them this art – if they desire to learn it – without fee and covenant; to give a share of precepts and oral instruction and all the other learning to my sons and to the sons of him who has instructed me and to pupils who have signed the covenant and have taken an oath according to the medical law, but to no one else.
>
> I will apply dietetic measures for the benefit of the sick according to my ability and judgment; I will keep them from harm and injustice.
>
> I will neither give a deadly drug to anybody if asked for it, nor will I make a suggestion to this effect. Similarly I will not give to a woman an abortive remedy. In purity and holiness I will guard my life and my art.

I will not use the knife, not even on sufferers from stone, but will withdraw in favor of such men as are engaged in this work.

Whatever houses I may visit, I will come for the benefit of the sick, remaining free of all intentional injustice, of all mischief and in particular of sexual relations with both female and male persons, be they free or slaves.

What I may see or hear in the course of the treatment or even outside of the treatment in regard to the life of men, which on no account one must spread abroad, I will keep to myself holding such things shameful to be spoken about.

If I fulfill this oath and do not violate it, may it be granted to me to enjoy life and art, being honored with fame among all men for all time to come; if I transgress it and swear falsely, may the opposite of all this be my lot.

Translated from the Greek by Edelstein.(3)

The Oath has since been modernized. Those who recite it no longer pledge their allegiance to the ancient Greek gods, and the increasing emphasis on separation of church and state in modern times has removed spirituality from most renditions.(1) Assisted suicide and abortion continue to be hot-button topics in bioethics, and cases of each frequent the legal system, calling into question the rights of patients, including the rights of the unborn.(1, 2) Today's surgeons are trained to "use the knife" to heal, contrary to the Oath in its original form, and patient confidentiality may need to be breached in certain circumstances, as when there is evidence of abuse or neglect.(1)

In spite of these alternations and regardless of its relevance to modern times, the tradition of the Oath has persevered along with its present day interpretation, *Do not harm*.(1)

1.1 The Development of Medical Paternalism

Do not harm gave birth to the concept of medical paternalism by ascribing the philosophy of doctor-knows-best to the physician and granting him the power to act upon this belief.(4–6) For instance, if sharing a diagnosis with a patient was thought to be detrimental to his health, then the physician had the right to withhold this information from the patient. Information withholding included terminal diagnoses, such as cancer. (5, 7, 8) A study by Donald Oken identified that nearly 90% of practitioners in the 1960s withheld this diagnosis.

Some physicians avoid even the slightest suggestion of neoplasia and quite specifically substitute another diagnosis. Almost everyone reported resorting to such falsification on at least a few occasions, most notably when the patient was in a far-advanced stage of illness at the time he was seen.(8)

It was believed that transparency in relaying a terminal diagnosis would extinguish hope and that lost hope might precipitate suicidal ideation.(9) It was thought to be kinder to allow patients to live with false hope rather than no hope at all. Physicians were, in a sense, privileged gatekeepers of information that could be withheld if doing so was deemed to be essential to the patient's physical and/or mental wellbeing.(10)

In addition to withholding information about death and dying, physicians also failed to communicate risks about medical and surgical procedures out of fear that "many people would refuse to have anything done, and therefore would be much worse off."(11) Patient autonomy was sacrificed for what was perceived to be clinical benefit.(4–6, 12)

Patient decision making was non-existent. Even guardians were not active participants in healthcare decisions of those under their care, including minors, such as newborns. Whether or not to initiate or continue life-saving measures was largely under the purview of doctors. Consider, for instance, early neonatal intensive care units and decision making about whether or not to resuscitate infants. Informed consent was rarely granted and physicians bore sole responsibility to make the call.

> At the end it is usually the doctor who has to decide the issue. It is … cruel to ask the parents whether they want their child to live or die …(13)

This attitude of paternalism was reinforced by the belief that "the healer has always been possessed of a body of knowledge and skills unavailable to his patient."(14) Because the physician was assumed to know more than the patient, he or she was expected to act on the patient's behalf to maximize wellbeing.(6, 9)

Case outcomes were therefore doctor-driven. The *good* doctor was one who orchestrated patient care behind-the-scenes to minimize physical harm or emotional trauma.(9) The *good* doctor made choices to protect the patient, in the way that he or she saw fit.(9)

This philosophical approach to medicine placed a heavy burden on the physician and his or her capacity to make life and death determinations about the welfare of the patient, without eliciting the patient's perspective on the matter.(9)

Physicians were expected to make decisions based upon sound evidence; yet decisions were often made based upon fear of how a patient might react: "I would be afraid to tell [a diagnosis that carried a poor prognosis] and have the patient in a room with a window."(8)

So, it was that, historically, clinical decisions and case outcomes were physician-driven. Patients were told what physicians felt they needed to know. In exchange, patients were expected to submit to physicians' orders and comply with the diagnostic and treatment plans that were prescribed.

Patient perspective was neither expressed nor welcomed. Patients did not have a say in their own care. Their experiences and insight took a backseat to the doctor-is-always-right attitude, and patients were frequently interrupted when the physician felt that it was time to move on.(15, 16)

Patients were pawns in the chess game of healthcare. They were trained to follow instructions, not to question them.(17) As a result, interpersonal communication was lacking to non-existent. The physician initiated dialogue that mirrored the sport of shot put: conversation was one-sided. The physician spoke, and the patient was expected to absorb, like a sponge, what limited information was provided.

1.2 The Limitations of Medical Paternalism

Paternalism was intended to benefit the patient. As a result, this model dominated human healthcare through the 1960s.(2) Physicians were authorized to make unilateral decisions about patient health based upon their own perceptions of what was best.(10, 18) However, research confirms that medical paternalism has the potential to adversely impact the physician–patient relationship. The following consequences have been highlighted in the medical literature as the direct result of paternalistic care.

* Patients are discouraged from sharing their story.(19)
* Many patient concerns are not voiced.(20)
* If patient concerns are voiced, they are rarely acknowledged and often dismissed.(21)
* Patients feel misunderstood.(15)
* Patients are frustrated by what they perceive to be their physicians' lack of empathy.(15)
* Consultations gather information that is inaccurate or incomplete.(22)
* The majority of presenting complaints are missed by physicians.(23)
* The majority of physicians and patients disagree on the primary problem.(24)
* Patients do not receive insight into that which they value most: information about what caused their condition and the prognosis for what ails them.(25)
* Patients are dissatisfied when they are dismissed from the examination room without being adequately informed.(26)
* Patients may feel uncertain about the diagnostic or treatment plan that has been prescribed; uncertainty is distracting and may detract from case outcomes.(27)
* Patients want more control over decision-making, but are prevented from doing so.(28)
* Patients end the consultation desiring more information than what was given.(29–31)
* Patients do not always understand or recall what has been shared after the fact.(32, 33)
* Patient compliance and adherence to medical recommendations is poor.(34, 35)
* The healthcare system is burdened by the cost of noncompliance.(36)
* Malpractice is a likely outcome when there is a breakdown in communication between physicians and patients.(37–41)

A primary downfall of medical paternalism is its assumption that the doctor knows best.(17) Medical paternalism assumes that the patient cannot, will not, or should not advocate for themselves.(17) Medical paternalism strips the patient of all rights and autonomy.(4) Patients are expected to be passive learners as opposed to active participants in decision making. Patients are expected to be on the sidelines instead of equal members of the medical team. This sidelining of patients is concerning because, in the words of John Gregory, a pioneer of medical ethics:

Every man has a right to speak where his life or his health is concerned, and every man may suggest what he thinks may tend to save the life of his friend. It becomes them to interpose with politeness, and a deference to the judgment of the physician; it becomes him to hear what they have to say with attention, and to examine it with candour; If he really approves, he should frankly own it, and act accordingly; if he disapproves, he should declare his disapprobation in such a manner, as shows it proceeds from conviction, and not from pique or obstinacy. If a patient is determined to try an improper or dangerous medicine, a physician should refuse his sanction, but he has no right to complain of his advice not being followed.(42)

1.3 The Evolution of Relationship–Centered Care

The paternalistic view of medicine, along with its "sage on the stage" approach to medical care, has largely fallen by the wayside as patients have grown to expect more from their medical care team.

As healthcare modernizes, patients want self-advocacy. Patients want to have a say in their medical care. Patients want to be determinants in their case outcomes.

While doctors may be experts in medical knowledge, patients are experts in what it is like to be them.(43) Only patients know what fits best into their lives and their expectations. So, it is that patients seek partnership rather than dictatorship; decisions rather than dictation. This is the foundation for so-called relationship–centered care.

Research has demonstrated time and again that patients who are granted a say in healthcare decisions have better clinical outcomes.(15)

- Patient satisfaction is improved when patients are invited to share their story.(44)
- Patients are happier when their expectations have been acknowledged and addressed. (45–47)
- Patients are more satisfied when their questions are elicited and their concerns are clarified.(48)
- Patients feel connected to physicians through non-verbal communication, particularly when eye contact, posture, and facial expressions confirm mutual understanding and that they have in fact been heard.(49–52)
- Patients that provide insight concerning their knowledge base, core beliefs, and concerns are more likely to comply with the medical team's recommendations.(53, 54)
- Patients want to share responsibility for decision making.(55)
- Patients who participate in decision making are more likely to adhere to treatment plans.(56)
- Patients are more likely to report shorter durations of illness and hastened recovery periods if they are involved in their own care plans.(57, 58)
- Patients are more likely to demonstrate buy-in that translates into better control of a disease process when they are allowed to ask clarifying questions and negotiate care.(59, 60)

- Patients are less anxious about treatment recommendations when they are granted a say in the design of their care plan.(61)
- Patient care is less costly when effective communication between patients and families during hospitalization stays is emphasized.(62)
- Patients are less likely to initiate litigation against practitioners with whom they have a good rapport.(40, 41)

Patients want to play a more active role in their care and clinical decision making. This desire is supported by the American Medical Association (AMA), which has revised its ethical codes for the practice of medicine.(10) In 1847, the AMA dictated that the patient be subordinate to the physician:

> The obedience of a patient to the prescriptions of his physician should be prompt and implicit. He should never permit his own crude opinions as to their fitness, to influence his attention to them. A failure in one particular may render an otherwise judicious treatment dangerous, and even fatal.(63)

By 1990, the AMA had overturned its view on the physician–patient relationship, in favor of a more patient–centered practice of medicine:

> The patient has the right to make decisions regarding the health care that is recommended by his or her physician. Accordingly, patients may accept or refuse any recommended medical treatment. (64)

Patient autonomy is now central to the practice of medicine in modern day healthcare. (10) Physicians are viewed as essential information providers; however, they no longer hold the authority to unilaterally dictate patient fates and clinical outcomes.(10) They are instead required to provide options and information that will facilitate decision making by the patient.(10) Collaborative efforts between both parties should ultimately lead to a patient-driven decision that will best serve the patient.(10)

1.4 The Modernization of Medicine Drives Relationship–Centered Care

The practice of medicine does not take place in a vacuum, but rather it continues to evolve as treatment options diversify approaches to care, and allow for medical and surgical recommendations to be tailored to the individual.(5) There is rarely just one effective treatment or one definitive cure.(5) As treatment options expand, patient-specific needs are more easily considered.(5) For instance, radiotherapy may provide voice-sparing options for those that require the ability to speak; and surgical options may be able to preserve the sense of taste for a chef who requires this special sense for his career.(5)

As medicine strays from a cookie-cutter approach – that is, a situation in which every patient receives the same care irrespective of patient-specific needs – physicians find that what is best is no longer the same for each patient. Each patient's version of what is "best" varies depending upon his or her own set of core beliefs, values, perceptions, and perspectives.(5) Patients may vary tremendously in terms of what they consider to be acceptable quality of life; terminal patients may not always agree that life-sustaining measures are "right" for them.(5)

Technological advances in medicine afford opportunities that did not exist previously, yet many require patients' active participation and involvement.(5) It is no longer as simple as getting a patient to take an oral prescription – and even that approach to medical care has its shortcomings. Many interventional therapies require patients to buy into their care and commit to taking the next steps in order to achieve the expected outcome.(5) If patients are not asked for input, they are less likely to participate in care. Without their commitment to the process, expected outcomes cannot be realized.(5) This increases the need to design treatment plans that involve patient participation if patients are to agree to engage in effective, efficient care.

Today's medical patients are not the same as those that presented for consultations decades ago. They are not blank slates onto which clinicians can write unilateral action plans. They are born into a society that offers increasing choice and consumerism.(65) They come armed with knowledge that is shaped by past experiences. They also have access to ever increasing sources of information that help to give them a voice when it comes to their medical care. The information that they access may or may not be accurate, but at least it provides common ground, a foundation upon which to build a collaborative effort.

Because patients have access to information, they expect to be in a position to share it. Patients may have personal experience with disease "X" or drug "Y." They may have experienced side effect "Z." They may know of someone with diagnosis "V" or prognosis "W." They may have firsthand or secondhand knowledge of a particular procedure or therapeutic option.

Even more importantly, they have their own set of core beliefs, cultural norms, and realities that define what is reasonable, what is desired, what is expected, and how they would like to proceed.

In other words, patients have the right to weigh in on their own care.

Ethics often dictate how patients respond to recommendations from the medical team. Patients may come to the table armed with preconceived views, for instance, on blood transfusions, organ donation, artificial organs, and dialysis. Terminal patients may elect palliative hospice care over more traditional life-prolonging measures. Patients may have their own opinions as to what constitutes a life worth living.

As patients are invited to share their insight and their experience with the rest of the medical team, the dynamic of the physician–patient relationship is forever changed. Today's patients care less about what the doctor knows – they can always research knowledge, after the fact. Instead, in the moment, at the time of the consultation, they care more about the physician's demeanor – how much they perceive him or her to be empathetic and how well the physician is able to communicate.(66) Trust, loyalty, and regard strengthen the doctor–patient relationship and improve the likelihood of a successful partnership.(67)

As the value of interpersonal communication between physician and patient increases, the shot put approach has fallen out of favor. Instead of a unilateral flow of information from the sender (the physician) to the recipient (the patient), the Frisbee approach to dialogue is preferred. Both parties, the physician and patient, now share an investment in the conversation. Both sides have a say.

Patients are allowed to ask questions – and may question physician recommendations or ask for clarification. Patients may research and propose alternatives to recommended care. Patients may even refuse care.

This shift in the power dynamic of the physician–patient relationship empowers the patient and offers a transformative approach to healthcare. The physician must be attentive and receptive to the patient, who is no longer an empty vessel to fill with knowledge.

As physicians learn to talk less and listen more, they need to consider the impression that they leave behind on their patients, as well as consider how much of the healthcare plan their patients actually understand.

1.5 The Concept of Health Literacy

In order for patients to make informed, educated decisions about their health, they need to have "the capacity to obtain, process, and understand basic health information and services."(68) This capacity is defined as health literacy, and it is influenced by the following patient-specific factors: (69, 70)

- culture
- language
- education
- cognition
- social skills
- socioeconomic background
- emotional state
- visual and auditory acuity.

Health literacy is not limited to print literacy, although that is often the first skill to come to mind.(69) Health literacy extends beyond reading, writing, and basic mathematics. Health literacy requires speech and speech comprehension.(69, 71) Both mediate interactions between healthcare provider and patient.(69) When both are intact and functionally sound, they facilitate the understanding and processing of health-related information and services.(69) Patients are able to make decisions that are appropriate for themselves based upon their needs and desires. In this respect, health literacy is the bridge between making medical recommendations and implementing them.(71)

Oral literacy facilitates the sharing of information, agreeing to action plans, and instituting change.(71, 72) It requires both parties to be literate.(71, 72) Patients must be able to present their symptoms in a way that is descriptive, logical, and clear so that they are understood. Providers, in turn, must be able to critically analyze the data, particularly that which is obtained through history taking. But analysis alone is insufficient. Providers must be able to take it a step further and articulate the findings in a way that is understood. In this way, proposed diagnostic and therapeutic plans are shared, mutually agreed to, and acted upon for the benefit of the patient, who has the final say in establishing the healthcare plan.(72–75)

Effective communication drives the success of healthcare:(72)

Medicine is an art whose magic and creative ability have long been recognized as residing in the inter-personal aspects of the patient–physician relationship.(76)

Unfortunately, what providers consider to be effective communication does not always align with or meet patient expectations. Consider, for instance, a 2005 study by the American Academy of Orthopedic Surgeons (AAOS) to evaluate communication skills of the healthcare team. From the surgeon's perspective, 75% of providers communicated effectively with patients.(77) By contrast, satisfactory communication was achieved in only 21% of encounters as determined by the patient's perspective.(77)

What constitutes this sizable divide? Physicians likely overestimate health literacy among patients, who leave the consultation room without fully understanding the discussions that providers felt were clear.(78–80) This overestimation may stem from misperceptions that someone's appearance translates into literacy level.(78, 81) Likewise, providers may overestimate a patient's health literacy based upon knowledge about his or her educational attainment.(82) The reality is that the highest grade level achieved in school does not set the bar for health literacy.(82–84)

Health literacy is globally limited among the general population, even among those in developed countries.(85, 86) It has been estimated that over one-third of adults in the United States alone have average to below-average health literacy.(16, 78, 87) Nearly one-fourth of Americans read at or lower than a fifth-grade level.(88) The average American reads at an eighth-grade level.(78, 89) However, over three-fourths of medical brochures for patients are written at a level that is appropriate for a high school or undergraduate reader.(78, 88)

Even those with intermediate health literacy may be challenged by what providers might consider to be simple tasks. For example, patients may not be able to understand what it means when a prescription dictates that medication be taken at mealtimes.(78, 90) Patients with intermediate health literacy cannot determine healthy weight ranges for people, based upon height, if given the appropriate graph.(78) They also cannot read a drug label to determine if they might be having an adverse reaction to an over-the-counter drug.(78)

When health literacy is poor, patients lack the knowledge and comprehension to advocate for their own healthcare.(85) Moreover, their lack of understanding handicaps their potential to achieve self-efficacy.(85) They lack the core belief in their abilities and right to advocate for themselves. As a result, they do not always make use of available health information or services.(85)

Poor health literacy is associated with poor health outcomes.(72) Those with poor health literacy are more likely to:(69, 72, 78, 88, 91–93)

- experience illness
- develop chronic disease
- skip immunizations
- decline cervical and colon cancer screening, and mammography
- frequent emergency rooms
- use preventative services
- be admitted to hospital
- experience medical errors
- misinterpret warnings on prescription labels
- misinterpret food labels
- misunderstand appointment slips and discharge instructions
- misread medical forms and informed consent documents
- misunderstand instructions on prescription medications
- confuse basic principles about their health conditions, pathophysiology, and treatment recommendations
- confuse what should be interpreted as worsening of symptoms
- misunderstand when recheck examinations are essential
- exhibit poor compliance and adherence to medical plans
- experience relapse or recurrence of medical ailments.

The use of medical jargon is corrosive to health literacy.(72) Patients do not always recognize medical terms. Even when they do, they are likely to misinterpret them. This leads to disconnects between providers, who think that both parties are following the conversation, and the patients, who became lost somewhere along the way. Consider, for instance, that patients of traumatic events often ask the medical team if they have sustained a fracture or a break.(72, 94) In a 1994 study by Peckham, the majority of patients believed that both terms were not synonymous, and 71% among these believed that a fracture was the preferred outcome.(94)

More than a decade later, the same confusion existed.(72, 95) Eight-four percent of patients surveyed believed there to be a difference between breaks and fractures, with 68% believing the latter to have a better prognosis.(95)

We as providers know that fractures and breaks are medically identical diagnoses. Why is it that our patients do not? Even when patients are given printed handouts that define key terms, confusion remains. Few read what is provided in print and those that do often fail to retain takeaway messages.(95) From the perspective of print literacy, efforts need to be taken to improve readability by addressing font size and style, layout, clarity, and visual appeal.(72, 96)

Oral literacy remains a significant barrier to successful healthcare outcomes.(72) For patients to be engaged in healthcare, they need a baseline of understanding. Providers cannot make assumptions about whether or not the baseline is there based upon a client's appearance, educational background, or career. Instead, they need to constantly assess the situation and tailor their approach to dialogue so that miscommunication and misunderstandings are reduced. Clients that do not share basic understanding cannot be expected to make sound, informed decisions about their health.(72)

Oral literacy is complicated by differences in medical specialties, particularly those that are encountered during emotional times. Consider, for instance, the emergency department at a hospital.(72) Triage and emergency settings do not lend themselves to slow, plodding conversation. Triage and emergency settings dictate expedience with care. These may overwhelm patients who already may have a difficult time following the flow of thoughts and ideas. Moreover, in an emergency setting, many patients lose the ability to comprehend complex words: hemorrhage is not understood to be synonymous with bleeding, and myocardial infarction is not taken to mean heart attack.(97)

Oral literacy is further compounded by language comprehension.(72, 88) Those for whom English is a second language may struggle to understand medical terms, yet embarrassment may silence their desire to ask clarifying questions.(72, 98)

When patients do not understand the information that has been presented to them, they may attempt to fill in the blanks for themselves with inaccurate, yet widely available resources, such as those that are accessible via the world wide web.(72) This information may dictate whether or not patients seek medical attention in the future, and whether or not they comply with recommendations that have been outlined by their primary care providers.(72)

How information is presented to patients is a key determinant in whether or not that communication is effective.(78) Because patients are unlikely to ask for clarification, it is important that providers communicate effectively from the start.(78, 99, 100) Even when communication is clear, there are limitations to patients' ability to recall what precisely was shared with them.(78, 99, 100) Only about 50% of the content of a clinical encounter is retained, on average.(78, 99, 100) This percentage is further reduced when communication is bogged down with the weight of medical terms that may be minimally understood.(78)

Additional barriers to provider–patient communication include: (78, 81, 101)

- fast-paced conversations
- inarticulate or otherwise poorly enunciated speech
- flowery prose that is difficult to follow because it lacks brevity
- content that is fact-rich and fails to limit itself to three key points
- complex recommendations that are ambiguous and/or lack concrete steps.

Consider, for instance, a provider's recommendation to eat a healthier diet. Which specific steps are the patient supposed to take in order to effectively make this happen? Has the plan been outlined? Is the patient's plan clear? Patients would be more likely to achieve success with this recommendation were it followed up with a concrete plan, for example, eating five servings of vegetables a day.(78) This is doable because it is tangible. The patient is able to grasp precisely what is required of him or her to achieve the end goal.

Likewise, consider the generic recommendation that a patient lose weight. Is this recommendation helpful? Not really. Generic recommendations, such as this, only raise more questions that all too often go unanswered. How much weight is to be lost and over how long of a time frame? How is weight loss to be achieved? How is weight loss to be sustained? Is the patient expected to lose weight simply by reducing caloric intake, or is the physician advocating that exercise(s) be undertaken? In the event of the latter, which exercises should be pursued initially (that is, high intensity vs low intensity) and what should the patient aim for in terms of duration and frequency?

If these answers are not provided to the patient at the time that services are rendered, then how likely is the patient to reach the end goal? Weight loss may be a reasonable recommendation, but without a concrete plan, providers unknowingly set up the patient for failure.

An additional obstacle to patient comprehension is when providers rely upon numerical data to guide healthcare decisions.(78) This data is usually presented in the form of statistics, which are intended to help patients make informed decisions and alter behaviors.(78) For example, a provider may relay to a smoker that cigarette smoking is a leading cause of preventable death, accounting for one in five deaths in the United States every year.(102) This is intended to effect change in the patient. The patient is supposed to want to stop smoking so as not to become another statistic.

The reality is that mathematics is not a strong suit for many Americans.(78, 103) Understanding what numbers, ratios, and percentages mean, and how to process that kind of data is challenging for those with low numeracy skills.(78, 103) A 2006 study of asthmatic patients confirmed that numbers do not necessarily mean the same thing to everyone: it was unclear to two-thirds of patients what 1% meant.(104)

Communication between patients and the healthcare team must transcend barriers such as these in order to be effective. If providers do not make an effort to adapt to their audience, then they have essentially lost their audience before being able to provide patients the high-quality healthcare that they deserve.

To facilitate communication, patients must have the opportunity to ask questions of the provider and clarify information to ensure that it was not misconstrued. Because not all patients feel comfortable expressing their confusion about a particular topic, the burden falls upon the provider to assess patient understanding.(78) Various strategies, such as the teach-back method, have proven to be successful in clinical practice. For example, diabetic patients that are asked by the provider to share what they understand, in their own words, are more likely to have improved glycemic control.(105)

Communication is thus essential to the clinical practice of medicine. It is a key determinant of health outcomes in that it influences whether or not mutual understanding is reached. Mutual understanding concerning the following topics is essential to the provision of care:

- patient history
- patient perspective

- expectations
- misconceptions
- concerns
- differential diagnoses
  - which diseases are possible?
  - which diseases are probable?
  - what might each disease process mean for the individual patient?
- diagnostic plan
  - which diagnostic tests are recommended?
  - what does diagnostic testing involve?
  - how are diagnostic test results interpreted?
  - what do diagnostic test results mean?
- diagnosis
- therapeutic plan
  - medical interventions
  - surgical interventions
  - potential benefits of therapies
  - complementary medicine
  - alternative approaches to treatment
  - anticipated treatment duration
  - potential for adverse effects
- expected outcome or prognosis
  - one-time event versus recurrence or relapse
  - acute versus chronic disease
  - curative versus palliative care.

1.6 How Do Health Literacy and Relationship–Centered Care Apply to Veterinary Medicine?

In Sections 1.1–1.5, effective communication was considered from the perspective of human healthcare. However, the provision of healthcare is not limited to human patients. The veterinary profession represents a unique segment of the medical field. Its providers care for non-human patients who cannot articulate their presenting complaints, expectations, and reservations about care in the same way that a human might. In this way, veterinary medicine bears striking resemblance to the practice of pediatric medicine in human healthcare.(106)

The veterinarian and pediatrician both engage in a tripartite relationship.(106–108) The veterinarian–client–patient and the pediatrician–parent–child relationships are unique.(106, 107) However, there is overlap in each caregiver's responsibilities to the patient. The veterinary client is responsible for the patient in the same way that the parent is responsible for the child.(106, 107) Both must advocate for decision making that will directly benefit the patient.(106, 107) Both are responsible for presenting the patient, relaying patient history, and initiating dialogue about a particular presenting complaint. (106, 107, 109, 110)

Veterinary clients are not all cut from the same cloth. That being said, many see themselves in the role of "pet parent."(108) As "pet parents", they are responsible for meeting the needs of those under their care.(108) In addition to providing the essentials – food, water, and shelter – they also need to call upon the advice of a veterinarian to provide medical and surgical services.(108) This requires "pet parents" to make informed decisions about healthcare.(108)

Decision making requires "pet parents" to gather information. "Pet parents" are hungry for information as veterinary consumers. Historically, they have not been well informed as to the types of healthcare services that are offered and how these services can meet the needs of the patient.(108, 111)

Being uninformed hinders the delivery of high quality healthcare. Clients do not understand why medication "X" was prescribed or why a follow-up examination in "Y" number of days or weeks is essential. Preventative care measures may not be taken, and client adherence to treatment recommendations is often poor.(108)

Why is this so? Why does compliance suffer?

Gaps in understanding corrode the veterinary–client–patient relationship. If the client does not understand the why factor, then how likely is follow-through?

The burden falls upon the veterinary team to educate the client as to what is best for the patient. However, education is a two-way street. The veterinarian may be the expert in the consultation room concerning medical knowledge and appropriate means of therapeutic intervention, but the client is the expert about that particular pet. The client must be allowed to educate the provider as to what is normal versus abnormal for that pet as well as which treatments are reasonable.

Clients need to be able to share the information that they have about the patient's presenting complaint. For instance, is the patient truly vomiting or is the patient regurgitating? Which action the pet is exhibiting confers a distinct set of differential diagnoses. The diagnostic investigation for each complaint is not necessarily one and the same.

Clients also require information from us about the following factors:

- anticipated cost of diagnostic work-up
- anticipated cost of care
- perceived benefits of diagnostic work-up
- perceived benefits of care
- potential risks associated with the diagnostic work-up
- potential risks associated with care
- treatment options
  - what is the best plan for the patient?
  - what is plan B?
- "best case" scenario

- "worst case" scenario
- urgency of care
  - when is care mandatory?
  - when is care urgent?
  - when is care elective?
- timeframe
  - is care required now?
  - can care be delayed?
  - if so, for how long?
- anticipated outcome.

When clients do not receive adequate information from the veterinary team or when they receive information that is inaccessible to them because of comprehension or language barriers, they will seek it elsewhere.(108)

The internet is frequented by pet-owners who are searching for information that is at their fingertips.(112) A 2012 study by Kogan et al. found that one-quarter of internet users search for pet health information monthly.(113) Just under 14% conduct weekly searches about pet health.(113) Half of these searches are performed for curiosity's sake; however, one-third are attempts by pet-owners to clarify information that was given to them by the veterinary team.(114)

Veterinarians report that two-thirds of clients bring internet-based resources into the consultation room.(112) Veterinarians are concerned about the accuracy of the material that is easily accessed by clients, and worry that it may confuse them.(112) Despite their concerns, veterinary practices rarely take the time to direct clients to vetted sites. (114, 115) Yet the validity of information that is accessible by clients on the internet is often questionable or incomplete.(116) Consider, for instance, the topic of veterinary anesthesia and breed-related risks. A 2008 study by Hofmeister et al. found that nearly 30% of websites that emphasized veterinary anesthesia espoused unfounded breed sensitivities to anesthesia.(116) Warnings were not evidence based.(116) They were purely anecdotal.(116) Yet these claims led veterinary clients to believe that Boxers, Afghan Hounds, Anatolian Shepherds, Border Terriers, and Tibetan Spaniels were predisposed to anesthetic reactions.(116)

The accuracy of information that is easily accessed by clients online is concerning to the practice of veterinary medicine. Veterinarians also acknowledge a growing trend that medical care is often delayed because of the internet. Clients may consult the internet first rather than make contact with the veterinary clinic to establish whether or not a sick or injured pet needs to be seen.(115)

It is a fair statement that the internet is here to stay. More clients are making use of it to conduct searches about health-related topics. Clients seek information when they perceive recommendations to be ambiguous. Clients also conduct internet searches so that they can be better informed.(112)

If clients do not find information that supports the veterinary team's recommendations, then they are not likely to comply with the prescribed care plan.

In general, compliance among veterinary patients is concerning. A 2003 study by the American Animal Hospital Association (AAHA) evaluated medical records from greater than 1400 companion animals (dogs and cats) from 240 practices.(117) An additional 1003 pet-owners were surveyed.(117) Compliance concerning the following content areas was explored:

- core vaccinations
- dental prophylaxis
- heartworm prophylaxis
- senior screenings
- therapeutic diets.

The following conclusions were made.

- Eight-three percent of dogs in endemic areas submit to heartworm testing; however, only 48% of dog-owners comply with recommendations that a preventative medication be administered.
- Approximately one-third of dogs and cats with at least grade 2 dental disease undergo dental work.
- Of those dogs and cats who do not undergo dental work, only one-third received specific recommendations from the veterinary team that supported a dentistry work-up.
- Only 19% of dogs and 18% of cats that are supposed to be fed a therapeutic diet are in compliance.

Although it is easy to blame the client that is armed with excuses for poor compliance, the reality is that blame may be better cast at the one who is making – or not making – the recommendation. Consider the following factors that are practice- and team-specific.

- Was a recommendation made?
- If so, was the recommendation vague or was it clear?
- Did the recommendation provide concrete and specific steps that could be taken to effect change?
- Did the recommendation provide a timeframe: when should change take place?
- Did the recommendation provide an explanation as to why it was being made? In other words, was the value of the recommendation conveyed?
- Were steps taken by the veterinary team to ensure mutual understanding?
- Did the client have ample opportunity to ask clarifying questions?
- Were the client's questions answered in a timely, appropriate, and sensitive manner?

Compliance breakdowns are common in veterinary practice. As is true of human healthcare, veterinary medicine is oftentimes bogged down by health literacy and its associated limitations. In addition, the following practice-driven factors may be responsible for reducing compliance.

- Information cramming, compounded by time limitations: veterinarians often feel that they have to deliver an exceptionally large amount of information to clients in a very small time window.(117)
- Lack of unconditional positive regard: the client may feel judged because of:
  - action: something that she or he did in an attempt to help the situation that turned out to be misguided, for example, the client administered acetaminophen to the family cat overnight because it seemed painful
  - finances: the client is unable to afford gold standard care
  - previous inaction: the client has historically not followed through on prior recommendations.
- Distractions within the consultation room.
  - The client's attention is often split between trying to hear what the veterinarian is saying and trying to maintain some semblance of control over the animal at the other end of the leash.(108)
  - The veterinarian's voice may be competing with the noise of vocalizing patients throughout the hospital, making it difficult for the client to concentrate.

The emotions that are inherently tied to veterinary practice also hinder compliance. Clients that are faced with unexpected bad news may not be ready to process additional information from the veterinary team.(108) Consider, for example, a client who presents a coughing dog for what he felt was the common cold. This client is not expecting to hear that his dog has congestive heart failure. When bad news comes as a shock, it may be difficult for the client to hear anything else. It is as if mental and emotional walls are put up to lessen the blow. These walls may prevent any additional information from breaking through. The clinical conversation may need to be tabled until the client has had time to come to terms with and accept the news.

The way in which bad news is delivered also may magnify the power of the blow. Many clinicians do not receive formal training in bad news delivery, including death notification.(118) Student doctors are more likely to observe what not to do rather than how to deliver bad news effectively.(118–120)

Clients need to feel supported by the veterinary team, in sickness and in health. In cases that involve the former, communication can either become the glue that bonds them to the veterinary team or the oil slick that creates a growing divide.

Effective communication is just as beneficial to the practice of veterinary medicine as it is to human healthcare. When communication is perceived to be effective in the client's eye, patient care benefits. Client adherence to treatment plans increases.(121, 122) Clients are seven times more likely to follow recommendations for care when they understand why it is essential.(121, 122)

Effective communication conveys consistency and reliability.(121) These attributes foster trust.(121) Trust is a practice-builder.(121, 123–126)

- Client loyalty to the practice is improved.
- Clients are more likely to be retained by the practice.

- Clients are more likely to return for follow-up care.
- Clients are more likely to refer others to the practice.

Today's veterinary clients are not afraid to pursue litigation when trust is breached. Poor communication is frequently cited in malpractice claims that fall upon the ears of veterinary licensing boards.(121, 127–129) The clinician may have delivered appropriate medical care to the patient, but if the way in which care was communicated was perceived as indirect, insensitive, substandard, or less than transparent, then clients are likely to take offense.(130)

Today's veterinary clients are more invested and more involved than past generations. As a whole, they expect to be asked about their past veterinary experiences.(121, 123, 131–133) They also want to be involved in decision making.(121, 123, 131, 134, 135)

In order to involve clients fully in healthcare decisions, veterinarians need to invest time and resources into developing a professional relationship with clients. Clients need to feel connected with and bonded to the practice. It is not the medical knowledge that provides this bond. It is the establishment of a mutual connection that can be achieved through effective, sincere, and grounded conversation.

Historically, communication was not taught to practitioners. It was viewed as a nice-to-have, but not essential, tool of the trade.(126) This viewpoint has since fallen out of favor in both human and veterinary fields as research has unearthed the science of communication and confirmed that it is in fact a teachable skill. Chapter 2 will outline some of this research in order to demonstrate that communication can – and should be learned. After all, veterinary medicine is above all else a people profession. Customer-service skills – or the clinician's lack thereof – is a critical barrier to career success in clinical practice.(136)

The purpose of this textbook as a whole is to explore how to make the most of clinical conversations such that communication is relevant and effective. Only by achieving both are we as practitioners able to deliver high-quality healthcare.

References

1. Markel H. "I swear by Apollo"—on taking the Hippocratic oath. N Engl J Med. 2004;350(20):2026–9.
2. Ogunbanjo GA, van Bogaert KD. The Hippocratic oath: revisited. South African Family Practice. 2009;51(1):30–1.
3. Edelstein L. The Hippocratic Oath: text, translation and interpretation. In: Temkin O, Temkin CL, editors. Ancient medicine: selected papers of Ludwig Edelstein. Baltimore, MD: Johns Hopkins University Press; 1967. p. 3–64.
4. McCullough LB. Was bioethics founded on historical and conceptual mistakes about medical paternalism? Bioethics. 2011;25(2):66–74.
5. Weiss GB. Paternalism modernised. J Med Ethics. 1985;11(4):184–7.
6. Tan NHSS. Deconstructing paternalism: what serves the patient best? Singapore Med J. 2002;43(3):148–51.

7. Veatch RM. Death, dying, and the biological revolution: our last quest for responsibility. New Haven, CT: Yale University Press; 1976.
8. Oken D. What to tell cancer patients – a study of medical attitudes. JAMA. 1961;175(13):1120–8.
9. Buchanan A. Medical paternalism. Philos Public Aff. 1978;7(4):370–90.
10. Chin JJ. Doctor–patient relationship: from medical paternalism to enhanced autonomy. Singapore Med J. 2002;43(3):152–5.
11. Malpractice Digest. 1977:6.
12. Miller TR. 100 cases of hemipelvectomy: a personal experience. Surg Clin North Am. 1974;54(4):905–13.
13. Shaw A. Dilemmas of "informed consent" in children. N Engl J Med. 1973;289(17):885–90.
14. Nuland SB. Autonomy run amuck: review of Patient Heal Thyself: How the 'New Medicine' Puts the Patient in Charge, by Robert M. Veatch. The New Republic. 2009;240(11):48–51.
15. Kurtz SM, Silverman J, Draper J, Silverman J. Teaching and learning communication skills in medicine. Second edn. Abingdon: Radcliffe Medical Press; 2005.
16. Beckman HB, Frankel RM. Training practitioners to communicate effectively in cancer care: it is the relationship that counts. Patient Educ Couns. 2003;50(1):85–9.
17. Hayry H. The limits of medical paternalism. London: Taylor & Francis; 2002.
18. McKinstry B. Paternalism and the doctor–patient relationship in general practice. Br J Gen Pract. 1992;42(361):340–2.
19. Byrne PS, Long BEL. Department of Health and Social Security. Doctors talking to patients: a study of the verbal behaviour of general practitioners consulting in their surgeries. London: HMSO; 1976. 195 p. p.
20. Barry CA, Bradley CP, Britten N, Stevenson FA, Barber N. Patients' unvoiced agendas in general practice consultations: qualitative study. BMJ. 2000;320(7244):1246–50.
21. Rogers MS, Todd CJ. The "right kind" of pain: talking about symptoms in outpatient oncology consultations. Palliat Med. 2000;14(4):299–307.
22. Platt FW, McMath JC. Clinical hypocompetence: the interview. Ann Intern Med. 1979;91(6):898–902.
23. Stewart MA, McWhinney IR, Buck CW. The doctor/patient relationship and its effect upon outcome. J R Coll Gen Pract. 1979;29(199):77–81.
24. Starfield B, Wray C, Hess K, Gross R, Birk PS, D'Lugoff BC. The influence of patient–practitioner agreement on outcome of care. Am J Public Health. 1981;71(2):127–31.
25. Kindelan K, Kent G. Concordance between patients' information preferences and general practitioners' perceptions. Psychol Health. 1987;1:399–409.
26. Hall JA, Roter DL, Katz NR. Meta-analysis of correlates of provider behavior in medical encounters. Med Care. 1988;26(7):657–75.
27. Adams CL, Kurtz SM. Skills for communicating in veterinary medicine. Oxford: Otmoor Publishing and Dewpoint Publishing; 2017.
28. Degner LF, Kristjanson LJ, Bowman D, Sloan JA, Carriere KC, O'Neil J, et al. Information needs and decisional preferences in women with breast cancer. JAMA. 1997;277(18):1485–92.
29. Beisecker AE, Beisecker TD. Patient information-seeking behaviors when communicating with doctors. Med Care. 1990;28(1):19–28.
30. Jenkins V, Fallowfield L, Saul J. Information needs of patients with cancer: results from a large study in UK cancer centres. Br J Cancer. 2001;84(1):48–51.
31. Waitzkin H. Doctor–patient communication. Clinical implications of social scientific research. JAMA. 1984;252(17):2441–6.

32. Dunn SM, Butow PN, Tattersall MH, Jones QJ, Sheldon JS, Taylor JJ, et al. General information tapes inhibit recall of the cancer consultation. J Clin Oncol. 1993;11(11):2279–85.

33. Tuckett D. Meetings between experts: an approach to sharing ideas in medical consultations. London: Tavistock; 1985. vii, 290 p. p.

34. Meichenbaum D, Turk DC. Facilitating treatment adherence: a practitioner's guidebook. New York: Plenum Press; 1987.

35. Butler C, Rollnick S, Stott N. The practitioner, the patient and resistance to change: recent ideas on compliance. CMAJ. 1996;154(9):1357–62.

36. Berg JS, Dischler J, Wagner DJ, Raia JJ, Palmer-Shevlin N. Medication compliance: a healthcare problem. Ann Pharmacother. 1993;27(9 Suppl):S1–24.

37. Levinson W. Physician–patient communication. A key to malpractice prevention. JAMA. 1994;272(20):1619–20.

38. Avery JK. Lawyers tell what turns some patients litigious. Med Malpract Rev. 1985;2:35–7.

39. Hickson GB, Clayton EW, Entman SS, Miller CS, Githens PB, Whetten–Goldstein K, et al. Obstetricians' prior malpractice experience and patients' satisfaction with care. JAMA. 1994;272(20):1583–7.

40. Adamson TE, Bunch WH, Baldwin DC, Jr., Oppenberg A. The virtuous orthopaedist has fewer malpractice suits. Clin Orthop Relat Res. 2000(378):104–9.

41. Levinson W, Roter DL, Mullooly JP, Dull VT, Frankel RM. Physician–patient communication. The relationship with malpractice claims among primary care physicians and surgeons. JAMA. 1997;277(7):553–9.

42. Gregory J. Lectures on the duties and qualifications of a physician. In: McCullough LB, editor. John Gregory's Writings on Medical Ethics and Philosophy of Medicine. Dordrecht: Kluwer Academic Publishers; 1998. p. 33–4.

43. Coulter A. Paternalism or partnership? Patients have grown up – and there's no going back. BMJ. 1999;319(7212):719–20.

44. Arborelius E, Bremberg S. What can doctors do to achieve a successful consultation? Videotaped interviews analysed by the "consultation map" method. Fam Pract. 1992;9(1):61–6.

45. Eisenthal S, Lazare A. Evaluation of the initial interview in a walk–in clinic. The patient's perspective on a "customer approach". J Nerv Ment Dis. 1976;162(3):169–76.

46. Eisenthal S, Koopman C, Stoeckle JD. The nature of patients' requests for physicians' help. Acad Med. 1990;65(6):401–5.

47. Korsch BM, Gozzi EK, Francis V. Gaps in doctor–patient communication. 1. Doctor–patient interaction and patient satisfaction. Pediatrics. 1968;42(5):855–71.

48. Shilling V, Jenkins V, Fallowfield L. Factors affecting patient and clinician satisfaction with the clinical consultation: can communication skills training for clinicians improve satisfaction? Psychooncology. 2003;12(6):599–611.

49. Larsen KM, Smith CK. Assessment of nonverbal communication in the patient–physician interview. J Fam Pract. 1981;12(3):481–8.

50. DiMatteo MR, Hays RD, Prince LM. Relationship of physicians' nonverbal communication skill to patient satisfaction, appointment noncompliance, and physician workload. Health Psychol. 1986;5(6):581–94.

51. Weinberger M, Greene JY, Mamlin JJ. The impact of clinical encounter events on patient and physician satisfaction. Soc Sci Med E. 1981;15(3):239–44.

52. Griffith CH, 3rd, Wilson JF, Langer S, Haist SA. House staff nonverbal communication skills and standardized patient satisfaction. J Gen Intern Med. 2003;18(3):170–4.

53. Inui TS, Yourtee EL, Williamson JW. Improved outcomes in hypertension after physician tutorials. A controlled trial. Ann Intern Med. 1976;84(6):646–51.

54. Maiman LA, Becker MH, Liptak GS, Nazarian LF, Rounds KA. Improving pediatricians' compliance–enhancing practices. A randomized trial. Am J Dis Child. 1988;142(7):773–9.

55. Gattellari M, Butow PN, Tattersall MH. Sharing decisions in cancer care. Soc Sci Med. 2001;52(12):1865–78.

56. Schulman BA. Active patient orientation and outcomes in hypertensive treatment: application of a socio–organizational perspective. Med Care. 1979;17(3):267–80.

57. Little P, Williamson I, Warner G, Gould C, Gantley M, Kinmonth AL. Open randomised trial of prescribing strategies in managing sore throat. BMJ. 1997;314(7082):722–7.

58. Stewart M, Brown JB, Donner A, McWhinney IR, Oates J, Weston WW, et al. The impact of patient–centered care on outcomes. J Fam Pract. 2000;49(9):796–804.

59. Kaplan SH, Greenfield S, Ware JE, Jr. Assessing the effects of physician–patient interactions on the outcomes of chronic disease. Med Care. 1989;27(3 Suppl):S110–27.

60. Rost KM, Flavin KS, Cole K, McGill JB. Change in metabolic control and functional status after hospitalization. Impact of patient activation intervention in diabetic patients. Diabetes Care. 1991;14(10):881–9.

61. Fallowfield LJ, Hall A, Maguire GP, Baum M. Psychological outcomes of different treatment policies in women with early breast cancer outside a clinical trial. BMJ. 1990;301(6752):575–80.

62. Ahrens T, Yancey V, Kollef M. Improving family communications at the end of life: implications for length of stay in the intensive care unit and resource use. Am J Crit Care. 2003;12(4):317–23; discussion 24.

63. Code of Ethics (1847).

64. Current opinions (1990).

65. Taylor K. Paternalism, participation and partnership – the evolution of patient centeredness in the consultation. Patient Educ Couns. 2009;74(2):150–5.

66. Frankel RM. Pets, vets, and frets: what relationship–centered care research has to offer veterinary medicine. J Vet Med Educ. 2006;33(1):20–7.

67. Chipidza FE, Wallwork RS, Stern TA. Impact of the doctor–patient relationship. Prim Care Companion CNS Disord. 2015;17(5).

68. Ratzan SC, Parker RM. Introduction. Bethesda, MD: National Institute of Health; 2000.

69. Health literacy: a prescription to end confusion. Washington, DC: Institute of Medicine; 2004.

70. Baker DW. The meaning and the measure of health literacy. J Gen Intern Med. 2006;21(8):878–83.

71. Kirsch IS. The framework used in developing and interpreting the International Adult Literacy Survey (IALS). Eur J Psychol Educ. 2001;16(3):335–61.

72. Kyle S, Shaw D. Doctor–patient communication, patient knowledge, and health literacy: how difficult can it all be? Ann R Coll Surg Engl (Suppl). 2014;96:e9–e13.

73. Bredart A, Bouleuc C, Dolbeault S. Doctor–patient communication and satisfaction with care in oncology. Curr Opin Oncol. 2005;17(4):351–4.

74. Duffy FD, Gordon GH, Whelan G, Cole–Kelly K, Frankel R, Buffone N, et al. Assessing competence in communication and interpersonal skills: the Kalamazoo II report. Acad Med. 2004;79(6):495–507.

75. Ha JF, Longnecker N. Doctor–patient communication: a review. Ochsner J. 2010;10(1):38–43.

76. Hall JA, Roter DL, Rand CS. Communication of affect between patient and physician. J Health Soc Behav. 1981;22(1):18–30.

77. Tongue JR, Epps HR, Forese LL. Communication skills. Instr Course Lect. 2005;54:3–9.

78. Hersh L, Salzman B, Snyderman D. Health Literacy in Primary Care Practice. Am Fam Physician. 2015;92(2):118–24.

79. Kelly PA, Haidet P. Physician overestimation of patient literacy: a potential source of health care disparities. Patient Educ Couns. 2007;66(1):119–22.

80. Rogers ES, Wallace LS, Weiss BD. Misperceptions of medical understanding in low–literacy patients: implications for cancer prevention. Cancer Control. 2006;13(3):225–9.

81. Weiss BD. Health literacy and patient safety: help patients understand. Chicago, IL: American Medical Association Foundation; 2007.

82. Chew LD, Bradley KA, Boyko EJ. Brief questions to identify patients with inadequate health literacy. Fam Med. 2004;36(8):588–94.

83. Baker FM, Johnson JT, Velli SA, Wiley C. Congruence between education and reading levels of older persons. Psychiatr Serv. 1996;47(2):194–6.

84. Meade CD, Byrd JC. Patient literacy and the readability of smoking education literature. Am J Public Health. 1989;79(2):204–6.

85. Nutbeam D. The evolving concept of health literacy. Soc Sci Med. 2008;67(12):2072–8.

86. Dewalt DA, Berkman ND, Sheridan S, Lohr KN, Pignone MP. Literacy and health outcomes: a systematic review of the literature. J Gen Intern Med. 2004;19(12):1228–39.

87. Paasche–Orlow MK, Parker RM, Gazmararian JA, Nielsen–Bohlman LT, Rudd RR. The prevalence of limited health literacy. J Gen Intern Med. 2005;20(2):175–84.

88. Safeer RS, Keenan J. Health literacy: the gap between physicians and patients. American Family Physician. 2005;72(3):463–8.

89. Wallace LS, Lennon ES. American Academy of Family Physicians patient education materials: can patients read them? Fam Med. 2004;36(8):571–4.

90. Kutner MA. The Health Literacy of America's Adults: results from the 2003 National Assessment of Adult Literacy. Washington, DC: U.S. Department of Education and the National Center for Education Statistics; 2006.

91. Coulter A, Ellins J. Effectiveness of strategies for informing, educating, and involving patients. BMJ. 2007;335(7609):24–7.

92. Wolf MS, Davis TC, Tilson HH, Bass PF, 3rd, Parker RM. Misunderstanding of prescription drug warning labels among patients with low literacy. Am J Health Syst Pharm. 2006;63(11):1048–55.

93. Williams MV, Baker DW, Honig EG, Lee TM, Nowlan A. Inadequate literacy is a barrier to asthma knowledge and self-care. Chest. 1998;114(4):1008–15.

94. Peckham TJ. "Doctor, have I got a fracture or a break?" Injury. 1994;25(4):221–2.

95. Kampa RJ, Pang J, Gleeson R. Broken bones and fractures – an audit of patients' perceptions. Ann R Coll Surg Engl. 2006;88(7):663–6.

96. Krass I, Svarstad BL, Bultman D. Using alternative methodologies for evaluating patient medication leaflets. Patient Educ Couns. 2002;47(1):29–35.

97. Lerner EB, Jehle DV, Janicke DM, Moscati RM. Medical communication: do our patients understand? Am J Emerg Med. 2000;18(7):764–6.

98. Bagley CH, Hunter AR, Bacarese-Hamilton IA. Patients' misunderstanding of common orthopaedic terminology: the need for clarity. Ann R Coll Surg Engl. 2011;93(5):401–4.

99. Crane JA. Patient comprehension of doctor–patient communication on discharge from the emergency department. J Emerg Med. 1997;15(1):1–7.

100. McCarthy DM, Waite KR, Curtis LM, Engel KG, Baker DW, Wolf MS. What did the doctor say? Health literacy and recall of medical instructions. Med Care. 2012;50(4):277–82.

101. Sudore RL, Schillinger D. Interventions to improve care for patients with limited health literacy.

J Clin Outcomes Manag. 2009;16(1):20–9.

102. Services USDoHaH. The health consequences of smoking – 50 years of progress: a report of the Surgeon General. Atlanta, GA: US Department of Health and Human Services, Centers for Disease Control and Prevention, National Center for Chronic Disease Prevention and Health Promotion, Office on Smoking and Health; 2014.

103. Lipkus IM, Peters E. Understanding the role of numeracy in health: proposed theoretical framework and practical insights. Health Educ Behav. 2009;36(6):1065–81.

104. Apter AJ, Cheng J, Small D, Bennett IM, Albert C, Fein DG, et al. Asthma numeracy skill and health literacy. J Asthma. 2006;43(9):705–10.

105. Schillinger D, Piette J, Grumbach K, Wang F, Wilson C, Daher C, et al. Closing the loop: physician communication with diabetic patients who have low health literacy. Arch Intern Med. 2003;163(1):83–90.

106. Englar RE. Common clinical presentations in dogs and cats. Hoboken, NJ: Wiley/Blackwell; 2019.

107. Shaw JR, Adams CL, Bonnett BN, Larson S, Roter DL. Use of the roter interaction analysis system to analyze veterinarian–client–patient communication in companion animal practice. J Am Vet Med Assoc. 2004;225(2):222–9.

108. Murphy SA. Consumer health information for pet owners. J Med Libr Assoc. 2006;94(2):151–8.

109. Gillis J. The history of the patient history since 1850. Bull Hist Med. 2006;80(3):490–512.

110. Gillis J. Taking a medical history in childhood illness: representations of parents in pediatric texts since 1850. Bull Hist Med. 2005;79(3):393–429.

111. Catanzaro TE. Promoting the human–animal bond in veterinary practice. Ames, Iowa: Iowa State University Press; 2001.

112. Kogan LR, Schoenfeld-Tacher R, Gould L, Hellyer PW, Dowers K. Information prescriptions: a tool for veterinary practices. Open Vet J. 2014;4(2):90–5.

113. Kogan LR, Schoenfeld–Tacher R, Viera AR. The internet and health information: differences in pet owners based on age, gender, and education. J Med Libr Assoc. 2012;100(3):197–204.

114. Kogan LR, Schoenfeld-Tacher R, Simon AA, Viera AR. The internet and pet health information: perceptions and behaviors of pet owners and veterinarians. Internet J Vet Med. 2010;8(1).

115. Kogan LR, Schoenfeld–Tacher R, Gould L, Viera AR, Hellyer PW. Providing an information prescription in veterinary medical clinics: a pilot study. J Med Libr Assoc. 2014;102(1):41–6.

116. Hofmeister EH, Watson V, Snyder LB, Love EJ. Validity and client use of information from the World Wide Web regarding veterinary anesthesia in dogs. J Am Vet Med Assoc. 2008;233(12):1860–4.

117. The path to high quality care: practical tips for improving compliance. Lakewood, CO: American Animal Hospital Association; 2003.

118. Englar RE. Using a standardized client encounter to practice death notification after the unexpected death of a feline patient following routine ovariohysterectomy. J Vet Med Educ. 2019:1–17.

119. Bowyer MW, Hanson JL, Pimentel EA, Flanagan AK, Rawn LM, Rizzo AG, et al. Teaching breaking bad news using mixed reality simulation. J Surg Res. 2010;159(1):462–7.

120. Fallowfield L, Jenkins V. Communicating sad, bad, and difficult news in medicine. Lancet. 2004;363(9405):312–9.

121. Show A, Englar RE. Evaluating dog and cat owner preferences for Calgary-Cambridge communication skills: results of a questionnaire. J Vet Med Educ. 2018:1–10.

122. Kanji N, Coe JB, Adams CL, Shaw JR. Effect of veterinarian–client–patient interactions on client

adherence to dentistry and surgery recommendations in companion-animal practice. J Am Vet Med Assoc. 2012;240(4):427–36.

123. Coe JB, Adams CL, Bonnett BN. A focus group study of veterinarians' and pet owners' perceptions of veterinarian–client communication in companion animal practice. J Am Vet Med Assoc. 2008;233(7):1072–80.

124. Brown JP, Silverman JD. The current and future market for veterinarians and veterinary medical services in the United States. J Am Vet Med Assoc. 1999;215(2):161–83.

125. Lue TW, Pantenburg DP, Crawford PM. Impact of the owner–pet and client–veterinarian bond on the care that pets receive. J Am Vet Med Assoc. 2008;232(4):531–40.

126. Englar RE, Williams M, Weingand K. Applicability of the Calgary-Cambridge guide to dog and cat owners for teaching veterinary clinical communications. J Vet Med Educ. 2016;43(2):143–69.

127. Martin EA. Managing client communication for effective practice: what skills should veterinary graduates have acquired for success? J Vet Med Educ. 2006;33(1):45–9.

128. Radford AD, Stockley P, Taylor IR, Turner R, Gaskell CJ, Kaney S, et al. Use of simulated clients in training veterinary undergraduates in communication skills. Vet Rec. 2003;152(14):422–7.

129. Robinsoin R. College of Veterinarians of Ontario (CVO); 2005.

130. Bonvicini KA, Cornell KK. Are clients truly informed? Communication tools and risk reduction. Compendium. 2008(November):572–6.

131. Stoewen DL, Coe JB, MacMartin C, Stone EA, Dewey CE. Qualitative study of the information expectations of clients accessing oncology care at a tertiary referral center for dogs with life–limiting cancer. J Am Vet Med Assoc. 2014;245(7):773–83.

132. Opperman M. The cost of a dissatisfied client. DVM Management Consultant's Report; 1990.

133. Heath TJ, Mills JN. Criteria used by employers to select new graduate employees. Aust Vet J. 2000;78(5):312–6.

134. Stoewen DL, Coe JB, MacMartin C, Stone EA, C ED. Qualitative study of the communication expectations of clients accessing oncology care at a tertiary referral center for dogs with life-limiting cancer. J Am Vet Med Assoc. 2014;245(7):785–95.

135. Shaw JR, Barley GE, Broadfoot K, Hill AE, Roter DL. Outcomes assessment of on-site communication skills education in a companion animal practice. J Am Vet Med Assoc. 2016;249(4):419–32.

136. Burge GD. Six barriers to veterinary career success. J Vet Med Educ. 2003;30(1):1–4.

Chapter 2

How Can We Help Our Clients to Understand?

The Emergence of Clinical Communication as a Teachable Science

Knowledge is the foundation of medical training. Human and veterinary medical doctors commit to years of formalized education to develop a clinically relevant understanding of anatomy, physiology, pathology, and pharmacology.

In addition, the veterinary surgeon must be able to translate textbook anatomy into procedural medicine on the operating room table to effect one or more of the following changes in their patients:

- biopsies – surgical sampling of tissues or organs in pursuit of histopathology to diagnose an ailment
- bowel resection and anastomosis
- fracture repair
- -ectomies – surgical removal of tissues or organs, as in ovariohysterectomy – removal of both ovaries and the uterus
- -otomies – surgically cutting into tissues or organs, as in cystotomy – the surgical entrance into a urinary bladder, as for the purpose of removing cystoliths (bladder stones).

The emphasis of human and veterinary medical training is on evaluating symptoms through pattern recognition to establish plausible diagnoses for each individual patient. The outcome of the diagnostic work-up dictates how the physician will proceed, factoring in patient response to treatment as a guide to subsequent interventions and future recommendations.

The clinical practice of medicine will always require a sound foundation of knowledge by the practitioner. However, the reality is that human patients and veterinary clients are preoccupied less about what their physician knows and more about how much she or he is perceived to care.(1, 2) This is consistent with the movement away from medical paternalism and the trend towards relationship-centered care.(1)

2.1 Connectivity and the Provider–Patient Relationship

The need for physicians to establish a connection with the patient is not a new concept. As early as the 1940s, the renowned internist and psychiatrist George Engel emphasized the need to prioritize the medical interview over technological advances and new medications because of its ability to connect to and better understand the patient.(3) After all, the medical interview is one of the most common procedures that a physician will perform in his or her lifetime.(1, 4) It has been estimated that over the course of a career, a physician conducts 120,000–160,000 consultations, and that among these, 80% of cases can be diagnosed based upon history alone.(1, 4) Moreover, when patient histories are incomplete or inaccurate, diagnostic errors are likely to occur.(5–7)

Engel's biopsychosocial vision highlighted a humanistic approach to medicine.(8) His work at the University of Rochester, New York, attempted to reduce the distancing of clinical care from the patient to facilitate interpersonal connections between patient and provider. Engel believed that connectivity was key to successful patient outcomes. (8) At the same time, connectivity fostered resilience and guarded against compassion fatigue.(8)

Engel's strong belief in clinical communication persisted as other physicians acknowledged the role that effective communication played in clinical outcomes. In the late 20th century, it was stated that "before anything else, a good doctor must be a good communicator."(9)

This perspective was more fully developed by the early 21st century:

> To attend those who suffer, a physician must possess not only the scientific knowledge and technical abilities, but also an understanding of human nature. The patient is not just a group of symptoms, damaged organs and altered emotions. The patient is a human being, at the same time worried and hopeful, who is searching for relief, help and trust. The importance of an intimate relationship between patient and physician can never be overstated because in most cases an accurate diagnosis, as well as an effective treatment, relies directly on the quality of this relationship.(10)

In the present day, patient-centeredness continues to be prized by human medical patients and veterinary clients alike. It has also been highlighted by the Institute of Medicine as an indicator for the practice of high-quality healthcare that is both safe and effective.(11)

Patient-centered clinicians are said to possess one or more of the following character traits: (12–14)

*   concern
*   empathy
*   regard
*   sensitivity
*   sincerity
*   warmth.

These traits have been collectively linked to bedside manner. Physicians with good bedside manner are said to demonstrate a kind and compassionate approach to the patient. Their attitude facilitates partnership, as compared to those with poor bedside manner, whose inability to connect with the patient detracts from the provider–patient relationship.

2.2 Past Assumptions about Relationship-Centered Care

Although patients have come to expect good bedside manner from their healthcare providers, the development of interpersonal skills was once strikingly absent from medical and veterinary curricula.(1) It was assumed that such attributes were innate to a fraction of the population: some people were born to be natural communicators.(12) It was therefore not seen as the responsibility or purview of medical educators to improve upon this competency.(12)

A student either possessed the ability to effectively communicate or did not.(12) If the student was taciturn, unwilling, or unable to articulate his thoughts coherently in a way that was conducive to patient care, then this was acceptable so long as he or she possessed the knowledge and clinical acumen to effectively diagnose.

2.3 Challenging Past Assumptions

Patients, physicians, and, ultimately, both medical and veterinary educators have only recently begun to challenge past assumptions about the role of communication in healthcare.(1, 15) These challenges have arisen from a growing body of literature that has linked provider attitudes and demeanor to patient outcomes.(2, 16)

Evidence-based studies have found that effective communication improves:(2, 17–22)

- accuracy of diagnosis
- interpersonal relationships and professional relationship-building, through which:(23, 24)
  - patients feel connected
  - patients feel understood
  - patients feel validated
- patient adherence to treatment plans
- patient compliance
- patient coping skills
- patient outcomes, including:(21, 22)
  - emotional health
  - function
  - mental health (acceptance of disease process, reduction of anxiety, and recognition of both treatment options and associated risks)

- ▪ physiologic health (blood pressure and blood sugar)
- ▪ symptom management, including pain
- ▪ symptom resolution
- patient satisfaction
- physician satisfaction.

Even better yet, effective communication reduces the risk of litigation: when patients are satisfied with the delivery of compassionate care, then they are less likely to submit malpractice claims to licensing boards.(2)

Despite the proven advantages of effective communication in the clinical consultation, educators were slow to incorporate this training into the classroom. Communication was still seen by many as a "soft skill" or part of the "informal" curriculum, meaning that it did not need to be referenced or addressed.(16, 22) Instead, it was thought that healthcare providers could develop communication skills during residency or clinical practice.(1, 22) Communication was, in other words, nice-to-have, but not essential. You could learn the art of communication through interactions with clients, but the discipline was not yet viewed from the lens of a legitimate science.(1, 16)

This perspective began to shift as new research unveiled that communication skills do not improve with time in those who graduate without formalized training.(16, 25) A study by Maguire et al. in 1986 demonstrated a paucity of communication skills among graduates who had been practicing medicine for 5 years and who had received no communication training. Graduates possessed the following deficiencies:(25)

- incomplete introductions of themselves to the patient
- tendency to ask the patient leading questions
- overreliance upon closed-ended questions during history taking
- difficulty with phrasing questions open-endedly to broaden history taking
- hesitation to ask questions that elicited the client's perspective or that could touch upon the patient's emotions
- reluctance to inquire if the patient's physical health had adverse effects on the patient's mental health
- failure to summarize and accuracy check data that was acquired during history taking
- failure to make concluding statements at end-of-visit
- tendency to be perceived by the patient to be less empathetic.

Maguire's team concluded that untrained graduates were apt to take incomplete patient histories that were "clinically inadequate."(25) This poor performance was disappointing.

A follow-up study by Maguire et al. evaluated the second half of the clinical consultation. The goal of this research was to explore how well physicians 5 years out in clinical practice could explain and discuss clinical findings and treatment options with patients. Maguire concluded that:

Though most gave simple information on diagnosis and treatment, few mentioned investigations, aetiology, or prognosis. Very few obtained and took any account of patients' views or expectations of these matters. Some young doctors do discover for themselves how best to give patients information and advice, but most remain extremely incompetent. This is presumably because they get no training as students in this important aspect of clinical practice. This deficiency should be corrected, and competence tested before qualification to practice.(25)

The viewpoint that communication training was not essential fell out of favor during the 1980s, as a growing body of research emerged in support of Maguire's claims.(16)

Governing bodies for medical colleges began to rethink their expectations of what constituted appropriate training, and communication was listed as a core competency.(16)

By 1992, the Canadian Medical Association (CMA) drafted requirements for teaching and assessing communication skills.(26) This philosophy was adopted by medical colleges throughout the UK. Standards were developed to train students how to lead patient-centered consultations.(27)

2.4 The Kalamazoo Consensus Statement and Relationship- Centered Care

In 1999, a joint conference was hosted in Kalamazoo, Michigan, by the Bayer Institute for Health Care Communication and the Fetzer Institute.(28) The conference sought to define the characteristics of effective communication between healthcare providers and patients.(28) Secondary aims were to establish how best to teach and assess clinical communication.(28)

The resulting Kalamazoo Consensus Statement emphasized the need for relationship building between the patient and healthcare provider.(28) To facilitate this development, physicians needed to not only understand the disease process, they needed to consider how disease "X" impacted the individual.(28) An essential part of relationship-centered care was allowing the patient to tell his or her story.(28) The patient's perspective was key to health outcomes.(28) To treat the entire patient, the physician had to elicit the patient's perspective and be open to hearing the patient's thoughts, feelings, ideas, and values.(28–31)

The delivery of relationship-centered care also required the physician to let go of sole authority to make decisions about patient care.(28) Patients needed to be welcomed as active participants of the healthcare team.(28) Patients' families and support networks were also to be considered as essential influencers of decision making and, by extension, health outcomes.(28)

The Kalamazoo Consensus Statement prioritized the following tasks as being essential to relationship-centered care and as such provided one of the first frameworks for teaching and assessing communication skills.(28)

- Allowing the patient to lead off the consultation with an uninterrupted opening statement.
- Eliciting the patient's perspective concerning beliefs, concerns, and expectations.
- Acknowledging and validating the patient's experience with disease "X" as being unique and tailoring the consultation to the patient accordingly.
- Structuring the consultation with an appropriate balance of open- and closed-ended questions.
- Using consistent, supportive, and non-judgmental non-verbal cues in support of oral statements.
- Referencing easy-to-understand language in lieu of medical jargon to facilitate comprehension.
- Allowing time for patient processing and clarifying questions.
- Summarizing and clarifying historical data and supporting details.
- Providing diagnostic and therapeutic options.
- Encouraging patients to actively participate in decision making.
- Identifying resources and strategies that will facilitate, rather than hinder, patient care.
- Contracting for the next steps by agreeing to follow-up.

2.5 The Changing Face of Medical Education

Regulatory bodies for medical institutions increasingly began to see the value in teaching interpersonal skills and training student doctors in clinical communication.(32) The following governing agencies subsequently developed guidelines for effective communication training:(16, 32–34)

- Institute for International Medical Education (IIME)
- General Medical Council (GMC)
- Liaison Committee on Medical Education
- Committee on Accreditation of Canadian Medical Schools (CACMS)
- Association of American Medical Colleges (AAMC)
- Association of Canadian Medical Colleges (ACMC).

In addition, several accrediting bodies require graduates to demonstrate competence in communication in order to receive certification. These include the:(16, 32)

- Accreditation Council for Graduate Medical Education (ACGME)
- American Board of Internal Medicine
- Canadian Medical Education Directions for Specialists
- Educational Commission for Foreign Medical Graduates (ECFMG)
- Royal College of Physicians and Surgeons of Canada.

The ACGME has since outlined specific communication skills that are considered "must haves" among practicing physicians:(22, 34)

- effective listening
- effective questioning to gather patient-specific data
- effective delivery of information during the explanation and planning portions of the consultation
- effective counsel of patients through the decision-making process
- effective decision making, which factors into consideration patient preference.

Communication is also testable as a core competency on the United States Medical Licensing Examination (USMLE) Clinical Skills Examination.(32)

2.6 The Changing Face of Veterinary Education

Although some veterinary programs have been teaching communication as early as the 1970s, the veterinary profession has been, on the whole, slower to embrace the necessity of communication skills training for clinical practice.(16, 35–38) Like human healthcare providers, veterinarians assumed that on-the-job training would provide for the development of essential interpersonal skills.(35)

Research to support this theory turned out to be no more promising than it had been in human healthcare.(16)

New graduates and practicing veterinarians were particularly vocal about content areas in which they felt inadequate.(1, 16) A 1999 survey confirmed that clinical communication was a self-reported weakness among new veterinary graduates.(1, 16, 39) Although graduates were armed with sufficient knowledge and technical skills, they did not feel equipped to handle life skills that were necessary to be successful in clinical practice.(16, 39–41) These skills included relationship-building with clients and navigating difficult conversations.

To be successful, veterinarians must obtain buy-in from their clients.(16) Buy-in is created by establishing interpersonal connections with clients.(16, 42–44) This connection must be maintained by effective, transparent communication.(16, 42–44)

New graduates recognized the need to communicate effectively with clients. However, they did not feel adequately prepared to meet the growing expectations of their consumer base.(16) New graduates also felt ill-equipped to meet employer expectations. (16) Much like their clients, veterinarians' employers also felt that new hires should be fluent in interpersonal skills.(16, 42, 45–47)

Research has demonstrated consistently that physician satisfaction is intimately tied to the interpersonal aspects of healthcare.(48, 49) If the same holds true for veterinary practitioners, then career satisfaction was at an all-time low.

Graduates continued to push for curricular revision and formalized training in interpersonal skills.(16, 50) At the same time, licensing boards began to recognize that the majority of complaints against veterinarians were communications based.(16, 51)

- A 2003 study found that 80% of veterinary negligence claims in the UK, as observed by the Veterinary Defence Society, involved ineffective communication. (52)
- A 2005 publication found that two-thirds of complaints that were filed with the College of Veterinarians of Ontario (CVO) involved miscommunication.(53)
- A 2010 review by the Queen Mother Hospital for Animals, a specialty practice associated with the Royal Veterinary College (RVC), confirmed that poor communication is a frequent source of client dissatisfaction.(54)

New graduates are most at risk of having a claim filed against them.(52) For 10% of these newly minted professionals, a claim arises during the first year of practice.(52)

Communication complaints are frequently the source of litigation. The most prevalent complaints that were reported to the CVO involved:(53)

- perceived lack of care
  - not asking for or using the patient's name
  - not speaking to the patient reassuringly
- perceived lack of professionalism
  - making inappropriate comments about the patient
  - making inappropriate comments about the client
  - making inappropriate comments about the client to other clinics
  - making inappropriate comments about other team members
  - breaching confidentiality
- perceived lack of transparency
  - not explaining procedural risks
  - not explaining test results
  - misrepresenting after-hours care
  - not obtaining consent for procedures
  - not painting an accurate picture of the patient's prognosis
- perceived lack of follow-up
  - not providing written or verbal instructions in the postoperative period
  - not providing copies of medical records upon request
  - not returning telephone calls in a timely fashion
  - not acknowledging or addressing client concerns
  - delegating follow-up to a staff member
  - not providing condolences after the death of a patient
  - not offering to perform a necropsy to establish cause of death.

Note that not one of the aforementioned complaints is about the veterinarian's lack of knowledge or medical expertise. All are related to the interpersonal skills that are the backdrop to the delivery of healthcare. None of these blunders are reflective of the veterinarian's competence, yet each blunder left a lasting mark on the client that detracted from the way in which care was perceived and/or received.

The power of communication failures cannot be understated. These blunders are corrosive to the veterinarian–client–patient relationship. Rather than building the relationship, they hinder it. The damage to the pre-existing relationship may or may not be repairable.

Each mistake is a reminder to veterinarians, new and old alike, that communication errors leave lasting impressions. It is not always about what you know. It is about how you present yourself.

Today's veterinary clients have high expectations for practicing veterinarians.(1, 2) These expectations center on whether or not the veterinarian appears to care.(1, 2)

Veterinary educators cannot necessarily teach students compassion or how to care. However, they can train students in interpersonal skills to soften the delivery of health-care in a way that is better received by the consumer.

New graduates expressed their desire for educators to impart these life skills. At the same time, veterinary clients were lobbying for the same attributes to be present among new graduates.(1, 50)

What once fell upon deaf ears was finally heard. Veterinary educators recognized that the deficit was real and could be best addressed by inserting communication training into the curriculum.(15) Change was slow to take hold, but one by one veterinary colleges saw a shift in their curricular emphasis.

In 2001, life skills were written into the list of attributes that the University of California, Davis, School of Veterinary Medicine expected of its graduates.(47) Having knowledge was no longer deemed adequate for professional success. Graduates were expected to pair knowledge with compassion, altruism, and skill.(47) Communication was implied, but not named.

In 2002, communication was recognized as being essential to the success of Australian veterinary graduates.(55) Its training was incorporated shortly thereafter into the professional practice program at the Faculty of Veterinary Science at the University of Sydney.(56)

Concurrently, communication training was beginning to seep into practice management curricula at various institutions, including North Carolina State University College of Veterinary Medicine.(57–59) Communication was taught along with relationship-building skills, such as teamwork.(59) Effective and empathic communication was conveyed as a life skill and an indicator of professional success.

In 2003, the desire to infuse communication training into the curriculum led to the development of the National Unit for the Advancement of Veterinary Communication Skills (NUAVCS) as a joint initiative between the Republic of Ireland and the UK.(60) Around the same time, the Atlantic Veterinary College of the University of Prince Edward Island began to offer an elective rotation in communication training during the senior year of clinical rotations.(61)

In the present day, communication is considered to be a Day One Skill by both the Ontario Veterinary College (OVC) and the Royal College of Veterinary Surgeons (RCVS).(16) Curricular revisions have also paved the way for communication training throughout veterinary institutions in the British Isles and in the Netherlands.(16, 52, 62)

The North American Veterinary Medical Education Consortium (NAVMEC) remains the driving force to effect change within the United States.(16) The organization's publication, the "Roadmap for Veterinary Medical Education in the 21st Century," is a testament to the perceived importance of clinical communication: it outlines guidelines for teaching and assessment.(16, 63)

The importance of clinical communication training is no longer questioned among academic circles. It has undergone immense transformation from being viewed as an option to a requirement.

2.7 Communication as a Teachable Skill

The focus of active investigation has shifted from whether or not communication should be taught to what are the best avenues for delivery and assessment of this skillset. There is immense variability in the way in which present-day human medical programs approach this content area.(36, 52, 64–68)

This section is not meant to be exhaustive, but rather to provide an overview as to the current training tools in existence.

Methodologies that are currently in use include:(36, 52, 64–71)

- didactic presentations as a platform for lecturing about communication
- communication checklists(34)
- educational modules, such as those created by the Institute for Healthcare Communication (IHC)
- interactive workshops
- leadership retreats
- mock interviews
- team-building exercises
- the incorporation of small-group discussions into the classroom
- the viewing of filmed skits, that is, simulated appointments
- videotape review of interactions with real patients
- student observations of live role-play between
    - students
    - support staff
    - faculty
    - support staff and faculty
- the opportunity for students to practice delivery of constructive feedback
- the opportunity to practice communication skills using role-play
    - student role-play with other students
    - student role-play with support staff
    - student role-play with faculty
    - student role-play with standardized patients (SPs) – or, as they are referred to in veterinary curricula, standardized clients (SCs)

- the review of audiovisual recordings of role-plays to encourage reflection about past performance and to engage in goal-setting for the next opportunity to practice
- objective structured clinical examinations (OSCEs)
- on-the-clinic-floor learning with real-life patients
- patient assessment of communication skills using surveys.

Didactic lectures were traditionally employed when communication training first entered into medical and veterinary curricula. However, most have been traded out for experiential learning opportunities when possible.(36, 65) The ability to observe, practice, and refine communication techniques results in improved skill performance over time.(36)

Communication training is not successful overnight. It takes time to develop, improve upon, and modify skills. Experiential learning opportunities that offer the chance for repeated practice are most beneficial to the learner, provided that the learner feels safe and supported through the process.(36)

Personal growth is facilitated when the learner is conditioned to both self-assess his or her performance and receive feedback from others. Feedback may come from a number of external sources, including:

- classmates
- the individual who assumes the role of the "patient" or "client"
- the instructor.

Feedback is most constructive when it is descriptive, specific, and non-judgmental. The learner who is receptive to feedback is most likely to grow. Word choice and delivery of feedback play pivotal roles in how it is received and whether or not it is ultimately considered.

Role-play has historically been of benefit in that it allows the learner to be on the receiving end of immediate feedback.(64, 68) The learner is also able to learn through practice and repetition without fear of harming an actual patient physically or emotionally, by saying the wrong thing at the wrong time.(36, 64, 72)

Yet there are limitations to the use of student–student role-play. Classmates already presumably know one another, both from in-class and outside-of-class interactions. Pre-existing relationships may color the way in which the students interact with one another. Interactions may progress easily if both parties are comfortable with one another. Although this is beneficial from the standpoint of comfort, it does little to simulate what it is like to engage a stranger.

At the other extreme, consider a class that is not particularly close-knit. Classmates may be inhibited because of fear of making a mistake in front of their peer group. If measures are not taken to create a safe, supportive environment, then students are set up for failure from the start. They may be less willing to engage in the simulation or less eager to share what it is that they want to say to their "client" if they feel that they are constantly under attack or being judged. They may also be reluctant to fully commit to the simulation if they fear that what is said in the consultation room will be taken out of context or shared with others who were not privy to the initial conversation.

Role-play with trained actors to simulate patients in medical and veterinary training programs revolutionized the way that communication could be taught.(64) Encounters of any variety could be scripted to train SPs and SCs to portray any role in any setting. (64) Their portrayal of the patient could be fine-tuned to reflect the emotional climate of the clinical case. They could be taught to act and react to a variety of statements in a way that would either facilitate or hinder the consultation, thus making the encounter more lifelike.

Encounters may focus on entry-level skills, such as:

- introducing the medical team
- eliciting the chief complaint
- history taking
- explaining and planning
  - diagnostic plan
  - diagnostic test results
  - diagnosis
  - therapeutic plan (curative, palliative, medical, and surgical)
- prognosticating
- summarizing
- concluding the visit.

As students develop clinical acumen, encounters may advance to content areas that are essential for sensitivity training, such as clinical communication that pertains to:(64, 68, 73–87)

- bad news delivery
- cardiopulmonary resuscitation (CPR)
- cultural competence
- discord within the medical team
- end-of-life
- interpersonal conflict
- medical error
- mental health awareness
- obstetrics
- pediatric medicine
- physical or sexual assault
- trauma
- triage
- unexpected death.

Additional content areas that have been explored in veterinary medical training include:(64, 69, 88)

- anesthetic death
- animal cruelty reporting
- animal husbandry
- animal neglect
- convenience euthanasia
- cost of care
- euthanasia
- herd health
- preventative medicine
  - canine
  - feline
- veterinary team disputes
  - doctor–employer
  - doctor–technician.

Method acting, cosmetics, prosthetics, and simulators – for instance, vests that are embedded with heart and lung sounds when the learner auscultates over the correct region – have all contributed to the realism of SP encounters. For instance, the following physical examination findings can now be realistically reproduced:(64, 68)

- adventitious lung sounds
- arrhythmias
- bradycardia
- bruising
- gut sounds
- jaundice
- tachycardia.

Live animals may or may not be used in veterinary simulations.(64)

2.8 Present-Day Challenges Associated with Teaching Communication

For communication training to be effective, there needs to be buy-in. Everyone who is involved in the program – students, support staff, faculty, SPs, SCs, and administration – must believe that communication is important and teachable. There needs to be a commitment to the cause, and recognition that effective communication is both practical and possible. It is not a soft and fluffy skill. It is not an option. It is essential.

As an essential skill, communication requires both practice and practical application. In colleges of veterinary medicine across the globe, other skillsets are practiced with repetition until they can be achieved with competence and proficiency. Consider, for example, the following skillsets:

- anesthesia
  - anesthetic protocol development
  - anesthetic protocol calculations
  - induction of anesthesia
  - intubation
  - maintenance of anesthesia
  - recovery from anesthesia
- surgery
  - aseptic technique
  - hand and instrument ties
  - instrument handling
  - instrument naming
  - instrument ties (suture handling and suture patterns)
  - patient prep
  - surgeon prep
  - tissue sampling
- miscellaneous
  - injections
  - intravenous catheterization
  - intravenous fluid administration
  - microscopy
  - necropsy
  - ophthalmoscopy
  - otoscopy
  - patient restraint
  - physical examination
  - radiographic interpretation
  - sample collection (bone marrow aspirates, fine needle aspirates, and venipuncture)
  - subcutaneous fluid administration.

Practice does not make perfect, but practice makes better. So, it is that we practice, and we practice, and we practice some more.

LeBlanc described this process eloquently in his treatise on communication skills training in the 21st century:

As a medical student in the early 2000s, we practiced physical examination maneuvers on each other first; we even learned to draw blood from each other's veins before anyone let us near a real patient, because simulation technology was not yet ready for prime time. Now there are central line insertion simulators and anesthesia simulators. We can practice doing airway intubations on test dummies and run mock "code blue" scenarios with realistic equipment that responds much as a patient might. These simulators allow trainees to practice the mechanics or a procedure or scenario outside the pressurized environment in which patients' lives are at stake. Building this "muscle memory" can serve us, and our patients, well.(89)

We would not expect a student to operate with finesse or give a student a live patient to operate on without first practicing these fundamental steps:

- hand hygiene
- gowning
- gloving
- draping
- how to hold the scalpel handle
- how to attach the scalpel blade
- how to recognize basic anatomical landmarks
- how to make an incision
- appropriate tissue handling
- hemostasis using proper instrumentation
- elimination of dead space
- skin and/or body cavity closure.

A surgeon must practice surgery to develop into an effective surgeon. Likewise, a clinician must practice effective communication to develop into an effective clinician.

LeBlanc explains:

Most people will … agree that trainees should practice using simulators first, before doing a risky procedure in real life on a real patient. This is hardly a controversial idea, and medical school curricula increasingly incorporate various types of simulation into their training … Allow me, then, to be a bit more controversial: I contend that we should take this logic a step further and extend it to the ways in which we communicate and interact with patients. After all, harm can come from words, too, or from body language, not just from the tip of an errantly placed needle or a mishandled scalpel. Simulation isn't just for procedures anymore; patient-doctor encounters can be simulated too.(89)

Practice takes time. Finding time in an already overloaded curriculum is challenging at best.(64, 90)

Content overload is a real phenomenon throughout veterinary curricula. In an attempt to prepare veterinary students for everything that they might encounter in practice, they are taught it all "just in case."(91–93) This philosophy leaves very little room for trimming. When students are faced with a full schedule of coursework, adding something new requires taking something out.

There is a palpable fear among educators of cutting out something that may be essential. The default has historically been to preserve content areas that are hard science at the expense of those that are "soft."

Communication has traditionally been viewed as a soft skill.(22) When cast in this light, communication training programs may struggle to find equal footing with other more prestigious disciplines. Time may ultimately be granted for communication training, but how much time and is it enough? Moreover, what does "enough" look like on paper? How is "enough" quantified? What data do educators need to collect to evaluate the strength and ultimately the success of communication curricula? Is there a baseline for comparison? Which approach to training communication is most effective? Why is it most effective, and how do we know this to be true? Questions beget questions.

In addition to curricular time constraints, communication programs require funding and a cohort of trained individuals.(90) It cannot be assumed that faculty have received training in communication. In fact, the majority have not. As a result, students have historically learned more about what *not* to say from faculty than *how* to communicate effectively.(69, 94, 95) This is especially true of clinical conversations that center on triage and emergency medicine, bad news delivery, and death notification.(69, 94, 95)

Train-the-trainers programs are essential so that teachers can model the very skills that students are being introduced to in the classroom.(96) Students need to witness communication skills in use within the classroom and throughout the clinic in order to recognize how effective communication facilitates clinical practice.

Students need to believe in communication training in order for it to be effective. (96–102) If they do not perceive a need for communication training, then they may not be open to learning it.(96)

2.9 The Future of Communication Training in Veterinary Curricula

Communication training in veterinary medicine is likely to evolve as each program establishes its own footing to emphasize key content areas that are particularly relevant to its student body.

Institutional flexibility allows each program to have autonomy.(103) This has allowed for novel approaches to implementing communication skills training, particularly among established universities, where time constraints require creativity and innovative ways to achieve curricular revision.

Newer veterinary programs are in a unique position to develop novel approaches to the teaching and assessment of communication skills by virtue of the fact that they are creating curricula from scratch. Consider, for instance, my role as founding faculty for Midwestern University (MWU) College of Veterinary Medicine (CVM) in Glendale, Arizona, between the years of 2014–2017. As founding faculty, I was in the unique position to design and implement one of the most extensive approaches to simulation-based education. This emphasis on clinical communication was made possible because, prior to the matriculation of the inaugural class of 2018, the MWU curriculum was a blank slate. Founding faculty were charged with customizing the curriculum based upon the perceived needs of the student body. Deficits in clinical communication as outlined by an extensive body of research, drove the curriculum in pursuit of the development of interpersonal skills. The result was that an expensive communication program was established at MWU CVM.

In total, 90 MWU CVM students of the class of 2018 participated in 27 SC encounters over eight consecutive quarters. Students' acquisition of communication skills and clinical communication confidence was tracked over time as one of the largest retrospective studies in this discipline. Students' performances were compared in the 1st and 27th encounters by evaluating their use of Calgary–Cambridge Guide (CCG) communication skills. These will be touched upon in Chapter 3.

Based upon self-reflective assessments and SC evaluations, students increased their use of all communication skills between the first and last encounter. Students were also more likely to take a complete and accurate patient history, and build rapport with the client. Mean scores for communication confidence, as self-reported by students, pre- and post-event, also increased. As was stated in the abstract:

> These findings support that an SC-rich curriculum facilitates student acquisition of communication skills and promotes confidence when students approach entry-level clinical tasks, such as history taking.(104)

Although not many universities are in the position to incorporate clinical communication training into the curriculum to this extent, MWU CVM set the stage for unique opportunities to test and subsequently share scripted encounters with colleagues.

Enthusiastic educators no longer have to reinvent the wheel. Resources that are designed to disseminate knowledge are increasingly accessible, both in print, through the *Journal of Veterinary Medical Education*, and by way of organizational events, such as the International Conference on Communication in Veterinary Medicine (ICCVM).

Much remains to be determined in terms of the impact that present-day communication training has on the success of recent graduates in the real world of veterinary practice. Further research is necessary to identify new deficits and/or previously unforeseen consequences of current curricular revisions. However, regardless of the direction in which clinical communication training moves towards, it is safe to say that the discipline has finally been accepted as a staple of the veterinary curriculum. As such, it is critical that students be trained in it as they would be for any other skill.

We train veterinary students to be successful surgeons by allowing them to practice tying square knots.

Why not do the same for communication?

Parts 2 and 3 of this textbook are designed to introduce entry-level communication skills to students of any institution to prepare them for success in clinical practice.

References

1. Frankel RM. Pets, vets, and frets: what relationship-centered care research has to offer veterinary medicine. J Vet Med Educ. 2006;33(1):20–7.

2. Stein TS, Nagy VT, Jacobs L. Caring for patients one conversation at a time: musings from the interregional clinician patient communication leadership group. Permanente J. 1998;2(4):62–8.

3. Engel GL. How much longer must medicine's science be bound by a seventeenth century world view? In: White KL, editor. The task of medicine: dialogue at Wickenburg. Menlo Park, CA: Henry J. Kaiser Family Foundation; 1988. pp. 133–77.

4. Lipkin MJ, Frankel RM, Beckman HB, Charon R, Fein O. Performing the interview. In: Lipkin MJ, Putnam SM, Lazare A, editors. The medical interview. New York: Springer-Verlag; 1995. pp. 65–82.

5. Bordage G. Why did I miss the diagnosis? Some cognitive explanations and educational implications. Acad Med. 1999;74(10 Suppl):S138–43.

6. Faustinella F, Jacobs RJ. The decline of clinical skills: a challenge for medical schools. Int J Med Educ. 2018;9:195–7.

7. Wiener S, Nathanson M. Physical examination. Frequently observed errors. JAMA. 1976;236(7):852–5.

8. Epstein RM. Realizing Engel's biopsychosocial vision: resilience, compassion, and quality of care. Int J Psychiatry Med. 2014;47(4):275–87.

9. Cohen-Cole SA. The medical interview: the three function approach. St. Louis, MS: Mosby Yearbook; 1991.

10. Hellin T. The physician–patient relationship: recent developments and changes. Haemophilia. 2002;8(3):450–4.

11. To err is human: building a safer health system. Washington, DC: Institute of Medicine; 2000.

12. O'Donnell M. The night Bernard Shaw taught us a lesson. BMJ. 2006;333(7582):1338–40.

13. Silverman JD, Kurtz SM, Draper J. Skills for communicating with patients. Oxford: Taylor & Francis; 2013.

14. Simpson M, Buckman R, Stewart M, Maguire P, Lipkin M, Novack D, et al. Doctor–patient communication: the Toronto consensus statement. BMJ. 1991;303(6814):1385–7.

15. Coleman GT, Salter LK, Thornton JR. What skills should veterinarians possess on graduation? Aust Vet Pract. 2000;30(3):124–31.

16. Englar RE, Williams M, Weingand K. Applicability of the Calgary–Cambridge Guide to dog and cat owners for teaching veterinary clinical communications. J Vet Med Educ. 2016;43(2):143–69.

17. Beckman HB, Frankel RM. The effect of physician behavior on the collection of data. Ann Intern Med. 1984;101(5):692–6.

18. Becker MH. Patient adherence to prescribed therapies. Med Care. 1985;23(5):539–55.

19. Coleman VR. Physician behaviour and compliance. J Hypertens Suppl. 1985;3(1):S69–71.

20. Garrity TF. Medical compliance and the clinician-patient relationship: a review. Soc Sci Med E. 1981;15(3):215–22.

21. Stewart MA. Effective physician–patient communication and health outcomes: a review. CMAJ. 1995;152(9):1423–33.

22. Travaline JM, Ruchinskas R, D'Alonzo GE, Jr. Patient–physician communication: why and how. J Am Osteopath Assoc. 2005;105(1):13–8.

23. Matthews DA, Suchman AL, Branch WT, Jr. Making "connexions": enhancing the therapeutic potential of patient–clinician relationships. Ann Intern Med. 1993;118(12):973–7.

24. Suchman AL, Matthews DA. What makes the patient–doctor relationship therapeutic? Exploring the connexional dimension of medical care. Ann Intern Med. 1988;108(1):125–30.

25. Maguire P, Fairbairn S, Fletcher C. Consultation skills of young doctors: I—Benefits of feedback training in interviewing as students persist. Br Med J (Clin Res Ed). 1986;292(6535):1573–6.

26. Cowan D, Danoff D, Davis A, Degner L, Jerry M, Kurtz S, et al. Consensus statement from the workshop on the teaching and assessment of communication-skills in Canadian medical schools. Can Med Assoc J. 1992;147(8):1149–50.

27. Tomorrow's doctors: outcomes and standards for undergraduate medical education. Manchester: General Medical Council; 2009.

28. Makoul G. Essential elements of communication in medical encounters: the Kalamazoo consensus statement. Acad Med. 2001;76(4):390–3.

29. Novack DH, Suchman AL, Clark W, Epstein RM, Najberg E, Kaplan C. Calibrating the physician. Personal awareness and effective patient care. Working Group on Promoting Physician Personal Awareness, American Academy on Physician and Patient. JAMA. 1997;278(6):502–9.

30. Makoul G, Curry RH, Novack DH. The future of medical school courses in professional skills and perspectives. Acad Med. 1998;73(1):48–51.

31. Makoul G, Schofield T. Communication teaching and assessment in medical education: an international consensus statement. Netherlands Institute of Primary Health Care. Patient Educ Couns. 1999;37(2):191–5.

32. Rider EA, Hinrichs MM, Lown BA. A model for communication skills assessment across the undergraduate curriculum. Med Teach. 2006;28(5):e127–34.

33. Batalden P, Leach D, Swing S, Dreyfus H, Dreyfus S. General competencies and accreditation in graduate medical education. Health Aff (Millwood). 2002;21(5):103–11.

34. Duffy FD, Gordon GH, Whelan G, Cole-Kelly K, Frankel R, Buffone N, et al. Assessing competence in communication and interpersonal skills: the Kalamazoo II report. Acad Med. 2004;79(6):495–507.

35. Latham CE, Morris A. Effects of formal training in communication skills on the ability of veterinary students to communicate with clients. Vet Rec. 2007;160(6):181–6.

36. Shaw JR, Adams CL, Bonnett BN. What can veterinarians learn from studies of physician–patient communication about veterinarian–client–patient communication? J Am Vet Med Assoc. 2004;224(5):676–84.

37. Reed CF, Koski GR, Baker BR. Use of simulated interview to teach doctor–client communication skills. J Vet Med Educ. 1974;1:9–10.

38. Horvatich PK, Meyer KB. Teaching client relations and communication skills: part II – a systematic approach. J Vet Med Educ. 1979;6:99–104.

39. Routly JE, Taylor IR, Turner R, McKernan EJ, Dobson H. Support needs of veterinary surgeons during the first few years of practice: perceptions of recent graduates and senior partners. Vet Rec. 2002;150(6):167–71.

40. Heath T. Teaching communication skills to veterinary students. J Vet Med Educ. 1996;23:2–7.

41. Heath T. The more things change, the more they should stay the same. J Vet Med Educ. 2006;33(2):149–54.

42. Case DB. Survey of expectations among clients of three small animal clinics. J Am Vet Med Assoc. 1988;192(4):498–502.

43. Antelyes J. Client hopes, client expectations. J Am Vet Med Assoc. 1990;197(12):1596–7.

44. Antelyes J. Difficult clients in the next decade. J Am Vet Med Assoc. 1991;198(4):550–2.

45. Coe JB, Adams CL, Bonnett BN. A focus group study of veterinarians' and pet owners' perceptions of veterinarian-client communication in companion animal practice. J Am Vet Med Assoc. 2008;233(7):1072–80.

46. Heath TJ, Mills JN. Criteria used by employers to select new graduate employees. Aust Vet J. 2000;78(5):312–6.

45

47. Walsh DA, Osburn BI, Christopher MM. Defining the attributes expected of graduating veterinary medical students. J Am Vet Med Assoc. 2001;219(10):1358–65.

48. Arborelius E, Bremberg S. What can doctors do to achieve a successful consultation? Videotaped interviews analysed by the 'consultation map' method. Fam Pract. 1992;9(1):61–6.

49. Bristol DG. Using alumni research to assess a veterinary curriculum and alumni employment and reward patterns. J Vet Med Educ. 2002;29(1):20–7.

50. Brown JP, Silverman JD. The current and future market for veterinarians and veterinary medical services in the United States – executive summary – May, 1999. J Am Vet Med Assoc. 1999;215(2):161–83.

51. Adams CL, Frankel RM. It may be a dog's life but the relationship with her owners is also key to her health and well being: communication in veterinary medicine. Vet Clin North Am Small Anim Pract. 2007;37(1):1–17; abstract vii.

52. Radford AD, Stockley P, Taylor IR, Turner R, Gaskell CJ, Kaney S, et al. Use of simulated clients in training veterinary undergraduates in communication skills. Vet Rec. 2003;152(14):422–7.

53. Miscommunication – always review the medical history. College of Veterinarians of Ontario (CVO); 2005.

54. Stell A. Communication skills training at the Royal Veterinary College (RVC): a review of undergraduate teaching and learning methods. London: Royal Veterinary College, University of London; 2010 [Available from: https://docplayer.net/11792503-Communication-skills-training-at-the-royal-veterinary-college-rvc-a-review-of-undergraduate-teaching-and-learning-methods.html].

55. Collins GH, Taylor RM. Attributes of Australasian veterinary graduates: report of a workshop held at the Veterinary Conference Centre, Faculty of Veterinary Science, University of Sidney, January 28–19, 2002. J Vet Med Educ. 2002;29(2):71–2.

56. Collins GH. The Professional Practice program in the University of Sydney curriculum. J Vet Med Educ. 2002;29(2):81–3.

57. Draper DD, Uhlenhopp EK. A veterinary business curriculum model. J Vet Med Educ. 2002;29(2):73–80.

58. Lloyd JW, Walsh DA. Template for a recommended curriculum in "veterinary professional development and career success". J Vet Med Educ. 2002;29(2):84–93.

59. Stell EJ, Price GS, Swanson C. Implementation and assessment of a career and life skills program for matriculating veterinary medical students. J Am Vet Med Assoc. 2000;217(9):1311–4.

60. Gray CA, Blaxter AC, Johnston PA, Latham CE, May S, Phillips CA, et al. Communication education in veterinary in the United Kingdom and Ireland: the NUVACS project coupled to progressive individual school endeavors. J Vet Med Educ. 2006;33(1):85–92.

61. Shaw DH, Ihle SL. Communication skills training at the Atlantic Veterinary College, University of Prince Edward Island. J Vet Med Educ. 2006;33(1):100–4.

62. Van Beukelen P. Curriculum development in the Netherlands: introduction of tracks in the 2001 curriculum at Utrecht University, the Netherlands. J Vet Med Educ. 2004;31(3):227–33.

63. Meehan MP, Menniti MF. Final-year veterinary students' perceptions of their communication competencies and a communication skills training program delivered in a primary care setting and based on Kolb's Experiential Learning Theory. J Vet Med Educ. 2014;41(4):371–83.

64. Englar RE. A novel approach to simulation-based education for veterinary medical communication training over eight consecutive pre-clinical quarters. J Vet Med Educ.44(3):502–22.

65. Kurtz SM, Silverman JD, Draper J. Teaching and learning communication skills in medicine. Grand Rapids, MI: Radcliffe; 2004.

66. Chun R, Schaefer S, Lotta CC, Banning JA, Skochelak SE. Didactic and experiential training to teach communication skills: the University of Wisconsin-Madison School of Veterinary Medicine collaborative experience. J Vet Med Educ. 2009;36(2):196–201.

67. Rickles NM, Tieu P, Myers L, Galal S, Chung V. The impact of a standardized patient program on student learning of communication skills. Am J Pharm Educ. 2009;73(1):4.

68. Barrows HS. An overview of the uses of standardized patients for teaching and evaluating clinical skills. AAMC. Acad Med. 1993;68(6):443–51; discussion 51–3.

69. Englar RE. Using a standardized client encounter to practice death notification after the unexpected death of a feline patient following routine ovariohysterectomy. J Vet Med Educ. 2019:1–17.

70. Veterinary communication. Institute for Healthcare Communication (IHC); 2019 [Available from: https://healthcarecomm.org/veterinary-communication/].

71. Egnew TR, Mauksch LB, Greer T, Farber SJ. Integrating communication training into a required family medicine clerkship. Acad Med. 2004;79(8):737–43.

72. Emanuel EJ, Emanuel LL. Four models of the physician–patient relationship. JAMA. 1992;267(16):2221–6.

73. Barrows HS. Simulated patients in medical teaching. Can Med Assoc J. 1968;98(14):674–6.

74. Karkowsky CE, Landsberger EJ, Bernstein PS, Dayal A, Goffman D, Madden RC, et al. Breaking bad news in obstetrics: a randomized trial of simulation followed by debriefing or lecture. J Matern Fetal Neonatal Med. 2016;29(22):3717–23.

75. McLaughlin S, Fitch MT, Goyal DG, Hayden E, Kauh CY, Laack TA, et al. Simulation in graduate medical education 2008: a review for emergency medicine. Acad Emerg Med. 2008;15(11):1117–29.

76. Okuda Y, Quinones J. The use of simulation in the education of emergency care providers for cardiac emergencies. Int J Emerg Med. 2008;1(2):73–7.

77. Kharasch M, Aitchison P, Pettineo C, Pettineo L, Wang EE. Physiological stress responses of emergency medicine residents during an immersive medical simulation scenario. Dis Mon. 2011;57(11):700–5.

78. Girzadas DV, Jr., Delis S, Bose S, Hall J, Rzechula K, Kulstad EB. Measures of stress and learning seem to be equally affected among all roles in a simulation scenario. Simul Healthc. 2009;4(3):149–54.

79. Clarke S, Horeczko T, Cotton D, Bair A. Heart rate, anxiety and performance of residents during a simulated critical clinical encounter: a pilot study. BMC Med Educ. 2014;14:153.

80. Brown RF, Bylund CL. Communication skills training: describing a new conceptual model. Acad Med. 2008;83(1):37–44.

81. Chumpitazi CE, Rees CA, Chumpitazi BP, Hsu DC, Doughty CB, Lorin MI. Creation and assessment of a bad news delivery simulation curriculum for pediatric emergency medicine fellows. Cureus. 2016;8(5):e595.

82. Contro N, Larson J, Scofield S, Sourkes B, Cohen H. Family perspectives on the quality of pediatric palliative care. Arch Pediatr Adolesc Med. 2002;156(1):14–9.

83. Meert KL, Eggly S, Pollack M, Anand KJ, Zimmerman J, Carcillo J, et al. Parents' perspectives on physician-parent communication near the time of a child's death in the pediatric intensive care unit. Pediatr Crit Care Med. 2008;9(1):2–7.

84. Park I, Gupta A, Mandani K, Haubner L, Peckler B. Breaking bad news education for emergency medicine residents: A novel training module using simulation with the SPIKES protocol. J Emerg Trauma Shock. 2010;3(4):385–8.

85. Ballman K, Garritano N, Beery T. Broadening the reach of standardized patients in nurse practitioner education to include the distance learner. Nurse Educ. 2016;41(5):230–3.

86. Hart JA, Chilcote DR. "Won't You Be My Patient?" Preparing theater students as standardized patients. J Nurs Educ. 2016;55(3):168–71.

87. Shirazi M, Labaf A, Monjazebi F, Jalili M, Mirzazadeh M, Ponzer S, et al. Assessing medical students' communication skills by the use of standardized patients: emphasizing standardized patients' quality assurance. Acad Psychiatry. 2014;38(3):354–60.

88. Englar RE. Using a standardized client encounter in the veterinary curriculum to practice veterinarian–employer discussions about animal cruelty reporting. J Vet Med Educ. 2018:1–16.

89. LeBlanc TW. Communication skills training in the twenty-first century. AMA J Ethics. 2015;17(2):140–3.

90. Communication skills: the case for early training. Vet Rec 2001;148:129–32.

91. Bushby PA. Tackling the knowledge explosion without overloading the student. Aust Vet J. 1994;71(11):372–4.

92. May SA, Silva-Fletcher A. Scaffolded active learning: nine pedagogical principles for building a modern veterinary curriculum. J Vet Med Educ. 2015;42(4):332–9.

93. Jackson EL, Armitage-Chan E. The challenges and issues of undergraduate student retention and attainment in UK veterinary medical education. J Vet Med Educ. 2017;44(2):247–59.

94. Bowyer MW, Hanson JL, Pimentel EA, Flanagan AK, Rawn LM, Rizzo AG, et al. Teaching breaking bad news using mixed reality simulation. J Surg Res. 2010;159(1):462–7.

95. Fallowfield L, Jenkins V. Communicating sad, bad, and difficult news in medicine. Lancet. 2004;363(9405):312–9.

96. Cushing A, Najberg E, Hajek P. Do medical students believe that communication skills can be learned? In: Scherpbier AJJA, van der Vleuten CPM, Rethans JJ, van der Steeg AFW, editors. Advances in medical education. Dordrecht: Kluwer Academic Publishers; 1997. p. 676–8.

97. Moral RR, Garcia de Leonardo C, Caballero Martinez F, Monge Martin D. Medical students' attitudes toward communication skills learning: comparison between two groups with and without training. Adv Med Educ Pract. 2019;10:55–61.

98. Langille DB, Kaufman DM, Laidlaw TA, Sargeant J, MacLeod H. Faculty attitudes towards medical communication and their perceptions of students' communication skills training at Dalhousie University. Med Educ. 2001;35(6):548–54.

99. Kaufman DM, Laidlaw TA, Macleod H. Communication skills in medical school: exposure, confidence, and performance. Acad Med. 2000;75(10 Suppl):S90–2.

100. Howley LD, Wilson WG. Direct observation of students during clerkship rotations: a multiyear descriptive study. Acad Med. 2004;79(3):276–80.

101. Humphris GM, Kaney S. Assessing the development of communication skills in undergraduate medical students. Med Educ. 2001;35(3):225–31.

102. Roter DL, Hall JA, Aoki Y. Physician gender effects in medical communication: a meta-analytic review. JAMA. 2002;288(6):756–64.

103. Kalet A, Pugnaire MP, Cole-Kelly K, Janicik R, Ferrara E, Schwartz MD, et al. Teaching communication in clinical clerkships: models from the macy initiative in health communications. Acad Med. 2004;79(6):511–20.

104. Englar RE. Tracking veterinary students' acquisition of communication skills and clinical communication confidence by comparing student performance in the first and twenty-seventh standardized client encounters. J Vet Med Educ. 2018;46(2):235–57.

Chapter 3

How Can We Structure the Consultation from the Vantage Point of Clinical Communication?

The Calgary–Cambridge Guide as a Blueprint for a Collaborative Consultation

Over the past 30 years, evidence-based research has made a compelling case that effective communication enhances the delivery of healthcare and patient outcomes.(1) Although knowledge forms a necessary foundation for medical training, clinical acumen is insufficient and may be inadequate without broadening the clinician's exposure to and development of interpersonal skills. The concept of what it means to be a good doctor is changing. The modernization of medicine, technological advances, and ubiquity of free and accessible healthcare information via the World Wide Web have altered consumer expectations. The provider's knowledge base is less important to today's veterinary client than knowing that the provider cares.(2, 3) This shift in consumer expectations has reshaped the doctor–patient relationship in human healthcare from one of medical paternalism to one of patient-centered care.

3.1 The Shift from Medical Paternalism to Relationship-Centered Care

In Western medicine, the "sage on the stage" physician has largely been replaced by the "guide on the side." In a sense, medicine has come full circle to revive the perspective of William Osler, a Canadian physician and a founding professor of Johns Hopkins Hospital. Osler received his medical degree in 1872 and was among the first faculty to teach students that patients had a voice in healthcare. Osler trained students at bedside and believed that there should be "no teaching without the patient for a text, and the best teaching is often that taught by the patient himself."(4)

Osler's perspective was in the minority during his career as an educator. However, his viewpoint is, in a sense, the heart of relationship-centered care. Relationship-centered care requires connectivity between two parties. This connectivity is grounded in mutual respect for one another, trust, and the belief in equality – that, while doctors may be experts in medical knowledge, patients are experts in what it is like to be them.(5)

Present-day patients are no longer just blank canvases for clinicians to paint as they see fit. Patients are individuals who require customized care that takes into consideration what they feel is best for them, given their unique circumstances. More than that, today's patients have the right "to considerate, respectful care from all members of the healthcare system at all times and under all circumstances."(6)

3.2 Relationship-Centered Care in Veterinary Medicine

The humanizing aspect of healthcare has trickled over into the veterinary sector, particularly in the realm of companion animal practice. Companion animals are now considered to be members of the family by 85% of pet owners.(7) This distinction emphasizes the importance that is placed upon dog- and cat-ownership. Pets are no longer considered, by the majority, to be property. They are part of the family. They are loved ones. Many would go so far as to say that they consider a pet to be a child. Just as a parent is responsible for a child, so, too, does the pet owner consider him/herself to be responsible for the cat or dog.(8, 9)

As the responsible agent, the veterinary client has risen to the role of advocate. The veterinary client must advocate for decision making that will be of direct benefit to the patient. (8, 9) This requires the veterinary client to take on a leading role in presenting the patient, relaying case history, and initiating dialogue about the chief complaint.(8–11)

As advocates for loved ones, pet owners expect healthcare to be delivered by veterinarians in such a way as to reflect the growing importance of the human–animal bond. (7, 12) An understanding of the human–animal bond is now essential to the practice of companion animal medicine.(12) Tending to the wellbeing of the pet must also, by default, include tending to the wellbeing of the person at the other end of the leash.(12, 13) Doing so requires investment in a two-way social interaction, in which history gathering, information processing, and decision making are joint efforts.(14) Decision making is thus shared, and the encounter is interactive.(14–16) To recognize and preserve this dynamic, various models for the medical consultation have been proposed.

3.3 The Development of Consultation Models

The delibery of primary care is exceptionally demanding in terms of what clinicians are expected to accomplish within a small window of time. Consider all that needs to transpire during a routine annual wellness visit. In what is typically a 10-minute time-slot, a human healthcare provider must:(17)

- greet the client
- make introductions
- maintain rapport
- establish the reason for the consult
- establish any pre-existing concerns
- establish patient expectations for the visit
- set the agenda for the visit
- gather history
- conduct a physical examination
- outline and address relevant findings
  - make recommendations
  - devise a diagnostic plan
  - develop a therapeutic plan
- contract for next steps
- make a plan for follow-up.

The content of the veterinary visit is strikingly similar, particularly if one were to compare the role of veterinarian to that of the pediatrician: both engage in a tripartite relationship.(8, 9, 18) The veterinarian and pediatrician both must rely upon a third party to provide valuable insight into the perceived health status of the patient and any apparent deviations from the norm.(8–11)

In order to get the most out of the clinical encounter, the clinician must find the proper balance between data mining and relationship building.(12) Both are assets to the developing provider–consumer relationship. The successful practitioner is mindful of this and obtains the information that is needed for clinical reasoning while remaining attentive to the partnership that she or he is attempting to build.(12)

Novices often focus on the content aspect of the consultation: "Doctors tend to see contact with patients as either getting information out of, or imparting advice to, sick people, and they therefore ignore a vital purpose of communication."(19) In so doing, they sacrifice any strides that would have been made towards collaboration.

Clients, on the other hand, may be "seeking a relationship as much or more than biological treatment." (20) "With … the medical system becoming increasingly impersonal, the modern day lament of patients is that physicians do not spend enough time with them, do not listen to them, and do not understand them." (21)

In other words, "they may want to air their troubles or vent their feelings; they may want instructions on how to relieve their suffering; they may want reassurance or information to calm their fears regarding their health."(20)

With each side focusing on their own needs, the healthcare provider and the patient risk missing the mark and passing each other by like two trains in the night. Each may attempt to understand the other with a near miss.

Evidence-based research suggests that in order to maximize patient satisfaction and outcomes, clinicians need to do their part to ensure that the patient's agenda is addressed. How can we, as providers, achieve just that, given the limited frame under which we operate?

A variety of consultation models have been developed to keep the clinician on track by providing a structured approach to the clinical interview.

In the early stages of medical education, this provides the learner with tangible steps and a logical order to the flow of the consultation. Learners may not be able to carry out all of the tasks for each step on account of limited knowledge and clinical acumen. However, they can at least make their way through the process to see how relationship building and content acquisition can be linked.

In the later stages of medical education, the learner can target key communication skills that she or he may personally find to be challenging and emphasize these in each encounter to improve clinical performance.(17)

Just as each clinician has his or her own communication style and clinical approach, there is no one right consultation model.(12) This is because there is no "gold standard" provider–consumer interaction.(12) Each interaction is unique by virtue of its participants and their respective needs. These needs may vary depending upon the clinical setting, situation, and underlying emotional currents.

For these reasons, several consultation models have been developed, each with the intention of highlighting, adapting, improving, and refining consultation skills. These include, but are not limited to, the following task-associated models:(17, 22)

- Balint model(23–25)
- Berne's model(26)
- Byrne–Long model(24, 25, 27, 28)
- Pendleton's model
- Neighbour's model(24, 29)
- Stott and Davis' model(30)
- Calgary–Cambridge model.(28, 31)

Proposed consultation models vary in terms of which aspect(s) of the consultation they emphasize. For instance, the Balint model concentrated on the psychological aspect of the consultation.(23–25) According to this model, the doctor is the most sought after and prescribed "drug."(17) The physician's ability to listen to his or her patients was in and of itself considered therapeutic. Balint proposed that active listening would make patients feel better irrespective of other treatment modalities.(17)

Proposed consultation models also vary in terms of patient-centeredness and their applicability to different clinical scenarios.(17) One model may be appropriate for one particular clinical scenario, but not for another.(12) Flexibility is essential so that care can be tailored to the individual patient in a manner that is genuine for the provider.(12)

Only the Calgary–Cambridge model will be discussed at length here. However, note that all models offer the healthcare team the potential to reinforce connectivity with clients.

3.4 The Calgary–Cambridge Model

The Calgary–Cambridge model is derived from a 1996 publication by Kurtz and Silverman that outlined the Calgary–Cambridge Referenced Observation Guides as a skills-based, patient-centered framework of the consultation.(17, 28, 31, 32)

Both Guides borrowed heavily from the model that was proposed by Riccardi and Kurtz in 1983.(32, 33) This model subdivided the consultation into five sequential tasks:(32, 33)

- initiating the session
- gathering information
- building the relationship/facilitating the patient's involvement
- giving information
- closing the session.

Kurtz and Silverman redefined the fourth task as explaining and planning.(32)

All five tasks were considered appropriate for every consultation.(32) Each task was associated with a subset of communication skills.

Guide One, Interviewing the Patient, concentrated on the first half of the consultation: history taking and data collection.(32)

Guide Two, Explanation and Planning with the Patient, was an attempt to flush out the second half of the consultation, which had been historically ignored in the training of new doctors by medical educators.(32, 34, 35) Despite recognition that explaining clinical findings is an essential part of the consultation, it was rarely discussed in the classroom or at the patient's bedside. This realization was summarized by the English medical educator and hematologist, Sir Ronald Bodley Scott:

> This transaction, [explanation and planning], is the doctor's quintessential function for it is a necessary preliminary to any treatment, [yet] we seldom discuss it with our students and never instruct them in its management.(34, 36)

Kurtz and Silverman felt that this omission was significant and led to incomplete consultations with potentially inaccurate outcomes. The consultation owed it to the patient and physician alike to be complete.

Thus the purpose of both Guides, collectively, was to provide a teaching tool for facilitators and a learning tool for students that provided a comprehensive, evidence-based approach to clinical communication training.(28, 31, 32, 37)

Prior to the Guides' development, faculty did not always feel comfortable with the subject, communication, or the science underlying it.(32) Kurtz and Silverman felt strongly that any communication program could not be successful unless its facilitators understood the "what" (the content) and the "how" (the process).(28, 31, 32, 37)

The Guides were an attempt to marry the two such that, moving forward, curriculum could be consistent and comprehensive.(31, 32, 37) In a sense, the Guides were the earliest rendition of train-the-trainer. They established which skills were deemed essential to the success of clinical conversations and how best to relate them to actual consultations.

Although several communication models had been developed prior to the Calgary–Cambridge Referenced Observation Guides, Kurtz and Silverman's approach was uniquely backed by research and theory.(32) Moreover, the Calgary–Cambridge Referenced Observation Guides were among the first to demonstrate a patient-centered approach to healthcare.(32)

This approach also strengthened the argument that physicians function not only to gather data, but to use that data for the purpose of explaining and planning.(32) Young doctors historically performed poorly in this aspect of the consultation, for lack of training.(34) Maguire et al. outlined their common failings in 1986 as such:(34)

- failure to summarize clinical problems or treatments
- failure to elicit the patient's perspective concerning diagnosis
- failure to elicit the patient's expectations for treatment
- failure to provide options for treatment
- failure to negotiate options for treatment with the patient
- failure to address prognosis
- failure to brainstorm with the client ways to improve compliance.

The Guides were an attempt to remedy these deficiencies by structuring the consultation. The resultant aide-mémoire was both concise and accessible. The basic framework allowed for consistency in one's approach to clinical communication for the first time in medical training.

The facilitator now had a foundation to refer students back to when they felt "stuck" in conversation with their patients. Even better yet, the facilitator could now reference key aspects of the model to help the learner answer the following questions.(32)

- Where are you in the interview?
- What are you trying to achieve here?
- Where do you want to get to?
- How do you get there?

Earlier versions of the Guides were piloted at the University of Calgary Medical School in Canada for 18 years prior to their publication in 1996.(32, 33, 38) Since then, the Guides have undergone several revisions. These revisions were intended to enhance the visual construct of the Calgary–Cambridge model for use in teaching. (28, 39)

The expanded framework integrates the process – what is happening in a medical interview, in the moment – with appropriate objectives for each task. For example, the task of initiating the session requires the clinician to achieve the following objectives:

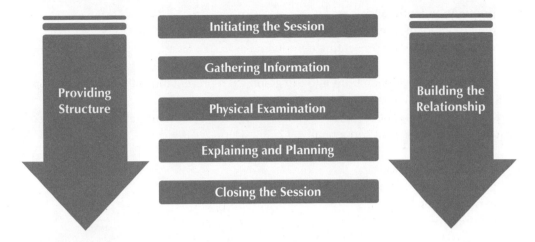

Figure 3.1 The basic framework of the Calgary–Cambridge model.
Reprinted with permission from the original work: Kurtz S, Silverman J, Benson J, Draper J. Marrying content and process in clinical method teaching: enhancing the Calgary–Cambridge guides. Acad Med. 2003;78(8):802–9. Reprinted with permission from the most recent work: Adams CL, Kurtz SM. Skills for communicating in veterinary medicine. Oxford: Otmoor Publishing and Dewpoint Publishing; 2017. p25.

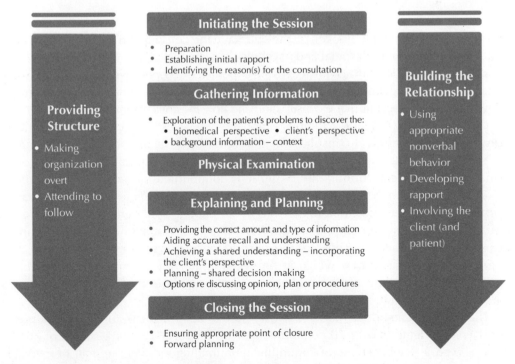

Figure 3.2 The expanded framework of the Calgary–Cambridge Guides.
Reprinted with permission from: Adams CL, Kurtz SM. Skills for communicating in veterinary medicine. Oxford: Otmoor Publishing and Dewpoint Publishing; 2017. p26.

- preparation for the visit
- development of rapport with the patient
- identification of the presenting complaint.

These objectives have been built into the graphical representations that were developed by Kurtz, Silverman, and Draper (see Figures 3.1 and 3.2).(31)

Kurtz, Silverman, and Draper's expanded model is consistent with the original construct's staging of the visit sequentially:(17, 28, 31)

- initiating the session
- gathering information
- explaining and planning
- closing the session.

Sandwiched in between the "gathering information" and the "explaining and planning" stages is the physical examination.(17, 28, 31)

Two additional tasks span all stages of the consultation: (17, 28, 31)

- building the relationship
- providing structure.

These tasks are essentially bookends: they package the consultation into an experience that blends medicine with social and psychological elements.(17)

Building the relationship acknowledges the importance of connectivity between provider and patient. Providing structure reiterates that both physicians and patients benefit from order; knowing what to expect from the consultation and how the consultation will flow.

Collectively, the Calgary–Cambridge model emphasizes the importance of clinical conversation. The clinical consultations that form the basis of relationship-centered care are intended to mirror a Frisbee toss rather than the shot put.(39) That is, relationship-centered care honors the belief that communication is a two-way street. Physicians rely upon the patient's contributions to gather complete and accurate data, from which they can make determinations about patient health and the likelihood of a disease state. However, physicians cannot and should not act on those determinations of their own accord. They are responsible for relaying information back to the client so that the client may weigh in on decision making. Compliance and adherence to treatment plans are both likely to be poor without mutual understanding, "buy-in," and commitment on the part of the patient.

The Calgary–Cambridge model is widely used to train medical students in the present-day, and identifies over 70 communication skills.(28, 31, 37, 40, 41) As of 2014, it has served as the backbone of communication training for over one-half of medical programs in the UK.(1, 42) The Calgary–Cambridge model is also popular in Canada and the United States.(1) It has been translated for use in undergraduate and postgraduate education throughout Europe.(1)

In addition to being a resource for the education of medical students, the Calgary–Cambridge model has been used to develop tools for formative assessments.(1) The performance of student doctors in the explanation and planning portion of the consultation, for instance, is commonly tested in OSCEs.(1, 43–45)

The use of the Calgary–Cambridge model in assessment has been validated.(1, 40, 46)

3.5 The Revised Calgary–Cambridge Model for Veterinary Patients

The veterinary profession is unique because it is grounded in a tripartite relationship: the veterinarian–client–patient is similar to, but not the same as the physician–parent–child. (8, 9, 18) There is significant overlap in that both parents and pet-owners see themselves in a guardian role. Both are responsible for those under their care, and want to be recognized for the role that each plays in advocating for patient welfare.(40, 47)

However, there are subtle distinctions between the human–animal and the parent–child bonds.(40, 48) The decision to treat or not to treat and how decision making unfolds in veterinary patients is unique.(40) Financial constraints often dictate the level of care that is provided, and, on account of cost, euthanasia may be performed out of necessity for a veterinary patient with otherwise curable disease.(40, 48)

It is critical that veterinarians develop strategies to navigate these communication challenges. Many of the same communication skills that are used in human healthcare are applicable to the veterinary profession. However, other veterinary scenarios may require additional skills and training that are beyond the scope of what a human physician might be expected to encounter in clinical practice.

To facilitate communication training by institutions outside of human healthcare, the Calgary–Cambridge model was adapted for use in veterinary medicine by Radford et al. in 2002.(40, 41, 44)

Radford recognized that, to be successful, communication training in veterinary institutions had to emphasize key features of the human–animal bond, with communication as the bridge that connected the dots within the veterinarian–client–patient relationship.

Through words and actions, the successful veterinarian needed to:(40, 44)

- acknowledge that the patient held value in the eyes of the client
- comfort the patient
- comfort the client
- interact with and connect to the patient
- allow the client to witness his/her interactions with the patient.

Being able to relate to the patient was a key determinant as to whether or not the veterinarian could build a relationship with the client.

In total, Radford's adaptation of the Calgary–Cambridge model for veterinary education and clinical practice outlines 54 communication skills.(40, 44) This veterinary version has become the backbone of communication training throughout the UK and much of Canada.(28, 40, 44, 49) Several institutions in the United States also make use of Radford's adaptation in the pre-clinical curriculum, including, but not limited to, Colorado State University College of Veterinary Medicine and Midwestern University College of Veterinary Medicine.(40)

Wording of the communication skills may vary based upon the innovation of each program and the lingo of its coordinators, however, the spirit of the original Calgary–Cambridge model remains intact.

The Calgary–Cambridge model provides learners and faculty alike with an opportunity to dissect clinical conversations into manageable tasks. Learners can select content areas to focus on to strengthen their performance, and facilitators can provide specific feedback concerning how successful they were in practice sessions. Practice is an essential part of communication training.

The Calgary–Cambridge model recognizes that need for practice and, in fact, is constructed to support that. After all, the reality is that "experience alone can be a poor instructor of communication skills."(39) The Calgary–Cambridge model provides for opportunity to view each encounter through a structured lens: one whose image can be refined with each reflection.

3.6 Limitations of Consultation Models

When I teach the Calgary–Cambridge model and the concept of clinical communication, students often challenge me with the question, "what if?"

Students are exceptionally good at finding holes in all-or-nothing, always-or-never statements. I know that to be true because I used to be one of them. When I am an attendee at continuing education conferences, I still am one among them.

I think that is what sets us apart as medical professionals. We have spent our whole lives training our clinical acumen; as educators, we spend our academic careers cultivating it in others.

Is it any surprise that students are constantly on a quest for answers, when we have provided them with the tools and the encouragement to embark on precisely that kind of search?

When I was an instructor at Cornell University, my colleagues had a knee-jerk response to students' incessant search for answers: "When you hear hoofbeats, think of horses, not zebras."

My colleagues did not invent this aphorism. I cannot even credit a veterinarian with it. Anecdotal evidence credits Dr. Theodore Woodward, a professor at the University of Maryland School of Medicine.

I heard this statement several dozen times in school; I have heard it several dozen times thereafter. I have wondered the same thing, each time I hear it: if we teach students how to find zebras, is it any wonder that students look for them?

"What if?" is not so much as a challenge to our expertise; it is a reasonable attempt on their part to find those long-awaited zebras, the ones that they know to be lurking if they just look hard enough for them.

When it comes to clinical communication, these "what ifs" weigh heavily on their minds. Inside and outside of the classroom, students have asked the following of me.

- What if you ask the client an open-ended question and she or he never stops talking?
- What if you are running behind on your appointments and you do not have the time you need to commit to patient-centered care?
- What if your client prefers medical paternalism?
- What if your client is not particularly chatty?
- What if your client does not appreciate your attempts to elicit his or her perspective?
- What if your client thinks that you are invading his or her privacy?
- What if your next appointment is an emergency instead of a wellness visit? Does a relationship-centered approach to care still apply? Or should you take on a more active role as leader?
- What if your patient is fractious and you only have so many minutes to complete the encounter before it runs out of "kitty minutes"? Is it appropriate to talk less to accomplish more?
- What if your patient was just hit by a car in front of the clinic and is rushed to the treatment area by your team for triage? Do you still need to take a history? You know what happened. Shouldn't you instead focus your efforts on reviving the patient?
- What if your patient is actively dying and you need to assist the transition between life and death with euthanasia solution, because the patient is now agonal? You do not have time to connect with the client. Communication isn't your primary focus. Your patient is.
- What if your client is responsible for the current state of the patient's health? Consider, for instance, the client who medicated the cat with over-the-counter acetaminophen. How can you be empathetic to the client's plight when they caused the cat's hepatopathy?
- What if you disagree with your client's assessment of the situation?
- What if your client declines your recommendations for care?

All of these "what ifs" are valid. I have experienced each in clinical practice. So, too, will my students, in due time.

What these "what ifs" have taught me – and what I now share with my students – is that the consultation does not always fit the mold. No model is a perfect representation of life in the consultation room. No single model can replicate every clinical scenario, with every client and every patient.

Not every consult will flow sequentially as implied by the Calgary–Cambridge model. Some consultations, by necessity, may flow out of order or may require the clinician to return to content areas that were previously discussed to check for understanding. Not every consult is appropriate for the Calgary–Cambridge model. There are, for example, instances in clinical practice when patient-centered care must take a backseat to triage and emergency medicine. It is not always appropriate to elicit the client's perspective when doing so takes away from the precious few seconds that a clinician has to save a patient's life.

Consider what transpires when a veterinary patient codes. To effectively act upon the code, the veterinarian must shift his role from being the relationship-driven "guide on the side" to "expert in charge." The veterinarian cannot delay treatment by asking open-ended questions of the client. The veterinarian does not have time, truly, to hear the answer. All the veterinarian needs to know, in the moment, is whether or not the client elects for the team to initiate cardiopulmonary resuscitation. There is no place for relationship building at that critical moment. A yes or no answer – and only that answer – is the driving force that determines how the veterinarian directs his team to react to the situation.

Emergencies do not negate the need for effective communication. However, they do require communication that is direct and often quite abrupt. That abruptness is essential in the moment to determine patient outcomes. That abruptness, however, does not and should not last. An attempt should be made to return towards patient-centered care once the figurative fire is put out. After the code, it may be appropriate to return to the Calgary–Cambridge model, but not during.

What all of this boils down to is that, yes, there are limitations to the Calgary–Cambridge model. It is not a "cure-all." It was never intended to be.

The Calgary–Cambridge model runs the risk of oversimplifying, but, by necessity, as a construct, it has to. If it did not limit itself to generalizations, then the model would grow so large it would become unwieldy and lose its value as a quick read, concise, easily accessible, go-to reference.

Therefore, the Calgary–Cambridge model is imperfect. It is not intended for every situation. It is not ideal for every client, patient, and clinician. Some will respond to it better than others. Some will dislike it. That is okay. At the end of the day, it is not about taking square pegs and forcing them into round holes. It is about adaptation.

The successful veterinarian is able to adapt to any given situation. How she or he is able to adapt is dependent upon his or her skillset. The Calgary–Cambridge model provides a solid toolbox with proven communication skills to facilitate most, but not all, consultations.

A second limitation of the Calgary–Cambridge model is that it was developed to guide face-to-face clinical conversations. The face of medicine is changing. Follow-up does not always happen face-to-face. Telephone and email are increasingly standard means for healthcare providers and consumers to connect. Moreover, as telemedicine becomes more prevalent, consultations are not necessarily conducted in person. Appointments may be conducted from afar, with the doctor and patient both seated in their respective living rooms. The changes in settings for consultations and the potential loss of face-to-face contact may challenge our relationship-building skills. Non-verbal cues, such as silence and hesitation, may be more likely to be missed.(17) Missed cues may lead to disconnects in the provider–consumer relationship. Missed cues may also lead to gaps in patient care.

As medicine modernizes and branches out into new avenues of healthcare, it is essential for models such as the Calgary–Cambridge construct, to adapt. Only time will tell whether revisions of the Calgary–Cambridge will be necessary to accommodate the changing face of healthcare. However, the core communication skills that the Calgary–Cambridge model outlines are still both accurate and relevant to the training of tomorrow's leaders.

Parts 2 and 3 of this text will expand upon a subset of communication skills that are essential to the veterinary–client–patient relationship, with emphasis on companion animal medicine.

References

1. Burt J, Abel G, Elmore N, Campbell J, Roland M, Benson J, et al. Assessing communication quality of consultations in primary care: initial reliability of the Global Consultation Rating Scale, based on the Calgary–Cambridge Guide to the Medical Interview. BMJ Open. 2014;4(3):e004339.
2. Frankel RM. Pets, vets, and frets: what relationship-centered care research has to offer veterinary medicine. J Vet Med Educ. 2006;33(1):20–7.
3. Stein TS, Nagy VT, Jacobs L. Caring for patients one conversation at a time: musings from the interregional clinician patient communication leadership group. Permanente J. 1998;2(4):62–8.
4. Bliss M. William Osler: a life in medicine. Oxford: Oxford University Press; 1999.
5. Coulter A. Paternalism or partnership? Patients have grown up-and there's no going back. BMJ. 1999;319(7212):719–20.
6. Stein K. Communication is the heart of provider–patient relationship. J Am Diet Assoc. 2006;106(4):508–12.
7. Brown JP, Silverman JD. The current and future market for veterinarians and veterinary medical services in the United States – executive summary – May, 1999. J Am Vet Med Assoc. 1999;215(2):161–83.
8. Englar RE. Common clinical presentations in dogs and cats. Hoboken, NJ: Wiley/Blackwell; 2019.
9. Shaw JR, Adams CL, Bonnett BN, Larson S, Roter DL. Use of the roter interaction analysis system to analyse veterinarian–client–patient communication in companion animal practice. J Am Vet Med Assoc. 2004;225(2):222–9.
10. Gillis J. The history of the patient history since 1850. Bull Hist Med. 2006;80(3):490–512.
11. Gillis J. Taking a medical history in childhood illness: representations of parents in pediatric texts since 1850. Bull Hist Med. 2005;79(3):393–429.
12. Shaw JR. Four core communication skills of highly effective practitioners. Vet Clin North Am Small Anim Pract. 2006;36(2):385–96, vii.
13. Blackwell MJ. Beyond philosophical differences: the future training of veterinarians. J Vet Med Educ. 2001;28(3):148–52.
14. Tarrant C, Stokes T, Colman AM. Models of the medical consultation: opportunities and limitations of a game theory perspective. Qual Saf Health Care. 2004;13(6):461–6.
15. Charles C, Gafni A, Whelan T. Shared decision-making in the medical encounter: what does it mean? (Or it takes at least two to tango). Soc Sci Med. 1997;44(5):681–92.

16. Elwyn G, Edwards A, Kinnersley P. Shared decision-making in primary care: the neglected second half of the consultation. Br J Gen Pract. 1999;49(443):477–82.

17. Denness C. What are consultation models for? InnovAiT. 2013;6(9):592–9.

18. Murphy SA. Consumer health information for pet owners. J Med Libr Assoc. 2006;94(2):151–8.

19. Persaud R. How to improve communication with patients. BMJ Career Focus. 2005;330:136–7.

20. Stiles WB. Discourse analysis and the doctor–patient relationship. Int J Psychiat Med. 1979;9(3–4):263–74.

21. Bub B. The patient's lament: hidden key to effective communication: how to recognize and transform. Med Humanit. 2004;30(2):63–9.

22. McKelvey I. The consultation hill: a new model to aid teaching consultation skills. Br J Gen Pract. 2010;60(576):538–40.

23. Balint M. The doctor, his patient and the illness. London: Churchill-Livingstone; 1957.

24. Moulton L. The naked consultation – a practical guide to primary care consultation skills. Oxford: Radcliffe Medical Press; 2007.

25. Tidy C, Huins H. Consultation analysis 2014 [Available from: http://www.patient.co.uk/doctor/Consultation-Analysis.htm].

26. Berne E. Transactional analysis: games people play. London: Penguin; 1970.

27. Gear S. The complete MRCP study guide. Oxford: Radcliffe Medical Press; 2005.

28. Silverman J, Kurtz S, Draper J. Skills for communicating with patients. Oxford: Radcliffe Medical Press; 2008.

29. Neighbour R. The inner consultation. Oxford: Radcliffe Medical Press; 1987.

30. Stott NC, Davis RH. The exceptional potential in each primary care consultation. J R Coll Gen Pract. 1979;29(201):201–5.

31. Kurtz S. Teaching and learning communication in veterinary medicine. J Vet Med Educ. 2006;33(1):11–9.

32. Kurtz SM, Silverman JD. The Calgary–Cambridge Referenced Observation Guides: an aid to defining the curriculum and organizing the teaching in communication training programmes. Med Educ. 1996;30(2):83–9.

33. Riccardi VM, Kurtz SM. Communication and counselling in health care. Springfield, IL: Charles C. Thomas; 1983.

34. Maguire P, Fairbairn S, Fletcher C. Consultation skills of young doctors: II – most young doctors are bad at giving information. Br Med J (Clin Res Ed). 1986;292(6535):1576–8.

35. Sanson-Fisher RW, Redman S, Walsh R, Mitchell K, Reid ALA, Perkins JJ. Training medical practitioners in information transfer skills: the new challenge. Med Educ. 1991;25:322–33.

36. Scott RB. The bedside manner. Trans Med Soc Lond. 1965;82:1–12.

37. Kurtz S, Silverman J, Benson J, Draper J. Marrying content and process in clinical method teaching: enhancing the Calgary–Cambridge guides. Acad Med. 2003;78(8):802–9.

38. Kurtz SM. Curriculum structuring to enhance communication skills development. In: Stewart M, Roter D, editors. Communicating with medical patients. Newbury Park, CA: SAGE Publications; 1989.

39. Kurtz SM, Silverman JD, Draper J. Teaching and learning communication skills in medicine. Grand Rapids, MI: Radcliffe; 2004.

40. Englar RE, Williams M, Weingand K. Applicability of the Calgary–Cambridge Guide to dog and cat owners for teaching veterinary clinical communications. J Vet Med Educ. 2016;43(2):143–69.

41. Adams CL, Ladner LD. Implementing a simulated client program: bridging the gap between theory and practice. J Vet Med Educ. 2004;31(2):138–45.

42. Gillard S, Benson J, Silverman J. Teaching and assessment of explanation and planning in medical schools in the United Kingdom: cross sectional questionnaire survey. Med Teach. 2009;31(4):328–31.

43. Howells RJ, Davies HA, Silverman JD, Archer JC, Mellon AF. Assessment of doctors' consultation skills in the paediatric setting: the Paediatric Consultation Assessment Tool. Arch Dis Child. 2010;95(5):323–9.

44. Radford A, Stockley P, Silverman J, Taylor I, Turner R, Gray C. Development, teaching, and evaluation of a consultation structure model for use in veterinary education. J Vet Med Educ. 2006;33(1):38–44.

45. Silverman J, Archer J, Gillard S, Howells R, Benson J. Initial evaluation of EPSCALE, a rating scale that assesses the process of explanation and planning in the medical interview. Patient Educ Couns. 2011;82(1):89–93.

46. Scheffer S, Muehlinghaus I, Froehmel A, Ortwein H. Assessing students' communication skills: validation of a global rating. Adv Health Sci Educ Theory Pract. 2008;13(5):583–92.

47. Rider EA, Volkan K, Hafler JP. Pediatric residents' perceptions of communication competencies: implications for teaching. Med Teach. 2008;30(7):e208–17.

48. Shaw JR, Adams CL, Bonnett BN. What can veterinarians learn from studies of physician–patient communication about veterinarian–client–patient communication? J Am Vet Med Assoc. 2004;224(5):676–84.

49. Radford AD, Stockley P, Taylor IR, Turner R, Gaskell CJ, Kaney S, et al. Use of simulated clients in training veterinary undergraduates in communication skills. Vet Rec. 2003;152(14):422–7.

Part II

Defining Oral Communication Skills as They Relate to the Veterinary Consultation

Chapter 4

First Impressions

Rapport building is the cornerstone of relationship-centered care.(1–6) It begins with first impressions, which set the tone of the consultation. A successful consultation recognizes the importance of first impressions and maximizes the opportunity to invest in the beginning of the encounter.(7–10) After all, clients are more likely to leave a practice on account of poor interpersonal skills than substandard medical care.(11, 12)

What we as veterinarians might consider to be relatively "small" or inconsequential aspects, the so-called "personal touches" of healthcare, are actually valued as completely different currency in the eyes of our consumers.(11)

4.1 Our Journey through Healthcare as Consumers

Consider yourself in the shoes of the consumer. That may be challenging because most of us are in the driver's seat at our own respective clinics. We rarely sit on the same side of the consultation room table as our clients. So let us step out of our comfort zone for a moment, and consider our own journey as a patient at any human healthcare facility.

Think about the last time that you went to see a new doctor for the first time – primary care, dentist, optometrist, chiropractor, physical therapist, specialist, etc.

- What did you notice about the practice right off the bat?
- Did your first impressions color your view of the practice?
- Did your first impressions facilitate or hinder your decision to return to the practice?

If you are like most human healthcare patients (and our veterinary clients!), your first impressions of the practice that you have in mind started long before you interacted with the medical team.

Consider how you felt upon arrival to the practice.

- Did you know where you were driving to?
- Was the practice easy to find?
- Was the practice signposted with branding?
- How easy was it to know that you had arrived at the correct facility?
- Was there parking?
- Was parking easy to find?

- Was there overflow parking?
- Was overflow parking labeled?
- Was the parking lot well maintained?
- From the parking lot, did the building appear to be well maintained?

Consider what your experience was like when you walked through the front door.

- Was the reception area cluttered?
- Was the reception area distracting?
- Was the reception area loud and noisy?
- Was the reception area overcrowded?
- Did the reception area have an odor?
- Was the reception area inviting?
- Did the reception area communicate who the practice is and what it stands for?
- Was it clear where to check in and with whom?

Now consider your check-in experience.

- Were staff wearing branded uniforms?
- Were you made to feel welcome?
- Were you greeted?
- Were you addressed by name?
- Were you interrupted by the receptionist so that she or he could answer a telephone?
- Was the average wait time stated?
- Was appropriate paperwork provided?
- Were instructions to complete the paperwork clear?

Consider your journey through the practice. Consider just how much your senses took in – sight, sound, smell – and the lasting impressions that this data made on you before you even reached the consultation room.

Recognize that your journey up to the consultation room matters.

I have been to healthcare offices that were a pleasure to work with, and I have been to healthcare offices that I hope never to experience again. If I am honest with myself and with my readers, for better or worse, much of my decision making as to whether or not I will return is based upon what I perceive to be the quality of my interactions with the team.

True, I could be having a bad day. Maybe my mood was already sour by the time I reached that front door. Maybe there was nothing that the team could have done to reverse my poor attitude. But what the team is responsible for is making sure that my experience, as a patient, does not go from bad to worse.

4.2 The Veterinary Client's Experience

Veterinary clients are just like us when we find ourselves in the role of consumer. They are quick to judge practices based upon quality of interactions with the veterinary team rather than the quality of medical attention that was received.(11)

A client of the average companion animal clinic is likely to formulate an opinion as to the caliber of the practice within the first 4 minutes of face time with team members. (11) In an avian-based exotic clinic, client perceptions take shape with even greater haste. Within the first 56 seconds of entry through a practice's front door, the client knows whether or not she or he will be coming back.(13)

It is therefore critical that we start the relationship off right. Failure to recognize the importance of first impressions makes our potential bond with clients that much more likely to be fleeting, when the goal is to create a lifelong connection.

When first impressions are positive, they plant a seed that develops into a relationship built on trust. Trust is an essential component of professional growth and success. (3–6, 14)

When first impressions are negative, clients may not feel appreciated nor valued. They may get the sense that the clinic practices assembly line medicine and that they are viewed as products rather than people. They may feel rushed or overlooked. These individuals are likely to leave the practice dissatisfied. They may feel disconnected from team members. This lack of connectivity jeopardizes their relationship with the practice and they are unlikely to be retained.

At the end of the day, the client's journey to the consultation room matters. The veterinarian plays a pivotal role in those interactions – she or he contributes to or reinforces client perceptions, good or bad – but she or he is not the only player on the team.

4.3 Starting the Client's Journey off on the Right Foot

To cement a positive client experience, what can we, as veterinarians, do?

For starters, we can prepare for the appointment, in advance, assuming that it is not a walk-in or emergency visit.(15) We can ask ourselves the following questions before we step into the consultation room.

- Do you have the right chart?
- Do you know who you are seeing, by name, in terms of the client?
- Have you seen this client before?
  - If yes, were there any previous problems with communication with this client?
  - If so, how will you avoid these issues today or make amends for past grievances?
- Do you know who you are seeing, by name, in terms of the patient?
- Have you seen this patient before?
- Do you know the patient's sex?
- Have you double-checked the patient's sex?

- ▪ Gender-neutral names, such as Bailey, Mackenzie, Madison, Coco, Reagan, Remy, Rory, Quinn, and Ryan, are prevalent in modern-day veterinary practice.
  - ▪ Clients are likely to take offense if you mistake their male dog for a female and vice versa.
- Do you know why the patient is being seen today?
- Do you know if the patient's presenting complaint is new? Or is it a recurring issue?
- Has past history been provided in the form of medical records, laboratory data, diagnostic images, or diagnostic test results?
  - ▪ What were the clinical findings?
  - ▪ What was the diagnosis?
  - ▪ Which treatment was prescribed?
  - ▪ What was the prognosis?
  - ▪ Was follow-up advised?
  - ▪ If so, within what time frame?

We have a tendency to make assumptions.

- How often are our assumptions correct?
- Is it worth risking an assumption that turns out to be wrong?

When in doubt, we need to clarify. We need to ask the client. We may be the expert in the room concerning medical care; however, our client is the expert in the room concerning his or her pet. We owe it to the client to allow him or her to elaborate.

4.4 Prep Work May Seem Silly, But ...

It was once said that "the art of consulting is often in doing the simple things extraordinarily well."(8)

Prep work is one of those simple things that often gets lost in the chaos of a busy day in clinical practice. Yet prep work is worth the initial investment. We can set ourselves up for success before we even enter the consultation room if we take the time to prepare.

Preparing means respecting your client's time by familiarizing yourself with the case as best as you can before you enter into the consultation. You would not sit for a test, cold. You would study first. Each consult is a test that can either make or break a client's relationship with the practice. Study for the test. Study the medical record.

Preparing also means setting aside distractions. Leave the last consultation behind you. That may mean taking a breath or a bathroom break. It may mean taking a walk down the hallway. It may mean sprucing up your attire and swapping a used or soiled white coat for a newly pressed one.

Do what self-care you can, in what time you're allotted, so that you can move on.

Preparation is key to starting the consultation off on the right foot. Preparation gets us in the right mindset. If you are preparing to visit with a new client and/or new patient, this pause grants the opportunity to "reset." When you enter into that consultation room, you want to present your very best self.

If you are instead prepping for a visit with a repeat customer, then this "reset" allows you to put aside past assumptions. For instance, just because the client has declined heartworm testing and annual preventative for 2 years in a row does not guarantee that today holds the same fate.

Preparation demonstrates that you are invested, both in the consultation and in building the relationship. When clients perceive a lack of preparation, they interpret this to be a poor reflection of the doctor's professionalism.(7, 16) A 1985 study in the human medical literature concluded that:

> Patients rated physicians who were unfamiliar with their cases or repeatedly referred to the chart during the encounter as less professional and as providing less satisfying care. Reviewing the case and planning the visit before entering the room is good practice. Saying explicitly, 'I've reviewed your record,' conveys some familiarity with the patient's history.(7, 16)

4.5 Greeting the Client: What the Veterinary Team Can Learn from Human Healthcare

Greeting the client in the consultation room is the clinician's first opportunity to connect with a client and to welcome him or her to the practice.(17–23) It may seem minor; however, a proper greeting sets the tone for the visit and increases the likelihood of establishing a positive, successful clinical relationship.(17, 24, 25)

The role of greetings has rarely been researched in veterinary medicine, so much of what is taught and practiced by veterinarians stems from that which has been reported in the human medical literature.

In traditional medical curricula, students are trained to complete the following actions as part of a standard greeting.(7, 9, 17–23, 26–28)

- Establish eye contact.
- Welcome the patient.
- Shake the patient's hand.
- Address the patient by name.
- Introduce yourself, stating your name and role.
- Find out who else is in the examination room and identify their relationship to the patient.
- Match your patient in terms of voice tone, language level, and posture.
- Build rapport through non-medical inquiries ("small talk").

Despite the emphasis on these tasks throughout medical training, there is little evidence about what patients want. To the author's knowledge, only one original investigation into this question has been published. A 2007 study by Makoul et al. obtained the following data on patient expectations for greetings:(17)

- handshake
    - 78.1% of 415 survey participants desire a handshake
    - older patients are less likely to prefer a handshake
- patient name
    - 50.4% want physicians to acknowledge them by first name (that is, "Hi John")
    - 23.6% want physicians to acknowledge them by first and last name (that is, "Hi John Smith")
    - 17.3% want physicians to acknowledge them by only their last name (that is, "Hi Mr. Smith")
- physician name
    - 56.4% want physicians to identify themselves by both first and last name (that is, "My name is Dr. Lowell Fox")
    - 32.5% want physicians to identify themselves by last name only (that is, "My name is Dr. Fox")
    - 7.2% want physicians to identify themselves by first name only (that is, "My name is Lowell").

Less than one-half of survey participants answered the question, "Is there anything else a doctor should do when meeting you for the first time?"(17) Of those who responded:(17)

- 23.2% of patients desired that their physician smile
- 19.2% of patients desired that their physician be "friendly, personable, polite, [or] respectful"
- 16.4% of patients wanted to be made to feel like a priority
- 13.0% of patients preferred eye contact.

The patient's desire for non-verbal cues, such as handshakes, smiling and eye contact, will be discussed at length in Chapter 7.

Makoul et al. went one step further. The research team compared what patients wanted by way of greeting with what patients received in the consultation room. One-hundred and twenty-three new patient visits were videotaped in order to characterize greeting patterns in clinical practice.(17) Data obtained from videotape analysis revealed that:(17)

- 82.9% of physicians shook the patient's hand
- 50.4% of physicians did not acknowledge the patient by name at all
- 11.4% of visits involved physicians who did not introduce themselves
- 0.81% of visits involved the physician asking the client how she or he preferred to be addressed.

There are obvious discrepancies between patient preferences and physician performance.

To the author's knowledge, there is no comparable study in the veterinary medical literature. However, a 2018 study by Stevens and Kedrowicz did explore fourth-year veterinary students' communication skills in the consultation room in an attempt to identify strengths as well as areas for improvement.(3) Videotape analysis was performed on 20 randomly selected veterinary–student–client interactions that took place between 2013–2015 as part of the clinical rotation through primary care.(3) When student performance was evaluated, coders found that 50% of students were deficient in:(3)

- greeting the client by name
- introducing themselves
- introducing their role.

What both studies – human and veterinary – demonstrate is that there is substantial room for improvement when physicians greet the client to initiate the session and to build rapport.

Greeting the client does not always align with client expectations. We may hit or miss.

In an attempt to be welcoming, we may in fact be off-putting. We may try to shake someone's hand who does not want to engage in a handshake. We may stumble over our words as we attempt to address the client by name. We may inadvertently make the consultation feel forced or rehearsed. This was acknowledged by Makoul et al.:(21)

> When asking patients how they would like to be addressed is an attractive and egalitarian strategy in the abstract, physicians may find it somewhat awkward in practice when meeting a patient for the first time. Indeed, this approach was evident in only 1 of the 123 videotaped encounters we studied, and seemed to be a result of confusion over different names in the chart rather than courtesy. When physicians ask how patients want to be addressed at the beginning of their encounter, patients may feel pressure to answer that the more familiar form of address is acceptable before rapport has been established. For some, this may increase a sense of familiarity; for others, it can exacerbate a sense of power imbalance, especially if physicians refer to themselves with formal titles (e.g., Dr. Jones).(17)

Building rapport is not an exact science. One client's preference may be another client's dislike.

It is difficult to guess how to interact with a single person in the consultation room, let alone when there are multiple individuals to acknowledge as an integral part of the patient's support network or care team.(29)

4.6 Greeting the Veterinary Client: Finding Common Ground

In veterinary medicine, just as in pediatric human medicine, there are often multiple people involved in the same patient's care. Sometimes these individuals are all present in the same consultation room. More often than not, follow-up care requires multiple conversations with contacts, who were not initially present in the exam room, to get everyone on the same page. This often requires the physician to repeat exam findings, diagnostic test results, and treatment options, and circle back in conversation to topics that once tabled, but now require revisiting.

Clients within the same household may be at odds over patient care or even the approach to patient care. Clients within the same household may have different wants and needs.

Communication is challenged by the physician's need to connect with those under his or her care in the way that is most likely to result in favorable outcomes.

It is impossible to please everyone, but it is good practice to do one's best to at least try. A good faith effort begins with introductions.

Taking into account what we have learned from the human medical literature, clients want to be made to feel welcome and secure within an established place of business. How can we achieve that?

- We can make eye contact.
- We can extend an arm to shake hands, when appropriate.
    - If a client is wrestling to maintain control over a leashed dog that is thrashing at the other end, then it is probably not appropriate to reach out to shake hands. The client already has his or her hands full.
    - Likewise, if a client is holding onto a cat carrier with both hands and/or toting the patient in his or her arms, then a handshake may be postponed so that the client does not have to rearrange him or herself or put him or herself in an awkward position.
- We can smile, when appropriate.
    - An emergency or a scheduled euthanasia are two common events in clinical practice when a different set of non-verbal gestures may be required.
- We can express an appropriate greeting.
    - "Hello."
    - "Hi."
    - "Good morning."
    - "Good day."
    - "Good afternoon."
    - "Good evening."
- We can acknowledge the client by name.
- We can acknowledge the patient by name.
- We can identify ourselves by name.
- We can identify our role.

The order in which each of the above occurs may vary from consultation to consultation and from clinician to clinician. Each clinician is likely to develop his or her own style. Styling of the consultation is to be encouraged. Just as no two clients are alike; no two clinicians are the same.

Greeting the client is not about creating cookie cutter medicine. It is about adapting our style to the consultation room in a way that feels genuine and welcoming. It is not always what we say; it is how we say it that counts.(9)

Whatever you do, be true to yourself in the consultation room. An ounce of sincerity is worth more than five pounds of disingenuity. Clients are very good at distinguishing that which is genuine from that which is fake.

If you are meeting a client for the first time, consider the following options for a greeting.

- "Hi there, Mr. Fox. It's a pleasure to be of service to you. My name is Dr. Ryane Englar and I will be Tango's veterinarian today."
- "Good afternoon, I'm Dr. Ryane Englar, an associate veterinarian here at Paws and Claws Clinic. Are you Rumba's owner, Lowell Fox?"
- "Good evening, [directing attention to the patient], you must be Foxtrot. Hi, I'm Dr. Ryane Englar, the owner of this practice, and [drawing attention back to the client] you must be Foxtrot's dad?"

If you are meeting a client for the first time and you are unsure how to pronounce the client's name, you might try one of the following.

- "Hello, sir, it's so nice to meet you and your cat, Waltz. I'm your veterinarian for today's visit, Dr. Ryane Englar. May I ask how to say your name?"
- "Hi, there, I'm Dr. Ryane Englar, the owner of the practice, and this must be your dog, Jive. I'm not sure how to pronounce your name and it's important to me that I not get your name wrong. Can you help me out?"
- "Good evening, miss. I see that you've brought your dog, Samba, in to see us. I'm Dr. Ryane Englar, the doctor on overnight emergency. May I ask how you would like to be addressed at this visit?"
- "Good morning. This must be your cat, Quickstep. I'm Dr. Ryane Englar, the doctor on emergency duty. May I ask your name?"

If you accidentally mispronounce the client's name and the client corrects you, do not beat yourself up about it. Accept responsibility for the error – you are only human. We all make mistakes. Apologize for the mistake and make amends. Be gracious about it.

When you make your next attempt at pronunciation, consider following it up with, "Did I get that right?" This demonstrates effort on your part to be attentive to detail and to consider the client as an individual.

If you are meeting a client for the first time and you are unsure of the pet's name, do not be afraid to ask. It is critical that the patient's identify be known from the get-go, particularly in multi-pet households, so that we know who received what care on which date. Patient identification constitutes an important part of the medical record. To clarify the patient's identify, consider the following examples.

- "Hi, Mr. Fox, it is good to meet you. And this is, [referring to the patient]?"
- "Good afternoon, Mr. Fox. Welcome to our clinic. Who did you bring in to meet us today?"
- "Good evening, Mr. Fox. I see that you've brought a new friend for us to meet. Who might this be?"

If you are meeting a client for the first time and you are unsure of the pet's gender, do not guess. Make an attempt to clarify as soon as you are able.

- "Hello, Mr. Fox. I see that I have the privilege of meeting your little one today. What a lovely name, Salsa. I bet there's a story there. May I ask if Salsa is a she or a he and what prompted you to select that name?"
- "Good day, Mr. Fox. This must be Pachanga. I was looking over your paperwork for today's visit and I didn't catch if Pachanga is a she or a he. Can you help me out?"

When customers return to the practice, it is not customary to go through the same extensive greeting process. This is particularly true if follow-up is recent or frequent. For example, the longstanding client with a chronic kidney disease (CKD) cat that presents every other week for assessment does not need a verbal reminder of team members' names, particularly if the care providers are consistent.

However, sometimes assumptions are made that the client remembers you. Just because you remember a client does not mean that the client remembers you. It may feel awkward to reintroduce yourself. However, it may be necessary to reestablish ties. Consider the following ways to make yourself and your role clear.

- "Hi, Mr. Fox, I don't know if you remember me from Bachata's annual wellness visit last year, but I am so excited to see you two back at our practice. I'm Dr. Ryane Englar."
- "Good afternoon, Mr. Fox. I don't know if we've ever formally met, but I remember Jitterbug well from the last time that he boarded with us. I'm Dr. Ryane Englar."
- "Good evening, Mr. Fox, it's good to see you again. I recall that we worked together years ago on Zouk's care, but I'm not sure if you remember me. I'm Dr. Ryane Englar."

If you have met the patient before, but not the family member who is here with the patient today, then it is important to acknowledge the new face and make him or her feel welcome.

- "It's so great to see Swing back for his follow-up visit. [Turning attention to the client] We didn't have the opportunity to meet in person last time. My name is Dr. Ryane

Englar. Whom am I speaking with?"

- "[Talking to the patient] Hi there, Peabody, it's so nice to see you again! And you've brought a new friend for me to meet! [Turning attention to the client] My name is Dr. Ryane Englar. It's a pleasure to meet you, sir/miss."

If there is no record of prior care and no mention of a prior relationship with this client in the medical record, but she or he looks familiar to you, you can always address the elephant in the room.

- "Mr. Fox, you look familiar, have we met before?"
- "I seem to remember you and Cha Cha. Have we worked with one another in the past?"

In my clinical experience, both in private practice and within the teaching hospital setting at academic institutions, roles of support staff and/or students are rarely clarified. This is a disservice to the client. Clients need to know who is involved in delivery of the patient's care.

Veterinary technicians – referred to as veterinary nurses in some programs – should be identified as such.

- "I see that you have already met Jennifer, Bolero's technician."
- "I would like to introduce you to Lowell, the technician who will be monitoring Paso Doble's anesthesia during his neuter today."
- "Gail, our technician, will need to borrow Polka to get started on his bloodwork."

Veterinary assistants and kennel attendants should also be named, particularly if they are entering the consultation room to collect a patient for intake.

- "This is Carolyn, the animal care attendant who will be caring for Lindy Hop during his hospitalization with us today."
- "Have you met Everett before? He is the veterinary assistant who will be handling Mambo during his blood draw. He's exceptionally good with cats and will do everything he can to keep Mambo comfortable."

Students often exclude themselves or are excluded from introductions by the veterinary team as if they are mere shadows or flies on the wall. In reality – and particularly at teaching hospitals – students function as the primary caregiver for inpatients. It is critical that we lead by example as attending physicians and model the behavior of making introductions.

There is no "I" in team – and the client benefits from putting a name to a face, especially if the patient needs to remain behind for diagnostic testing or initiation of treatment.

Teach students to make themselves. Each institution is likely to have their own protocol for how students should address the client. However, consider the following examples.

- "Hi, Mr. Fox. My name is Alyssa Show and I am the fourth-year veterinary student who is working with Dr. Englar."
- "Hi, Mr. Fox. We have not yet met before, but I am the senior veterinary student who is working on Tango's case with Dr. Englar. My name is Alyssa Show."
- "Hi, Mr. Fox. I am one of two students who are taking care of Tango with Dr. Englar. My name is Alyssa Show, and this is my colleague, Andy Burch."

Interns and residents should also identify their role. Although it is unlikely that clients will recall everyone's name, especially after only hearing it once, clients are more likely to feel secure in leaving their animal behind when they know who is responsible for the pet's care.

It also helps clients to recognize that care is extensive, and that there is an entire team working behind the scenes to help their animal.

Clients do not often know the extent to which we care for their pets, or the amount of work that is put into daily treatments. We assume that they know the value of healthcare; however, all they may see is cost.

Greetings are one of the little things that we can do to acknowledge that healthcare is a team effort and to connect the client to the patient care team.

4.7 Attending to the Client's Comfort

The veterinary field is a customer service industry.

I often interview applicants for matriculation into veterinary programs. As part of the interview process, we often ask the question, "Why do you want to become a veterinarian?"

I worry when applicants respond that they prefer animals to people. The truth is that veterinary medicine is about people. Unless you are going to work at an animal shelter, with patients that do not have guardians, the reality is that patients come with clients attached.

At the other end of the leash is a client. At the other end of the carrier is a client. Ultimately, it is the client, not the patient, who decides to schedule an appointment when a pet needs to be seen for examination. It is the client, not the patient, who determines if the patient will present, as a walk-in, on an emergency basis. It is the client, not the patient, who consents to and ultimately finances care. It is the client, not the patient, who determines the success of compliance, adherence, and follow-up. It is the client, not the patient, with whom we need to establish 'buy-in'. Therefore, the comfort of the client is critical to rapport building.

When you walk into the consultation room, the comfort of the client can facilitate partnership or hinder it.

- Is the consultation room private?
    - If doors to the consultation room are open, can they be closed?

- Is the consultation room quiet?
  - Is the client able to focus on the patient?
  - Is the client able to focus on you?
  - Is the client able to hear what you are saying?
- Is the consultation room odor-free?
  - Is the consultation room well-ventilated?
  - Has the room been soiled?
  - If so, can the room be cleaned?
  - Are cleansers associated with noxious fumes?
  - Are cleansers free from perfumes?
- Is the consultation room thermally neutral?
  - Is the consultation room too hot?
  - Is the consultation room too cold?
  - Was the consultation room "just right" before it was filled with two clients and a panting dog, and now it is uncomfortably warm and stuffy?
- Is there seating available to the client?
  - Is there adequate space for the client to be seated and maintain control over his or her pet?
- Is the lighting adequate?
  - Is the examination room too dark?
  - Is the examination room too bright?
- Are there examination room windows?
  - If so, are these contributing to glare?
  - Is the client able to see you, the veterinarian, as you are conversing?
  - Does the client have to avert his or her gaze in order to focus?
- Is there room for you to seat yourself at a knee-to-knee angle relative to the client?

There are occasions when client comfort cannot be helped. Perhaps there is overcrowding of the consultation rooms and/or appointments are running behind schedule. Clients may be forced to have conversations in waiting areas or in corridors. Patients may soil rooms that cannot be cleaned before the doctor initiates the consultation due to lack of staffing. Patients may present on emergency and have to be rushed to the treatment area, with or without their owners.

These circumstances require flexibility on the part of the veterinary team and client. Most of the time, clients will be understanding of this. To improve the likelihood, be transparent.

If the veterinarian is running behind, set that expectation for the client at time of check-in. Explain why, whenever possible, without breaking the trust and/or confidentiality or other clients. Provide clients with options when unforeseen obstacles present themselves:

- Does the client wish to reschedule?
- Does the client want to stage the appointment?

- Does the client want to sign the patient over as a drop-off?

Options convey to the client that the veterinary team respects his or her time.

4.8 Acknowledging and Attending to the Patient

In addition to client comfort, the veterinary team must also connect to and comfort the patient.

Traditionally, the approach to pet care was "get it done." When I was a kennel attendant and, later, a veterinary assistant, I was regretfully trained in this manner. If it took four people to hold down the dog to get the dog's nails trimmed, then it took four people. Checking tasks off of a 'to do' list took precedence to the patient's mental health.

As a result, patient anxiety in the veterinary clinic was commonplace.(30) A 2009 study by Döring et al. found that 78.5% of clinically healthy dogs were fearful on the examination room table at a primary care practice in Germany.(31) Less than one-half of these dogs were calm walking through the clinic doors, and 13.3% of the dogs required assistance to force their entry, either through being dragged or being carried.(31)

Routine veterinary care that incites stress is detrimental to patient wellness.(30) As early as the first puppy or kitten visit, patients can be scarred by one or more of the following variables:(30, 32–35)

- auditory stimulation
- olfactory cues
- physical, visual, or temporal separation
  - from the client
  - from conspecifics
- interactions between patients
- interactions with the healthcare team
- lack of analgesia.

It used to be seen as "normal" for the veterinary patient to be afraid of the clinic.(30) This is no longer believed to be true.

In fact, inciting anxiety in our patients may actually precipitate a lifetime of fear-based responses.(30, 36) In 2011, Godbout and Frank demonstrated that fearful signs in 2- to 4-month-old pups in the veterinary clinic repeated themselves when the same pups were reintroduced to the clinic 12 months later.(36)

Fear at an earlier age does not translate into patient acclimatization. If anything, fear potentiates fear. The persistence of fear and the potential for adverse effects that persist into adulthood is concerning to the veterinary profession.

The veterinary team does not want to create anxiety. In fact, having to handle anxious patients triggers its own anxiety in the veterinary team. Anxiety in our patients sets the stage for a vicious cycle in which patients are labeled "difficult" and become increasingly difficult over time.

However, patient anxiety does not just impact the patient or the veterinary team. Patient anxiety about veterinary care is also a stressor for clients.(37) When clients witness the anxiety that veterinary visits cause their pets, they are less likely to return to the clinic for follow-up.(37)

Follow-up is further hindered in cats because feline anxiety often persists for several days after the veterinary visit.(30, 37) In 2011, Volk et al. published an Executive Summary of the Bayer veterinary care usage study:

> Many cat owners in the study indicated that their cats acted remote and unfriendly for several days after returning home, which is particularly undesirable in sick or recovering animals.(30)

As a result of empirical data about patient stress and animal welfare, there has been a movement towards so-called low-stress or fear-free veterinary practice.(30) Today's veterinary schools areintroducing students to this mindset with the hopes that it will trickle into modern-day practice. "Brudacaine" is being sidelined for the sake of animal welfare as research demonstrates the importance of low stress handling.(30, 38–43)

Low-stress or fear-free practice aims to:(30, 41, 44)

- detect anxiety, fear, and pain so that early interventions are possible
- reduce anxiety, fear, and pain for patients, clients, and the veterinary team
- reduce patient and veterinary team injuries that result from escalating anxiety
- improve the veterinary team-client-patient relationship
- make follow-up less stressful on the patient and client, thereby improving compliance
- increase job satisfaction for the veterinary team.

Low-stress or fear-free practice requires both an understanding of patient behavior and attentiveness to our own body language, so that the veterinary team conveys the message that we are not a threat.(30) These signals are beyond the scope of this text, which concentrates on oral communication between people. However, we need to be aware that the way in which we greet our veterinary patients can incite stress.

To reduce the likelihood that our greeting will be perceived as a threat by canine and feline patients, consider the following.(30, 40, 41, 44, 45)

- Avoid towering over, leaning on, reaching over, and reaching for the patient.
- Avoid facing the patient head-on with a direct gaze.
- Avoid sudden hand motions or movements, particularly near the patient's face.

Instead:(30, 40, 41, 44, 45)

- be prepared: anticipate what you will need before the visit
- be observant: pay careful attention to the patient's trends in:
  - posture

- shifting weight
- eyes (is the patient demonstrating "whale eye"?)
- ear position
- brow position
- position of the whiskers
- facial expressions
- lip curl and exposure of the teeth
- piloerection of the coat
- tail carriage
- vocalizations

- move slowly and deliberately: you must "go slow to go fast"(41)
- be deliberate with body actions: be smooth rather than jerky
- squat, sit, or stand sideways relative to the patient
- use peripheral vision rather than direct eye contact to visualize the patient.

For more information, consult appropriate veterinary behavior reference texts.

References

1. Kurtz SM, Silverman JD, Draper J. Teaching and learning communication skills in medicine. Grand Rapids, MI: Radcliffe; 2004.
2. Kurtz SM, Adams CL. Essential education in communication skills and cultural sensitivies for global public health in an evolving veterinary world. Rev Sci Tech Off Int Epiz. 2009;28(2):635–47.
3. Stevens BJ, Kedrowicz AA. Evaluation of fourth-year veterinary students' client communication skills: recommendations for scaffolded instruction and practice. J Vet Med Educ. 45(1):85–90.
4. Kedrowicz AA. Clients and veterinarians as partners in problem solving during cancer management: implications for veterinary education. J Vet Med Educ. 2015;42(4):373–81.
5. Arborelius E, Bremberg S. What can doctors do to achieve a successful consultation? Videotaped interviews analysed by the 'consultation map' method. Fam Pract. 1992;9(1):61–6.
6. Little P, Everitt H, Williamson I, Warner G, Moore M, Gould C, et al. Preferences of patients for patient centred approach to consultation in primary care: observational study. BMJ. 2001;322(7284):468–72.
7. Frankel RM, Stein T. Getting the most out of the clinical encounter: The Four Habits Model. The Permanente Journal. 1999;3(3):79–88.
8. Manning P. Veterinary consultations: the value of reflection. In Practice. 2008;January:47–9.
9. Ranjan P. How can doctors improve their communication skills? J Clin Diagn Res. 2015;9(3):1–4.
10. Corsan JR, Mackay AR. The Veterinary Receptionist: Essential Skills for Client Care. China: Elsevier, Ltd; 2008.
11. Goldstein SA, Burkgren T. Client relations. IA State Univ Vet. 1993;55(2):75–7.
12. McCurnin D. Veterinary Practice Management. Philadelphia, PA: J.B. Lippincott Co.; 1988.
13. Fiskett RAM. That First Impression. J Exotic Pet Medicine. 2006;15(2):84–90.
14. Grand JA, Lloyd JW, Ilgen DR, Abood S, Sonea IM. A measure of and predictors for veterinarian

trust developed with veterinary students in a simulated companion animal practice. J Am Vet Med Assoc. 2013;242(3):322–34.

15. Mossop L, Gray C. Teaching communication skills. In Practice. 2008;June:340–3.

16. Inui TS, Carter WB. Problems and prospects for health services research on provider–patient communication. Med Care. 1985;23(5):521–38.

17. Makoul G, Zick A, Green M. An evidence-based perspective on greetings in medical encounters. Arch Intern Med. 2007;167(11):1172–6.

18. Silverman J, Kurtz S, Draper J. Skills for communicating with patients. Oxford: Radcliffe Medical Press; 2008.

19. Thompson TL. The initial interaction between the patient and the health professional: communication for health professionals. Lanham, MD: Harper and Row Publishers; 1986.

20. Zeldow PB, Makoul G. Communicating with patients. In: Wedding D, Stuber ML, editors. Behavior and medicine. Cambridge, MA: Hogrefe and Huber Publishers; 2006. pp. 201–18.

21. Lipkin M, Frankel RM. Performing the interview. In: Lipkin M, Putnam SM, Lazare A, editors. The medical interview: clinical care, education, and research. New York: Springer-Verlag NY Inc.; 1995. pp. 65–82.

22. Coulehan JL, Block MR. The medical interview: mastering skills for clinical practice. Philadelphia, PA: FA Davis Co Publishers; 1997.

23. Makoul G. The SEGUE Framework for teaching and assessing communication skills. Patient Educ Couns. 2001;45:23–34.

24. Comstock LM, Hooper EM, Goodwin JM, Goodwin JS. Physician behaviors that correlate with patient satisfaction. J Med Educ. 1982;57(2):105–12.

25. Makoul G. The interplay between education and research about patient–provider communication. Patient Educ Couns. 2003;50(1):79–84.

26. Billings JA, Stoeckle JD. The clinical encounter: a guide to the medical interview and case presentation. St. Louis, MO: Mosby Year Book Inc.; 1999.

27. Lloyd M, Bor R. Communication skills for medicine. New York: Churchill Livingstone, Inc.; 1996.

28. Smith RC. The patient's story: integrated patient–doctor interviewing. Boston, MA: Little Brown and Co, Inc.; 1996.

29. Williams D, Jewell J. Family centred veterinary medicine: learning from human paediatric care. Vet Rec. 2012;170(3):79–80.

30. Lloyd JKF. Minimizing stress for patients in the veterinary hospital: why it is important and what can be done about it. Vet Sci. 2017;4(2):22.

31. Döring D, Roscher A, Scheipl F, Kuchenhoff H, Erhard MH. Fear-related behaviour of dogs in veterinary practice. Vet J. 2009;182(1):38–43.

32. Overall KL. Fear factor: is routine veterinary care contributing to lifelong patient anxiety? DVM360; 2013 [Available from: http://veterinarynews.dvm360.com/fear-factor-routine-veterinary-care-contributing-lifelong-patient-anxiety].

33. Overall KL. Facing fear head on: tips for veterinarians to create a more behavior-centered practice. DVM360; 2013 [Available from: http://veterinarynews.dvm360.com/facing-fear-head-tips-veterinarians-create-more-behavior-centered-practice].

34. Overall KL. Karen Overall on the effects of fear on veterinary patients. DVM360; 2014 [Available from: http://veterinarynews.dvm360.com/karen-overall-effects-fear-veterinary-patients].

35. Dawson LC, Dewey CE, Stone EA, Guerin MT, Niel L. A survey of animal welfare experts and practicing veterinarians to identify and explore key factors thought to influence canine and

feline welfare in relation to veterinary care. Anim Welfare. 2016;25(1):125–34.

36. Godbout M, Frank D. Persistence of puppy behaviors and signs of anxiety during adulthood. J Vet Behav. 2011;6:92.

37. Volk JO, Felsted KE, Thomas JG, Siren CW. Executive summary of the Bayer veterinary care usage study. J Am Vet Med Assoc. 2011;238(10):1275–82.

38. Hewson C. Stress in small animal patients: why it matters and what to do about it. Irish Vet J. 2008;61(4):249–54.

39. Hewson C. Why are(n't) you using pheromones in your hospital ward? There's more to reducing patient stress. Vet Ir J. 2012;2:84–90.

40. Yin S. Low stress handling, restraint and behavior modifications of dogs and cats: techniques for patients who love their visits. Davis, CA: CattleDog Publishing; 2009.

41. Rodan I, Sundahl E, Carney H, Gagnon AC, Heath S, Landsberg G, et al. AAFP and ISFM feline-friendly handling guidelines. J Feline Med Surg. 2011;13(5):364–75.

42. Lloyd J, editor. Behaviour and welfare – minimizing stress for patients in the veterinary hospital. Proceedings of the Australian Veterinary Association North Queensland Branch Conference; 2014 August 22–24; Townsville, Queensland, Australia.

43. Harvey A, editor. A cat friendly clinic – why do you need it and how do you do it? Proceedings of the Feline Medicine Seminar; 2016 November 12–13; Townsvillege, Queensland, Australia.

44. Hammerle M, Horst C, Levine E, Overall K, Radosta L, Rafter-Ritchie M, et al. 2015 AAHA canine and feline behavior management guidelines. J Am Anim Hosp Assoc. 2015;51(4):205–21.

45. Yin S. Low stress handling of dogs and cats. Davis, CA: CattleDog Publishing; 2012.

Chapter 5

Defining Entry-Level Communication Skills

Reflective Listening

As discussed in Chapter 4, first impressions are essential. They set the tone for the clinical consultation. When done poorly, first impressions take away from the veterinarian–client relationship. When done properly, they convey to the client a sense of value. First impressions are a means by which the veterinarian communicates to the client that:

- "I am here for you"
- "I care about you"
- "I am listening to you"
- "I hear you"
- "I care about what you have to say"
- "I am ready to help"
- "I am invested in this relationship."

First impressions are the first step towards establishing a connection between two people.

First impressions plant a seed that has the potential to develop into a lifelong working relationship. That seed can only take root if first impressions are maintained throughout the clinical consultation. In other words, it is not appropriate to greet the client properly, only to abandon social graces for the remainder of the visit. To build a relationship, the veterinarian must work at it.

The veterinary profession is a customer service industry. Clients expect to contribute to the health of their pets, as partners in the delivery of care. Clients are not empty vessels that come to us to be filled. Clients bring a host of knowledge and past experiences with them to share with the veterinary team. In this way, clients represent untapped potential. They are poised and eager to share, but for them to be able to do so, they must feel that they have a place at the table.

In exchange for their time and perspective, clients want to be heard, served, respected, and cared for, for the benefit of the patient that is being presented. The veterinary client of the past is not the veterinary client of today.(1) Today's veterinary client expects to be engaged in conversation with us, not talked at.(1) This is consistent with the movement away from medical paternalism and the trend towards relationship-centered care.(2–5)

Communication is the vehicle that drives relationship-centered care. Although knowledge comprises the backbone of the competence and proficiency of the veterinarian, knowledge alone cannot determine patient outcomes. Communication does.

How effective we are at communication determines:

- whether or not our client feels safe to share his/her perspective with the veterinary team
- whether or not our client understands what we are saying
- whether or not our client will agree to healthcare recommendations
- whether or not our client will comply and adhere to healthcare recommendations
- whether or not our client will return for the patient's follow-up care
- whether or not our client will refer others to the practice.

At the end of the day, communication is responsible for everything we do in the practice of veterinary medicine. Communication is how we get things done. To be an effective practitioner, we can no longer ignore the role that communication plays in the consultation room.(3, 6–8)

To be successful, we need to draw upon four entry-level communication skills.(3) These communication skills can be recalled by the mnemonic, RENO:

- R – reflective listening
- E – empathy
- N – nonverbal cues
- O – open-ended questions.

5.1 Introduction to Reflective Listening

Within the consultation room, student doctors often act as though clinical communication is a monologue. This is not surprising when you consider how most students are assessed in their formative years. Student doctors are so used to being graded on what they know and how much they can regurgitate on paper that they often forget their place as they transition into the role of doctor.

Today's doctor is not the "sage on the stage." This paternalistic view of medicine has largely fallen by the wayside as human patients and veterinary clients have grown to expect more from their medical care team.

Today's doctor is a "guide on the side." This role makes room for partnership in the veterinarian–client relationship and acknowledges that the most effective clinical consultations are not monologues; they are *conversations*.

5.2 Clinical Conversations, Defined

A conversation implies *dialogue*. There is information transfer both ways: doctor–patient and patient–doctor. Ideas are exchanged, clarified, and/or amended. Communication thus becomes a feedback loop. One or more rounds of conversation may be necessary to attain mutual understanding and to make informed decisions concerning healthcare.

The benefit is that both parties have a say in decision making. Because each person is able to weigh in and share his or her perspective, both sides are more likely to be invested in the end product. Client compliance and adherence are expected to be high because the client helped to determine the diagnostic and/or treatment plan.

In order for this Frisbee approach to be effective in practice, each party must take turns being the sender of information and the recipient. In other words, one side must *listen* when the other side is speaking, and roles will reverse. The sender is not the sender forever, just as the receiver is not the receiver forever. Each has an opportunity to speak. However, it is most important that each fine-tune the art of how to be a better listener.

5.3 Why Should Healthcare Providers Listen?

Listening is an essential skill for any form of human interaction, not just that which occurs within the boundaries of the healthcare industry.(9) Listening is the glue that bonds people to one another as they open themselves up to sharing thoughts, feelings, ideas, and information.(9)

Like first impressions, listening conveys to the speaker that the recipient values what she or he has to say.(9–11)

Listening denotes respect and investment.

- "I am willing to invest in your ideas because they matter."
- "Your voice counts."
- "You matter."

Despite over 40 years of research into communications skills training in human health-care, the role of listening and what listening means to the healthcare consumer continue to be underplayed in both education and clinical practice.(3, 8, 9, 12–21)

Yet, listening is powerful:

> By engaging in the simple yet complex act of listening, the physician can provide a safe haven for the patient's fears and anxieties – a trustworthy container for all the shifting emotions borne from the experience of illness. S/he provides that which medical technology can never provide – a human touch. It is the kind of connection that comes from being present with another, from giving our full attention so that we may listen not only with our minds, but with our hearts as well.(22)

Listening is desired by our consumers. Our consumers want to feel valued. They want to feel heard:(15, 23)

> Patients long for doctors who comprehend what they go through and who, as a result, stay the course with them through their illnesses. A medicine practiced without a genuine and obligating awareness of what patients go through may fulfill its technical goals, but it is an empty medicine, or, at best, half a medicine ...(24)

Many healthcare providers equally yearn for the kind of connectivity that effective listening provides. Human physician Pamela Wible explained this quite eloquently:

> The most important therapy I deliver is a human relationship ... I want my patients' passions listed on their charts. Because if that's not there, then the only thing I read is "endometrial cancer", carpal-tunnel syndrome, fibromyalgia, chronic fatigue, and mother died when she was 40 of breast cancer. I don't want to look at this person and simply think, she's *doomed*. I want to know what her passion is in life. Who is this person sitting in front of me? ... People come to the doctor for care and end up with a prescription. We need to get rid of this idea of professional distance and let physicians be vulnerable.(25)

Listening humanizes medicine. Listening also allows healthcare providers to deliver higher quality care because we are able to:

- establish patient presenting complaints early on in the encounter
- gather appropriate data
- hear the client articulate his or her needs
- process what the client has shared
- clarify that our understanding of the situation is accurate
- correct misperceptions.

Despite its importance to the healthcare industry, care providers often lack basic listening skills.(12) Some overrate their ability to listen.(12, 26) Others are surprised to find lapses in this skillset during training exercises.(12, 26)

5.4 Why Is Effective Listening such a Difficult Task?

Effective listening is so hard for so many of us because, in clinical consultations, it cannot be a passive process. As doctors, we need to pay attention in order to hear what is being said. However, paying attention requires active effort on our part.(12) Effort is required in order to:(12, 27–29)

- set aside our own agenda
- table our own words so that we can hear another's
- place another's needs before our own
- invest in what the other person is saying
- consider what the other person is sharing and why it is being shared
- reflect upon how it might feel to be that other person, in the moment
- curb judgments about what is being shared because biases limit our understanding.

Because listening requires effort on the part of the listener, it is often referred to in clinical practice as the communication skill of active, or reflective, listening.

5.5 Active or Reflective Listening, Defined

Conceptually, active listening can be traced back to the humanistic approach to psychology that was inspired by Carl Rogers in the 1950s.(30, 31) Rogers' concept was intimately connected with empathy, which will be discussed at length in Chapter 6. He believed strongly in a client-centered approach to therapy. Clients benefited from being accepted unconditionally. More than that, they needed to be understood without judgment. This required the listener to put him- or herself in the speaker's shoes, to gain an understanding of what life was like for the speaker without "the listener's own interpretive structures intruding on his or her understanding of the other person."(30)

By 1975, the term, "active listening," was applied to parenting.(30, 32) Its use has since expanded into the classroom, as well as into virtually every field of communication skills training, from commercial sales representatives to marriage and crisis counsellors, non-medical caregivers to medical support staff.(30, 33–38)

Today, active listening is outlined in virtually all interpersonal communication textbooks, medical and veterinary.(6–8, 30, 39–44) Active listeners aim to answer the following questions by the conclusion of every consultation. (9)

- Did I hear the message that my client wanted to share with me?
- I know what my client said, but what exactly did she or he mean?
- How do I know that I heard the message correctly?

Answering these questions requires three elements or basic steps.(30, 41, 42, 45, 46)

1. Non-verbal communication by the listener that the speaker has undivided attention. Alternatively, the listener may provide minimal feedback responses to convey attentiveness, such as "hmh," "uh-huh," "yeah," "ok," and "right."
2. Paraphrasing, restating, or otherwise reflecting back what the speaker shared to check for clarity and accuracy of understanding.
3. Inviting the speaker to elaborate his or her perspective and to share additional details.

5.6 Active Listening Requires Preparation

To be an effective active listener, you need to prepare yourself for the task ahead. You need to be ready to listen. This requires you to attend to your physical needs before you are prepared to invest fully in the conversation. Doing so is not always possible in a busy clinical practice. However, take advantage of these opportunities when you can so as to improve the capacity with which you listen.

- Use the restroom rather than entering a consultation room on a full bladder.
- Take scheduled meal breaks when possible, so that an empty stomach does not distract during your next consultation.
- Listen to your body: if you are in pain, find a way to alleviate or reduce pain before investing in a conversation. For example:
  - if you have an injured foot, consider listening from a seated position rather than standing
  - if you have a strained neck, avoid twisting it to make eye contact with your client; position yourself instead so that you are comfortably able to access your client.

To be an effective active listener, you also need to be mentally prepared to hear what is being shared. Mental preparation may mean that you:

- take a deep breath
- close your eyes for a moment, to shut out distractions, before entering the examination room
- picture yourself leaving other tasks behind so that you can start anew with the next consultation.

Without physical and mental preparation, active listening is difficult to sustain.(12)

Active listening requires your entire body to be present in the moment. Nowhere is this better depicted than in the traditional Chinese character for listening: (9)

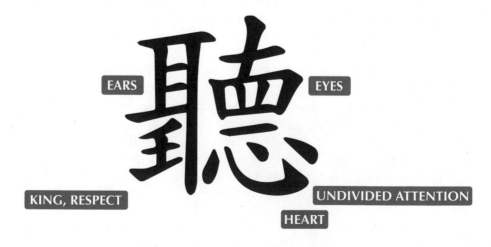

EARS — EYES — KING, RESPECT — UNDIVIDED ATTENTION — HEART

Active listening requires you to listen with your eyes, ears, and heart. The customer is "king." Demonstrate respect by giving all of yourself to him or her, meaning your undivided attention.

5.7 Active Listening in Veterinary Practice

Active or reflective listening is an essential skill in veterinary practice. The veterinary profession represents a unique segment of the healthcare industry. Its providers oversee the care of non-human patients who cannot articulate their presenting complaints, expectations, and reservations about care in the same way that a human might.

Because veterinary patients cannot speak our language to share their own story with us, we have to rely heavily upon the client's perspective to gain insight into the patient's presenting complaint.

True, we are able to examine the patient to build onto our understanding of the patient's health status. However, we are largely dependent upon the details that the client provides. The veterinary client is responsible for the patient, much as a parent is responsible for a child.(47, 48) This results in a tripartite relationship between the veterinarian, client, and patient.(47–49)

It is up to us to extract the right amount of information at the right time if we are going to be successful in decision making about diagnostics and therapeutics, and forward planning.

When speaking with the client, we need to be sure of the following.

* We have all the facts we need.
* We understand the facts, including what happened, when it happened, where it happened, how it happened, and perhaps even why it happened.
* We understand the timeline of events.
* We understand the client's chief concern(s).

If there is confusion about what happened or the timeframe, then we need to be able to:(3)

* check in
* confirm our understanding
* ask questions
* clarify and/or correct our understanding
* restate what we think we understand to be correct.

Reflective listening is the communication tool through which we are able to achieve all of the above to enhance the accuracy of data collection.

5.8 Examples of Active Listening Statements in Veterinary Consultations

Reflective listening often takes the form of certain words or phrases that you, the veterinarian, relay back to the client after the client has spoken.

- "It sounds like …"
- "It sounds to me as if …"
- "It sounds to me that …"
- "What I'm hearing you say is …"
- "What I think you're saying is …"
- "So, if I understand this correctly …"
- "So, you're saying that …"
- "If I have this correct, then …"
- "It seems to me that …"
- "I get the impression that …"
- "I sense that …"
- "You are wondering if …"
- "So, you are concerned about …"
- "So, you aren't sure if …"
- "So, your primary concern is …"
- "So, you are worried that …"

These are simply examples for the novice to make use of while she or he is learning which words and/or phrases seem most genuine. Every one of us practices medicine in a slightly different manner, and that extends to our choice of words that we use to engage our clients in conversation. You may find your own version of an active listening statement that is more natural to you. That is great. In fact, I encourage it. In order for communication to be effective, it must be sincere. You need to feel that you are not just playing a part when you make use of this skill; you are actually making use of this skill for a reason. That reason is often to clarify what you think you heard your client say to you. Consider, for example, the following clinical vignette.

A 15-year-old female spayed Burmese cat, Tango, is presented by her owner, Mrs. Smith, a long-term client of yours, with a 3-day history of inappropriate urination. Tango is the only cat in a single pet household.

In response to your initial statement, "Tell me what's been going on with Tango", the client shares the following:

Gosh, what hasn't been going on? … It's been a crazy summer – my work schedule changed and has me travelling all over the place; I'm barely home. When I am, I'm usually sound asleep. I haven't been able to pay attention to Tango like I have in the past. It hasn't helped that our lives were thrown upside down since the divorce. With

John gone, we had to downsize. We moved six weeks ago to a new apartment; it's small. I hate it. I wouldn't be surprised if she does, too. There's no porch for her to enjoy. There aren't bird feeders to watch through the windows. The neighbors are loud. We can hear their dog through the walls. And now, just when things can't get any worse, Tango's peeing on the carpet. It looks pink – I don't know, could it be blood? – and that has me worried because, well, you know, doc, she's old – and my friend said that peeing blood could mean bladder cancer. I don't know what to do, it's just a lot to take in all at once.

Your client has just shared a significant amount of information with you about both Tango and her situation. From what she stated above, we can extract the following facts about this client–cat duo:

- recently divorced – John is no longer in the picture
- downsized 6 weeks ago
- apartment is small, no porch, no birdwatching
- loud neighbors, dog barking through the walls
- 3-day history of inappropriate urination, possibly hematuria
- client is concerned about bladder cancer.

There are a large number of opportunities for reflective listening here.

1. Reflective listening could be used to acknowledge what it is that you think the client is feeling: stressed, overwhelmed, and worried. For example:
   - "It sounds like you have a lot going on at home that is outside of your control."
   - "It sounds like you and Tango have been through more than your share this summer."
   - "It sounds like between the divorce, downsizing, and your work, you can't catch a break."
   - "I sense that you've been through quite a lot."
2. Reflective listening could be used to address and validate the client's concerns about the patient' presenting complaint. For example:
   - "It sounds like you're not sure where to go from here."
   - "You're concerned that if there is blood in Tango's urine, then she might have cancer?"
   - "You're worried that Tango could have bladder cancer?"
3. Reflective listening could be used to clarify the patient's clinical signs. For example:
   - "So, Tango began to pee outside of the litter box three days ago?"
   - "So, if I understand this correctly, Tango's urine may have blood in it?"

Reflective listening allows the clinician to check in with the client, to see if what she or he heard was correct. When the clinician is able to demonstrate that she or he understood the client, the client feels heard.

Consider, for example, your statement to the client, "It sounds like you and Tango have been through more than your share this summer."

This statement is powerful because it acknowledges what the client shared and validates her experience. The client may respond with:

- "For sure, it's been so hard."
- "Indeed, I don't really know how I'm juggling it all."
- "I'm just waiting for the other shoe to drop."

Or the client may respond with: "You have no idea."

Unless you've been in the client's shoes, that's probably well stated and very true, in which case it would be appropriate to reflect that back to her: "You know what, you're right, I don't. What can I do to help?"

You are supporting the client by acknowledging her plight, and you are investing in the relationship by making strides to build rapport and trust.

On other occasions, you may need to make use of reflective listening because you are not sure that you've gotten an understanding of the complete picture. Maybe the client's story is difficult to follow or changes over time. Maybe the timeline is unclear. Maybe you need additional details to fill in the complete picture.

Consider the following clinical vignette.

> A 5-year-old intact female Basenji dog, is presented by her owner, Mr. Wolf, a brand new client, with a vague history of protracted vomiting.
>
> In response to your initial statement, "Tell me what's been going on with Jive", the client shares the following:
>
> Jive threw up four days ago. Just froth and foam, nothing much. I didn't think anything of it. She acted fine. Then yesterday she wouldn't eat. She threw up food from the night before. No, that was this morning – so maybe the food just sat in her stomach and didn't really go anywhere? I don't know. I've racked my head, but I don't see that she could have gotten into anything. Oh yeah, and now there's diarrhea, too.

Your client has provided an abbreviated clinical history. In his haste to share this history with you, some of the facts are a little hard to wrap one's head around. For example, the timeline gets a bit jumbled.

It is important for you to know when the vomiting started relative to the diarrhea. The timeline is essential.

Reflective listening statements provide an opportunity to clarify your understanding of the client's history:

- "So, let me see if I've got this right: Jive threw up foam four days ago, wouldn't eat yesterday, then threw up food this morning that she ate two days ago?"

- "So, you're saying that Jive had a good appetite until yesterday?"
- "And the diarrhea started today?"

Reflective listening gives the client the chance to clarify his or her message. It gives the client a chance to say, "No, you got it wrong, *this* is what I was trying to say…"

Maybe the diarrhea did not start today. Maybe the diarrhea started yesterday. Maybe it is not until you restate the client's story that he realizes it came out wrong, or maybe he had remembered it wrong. Maybe you misheard. Or maybe what you thought you heard was actually somewhat different.

At the end of the day, it is not about being right or wrong. It is not about whether we heard right, but the story was wrong; or we heard wrong, but the story was right. It is about clarifying so that both of us are on the same page at the end of history taking and data gathering.

Reflective listening gives the client the opportunity to correct the message. In the process, the client may remember important details that had otherwise slipped his mind. Maybe the client now recalls that there were four episodes of diarrhea this morning. Maybe the client now remembers its color or consistency, its volume or odor.

Clarification is essential because we cannot ask the dog what happened. We can only ask the owner.

Doing so requires us to be both patient and flexible. The story might change, and when it does, it is not usually done out of malice to trip us up. It's because as we give the client the chance to communicate with us, and as we play Frisbee with our words, the client has an opportunity to reflect upon what she or he shared. The client has an opportunity to recall a more complete story, rather than just a few snippets here and there.

In many disease presentations, clarification can make the difference between life or death and a medical or surgical emergency. For instance, it matters whether the patient vomited two or ten times or whether a male cat has or has not been able to urinate. If we misinterpret the history that is shared by the client, the results may be catastrophic.

So, get comfortable with reflective listening. Understand that it is okay to double-check details and to clarify the patient's history. Remember that at the end of the day, it is not about being right or wrong. It is about getting the information that you need to manage the patient's care in the best way possible.

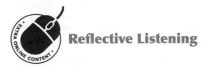 **Reflective Listening**

References

1. Blackwell MJ. Beyond philosophical differences: the future training of veterinarians. J Vet Med Educ. 2001;28(3):148–52.
2. Frankel RM. Pets, vets, and frets: what relationship-centered care research has to offer veteri-

nary medicine. J Vet Med Educ. 2006;33(1):20–7.

3. Shaw JR. Four core communication skills of highly effective practitioners. Vet Clin North Am Small Anim Pract. 2006;36(2):385–96, vii.

4. Brown JP, Silverman JD. The current and future market for veterinarians and veterinary medical services in the United States. J Am Vet Med Assoc. 1999;215(2):161–83.

5. Roter D. The enduring and evolving nature of the patient–physician relationship. Patient Educ Couns. 2000;39(1):5–15.

6. Adams CL, Kurtz SM. Skills for communicating in veterinary medicine. Oxford: Otmoor Publishing and Dewpoint Publishing; 2017.

7. Kurtz SM, Silverman JD, Draper J. Teaching and learning communication skills in medicine. Grand Rapids, MI: Radcliffe; 2004.

8. Silverman J, Kurtz S, Draper J. Skills for communicating with patients. Oxford: Radcliffe Medical Press; 2008.

9. Van Dulmen S. Listen: When words don't come easy. Patient Educ Couns. 2017;100(11):1975–8.

10. Langewitz W, Denz M, Keller A, Kiss A, Ruttimann S, Wossmer B. Spontaneous talking time at start of consultation in outpatient clinic: cohort study. BMJ. 2002;325(7366):682–3.

11. Marvel MK, Epstein RM, Flowers K, Beckman HB. Soliciting the patient's agenda: have we improved? JAMA. 1999;281(3):283–7.

12. Nemec PB, Spagnolo AC, Soydan AS. Can you hear me now? Teaching listening skills. Psychiatr Rehabil J. 2017;40(4):415–7.

13. Jagosh J, Donald Boudreau J, Steinert Y, Macdonald ME, Ingram L. The importance of physician listening from the patients' perspective: enhancing diagnosis, healing, and the doctor–patient relationship. Patient Educ Couns. 2011;85(3):369–74.

14. Boudreau JD, Cassell E, Fuks A. Preparing medical students to become attentive listeners. Med Teach. 2009;31(1):22–9.

15. Fassaert T, van Dulmen S, Schellevis F, Bensing J. Active listening in medical consultations: development of the Active Listening Observation Scale (ALOS-global). Patient Educ Couns. 2007;68(3):258–64.

16. Snyder U. The doctor-patient relationship II: not listening. Medscape J Med. 2008;10(12):294.

17. Snyder U. The doctor-patient relationship III: a way of listening – the Balint group revisited, 2008. Medscape J Med. 2009;11(1):2.

18. Steele DJ, Marvel K. Listening, talking, relating: the state of the art and science of the doctor-patient relationship in family medicine education. Family Medicine. 2002;34(5):310–1.

19. Anderson LA, Zimmerman MA. Patient and physician perceptions of their relationship and patient satisfaction – a study of chronic disease management. Patient Educ Couns. 1993;20(1):27–36.

20. Frederikson LG. Exploring information-exchange in consultation: the patients' view of performance and outcomes. Patient Educ Couns. 1995;25(3):237–46.

21. Ong LM, de Haes JC, Hoos AM, Lammes FB. Doctor–patient communication: a review of the literature. Soc Sci Med. 1995;40(7):903–18.

22. Shannon MT. Please hear what I'm not saying: the art of listening in the clinical encounter. Perm J. 2011;15(2):e114–7.

23. Steine S, Finset A, Laerum E. What is the most important for the patient in the meeting with a general practitioner? Tidsskr Nor Laegeforen. 2000;30:349–53.

24. Charon R. Narrative medicine. New York: Oxford Press; 2006.

25. Passaro J. Who will heal the healers? The Sun Magazine. 2009:6, 10, 1.

26. Walfish S, McAlister B, O'Donnell P, Lambert MJ. An investigation of self-assessment bias in mental health providers. Psychol Rep. 2012;110(2):639–44.

27. Rogers CR, Roethlisberger FJ. Hbr classic – barriers and gateways to communication Harvard Bus Rev. 1991;69(6):105–11. (Reprinted from Harvard Business Review, July August, 1952.)

28. Bodie GD, Vickery AJ, Gearhart CC. The nature of supportive listening I: exploring the relation between supportive listeners and supportive people. Int J Listening. 2013;27:39–49.

29. Rogers CR, Farson RE. Active listening. Chicago, IL: University of Chicago Industrial Relations Center; 1957.

30. Weger H, Castle GR, Emmett MC. Active listening in peer interviews: the influence of message paraphrasing on perceptions of listening skill. Int J Listening. 2010;24:34–49.

31. Rogers CR. Client-centered therapy. Boston, MA: Houghton-Mifflin; 1951.

32. Gordon T. P.E.T.: parent effectiveness training. New York: New American Library; 1975.

33. Comer LB, Drollinger T. Active empathetic listening and selling success: a conceptual framework. J Personal Selling & Sales Management. 1999;19:15–29.

34. Cole CL, Cole AL. Marriage enrichment and prevention really works: Interpersonal competence training to maintain and enhance relationships. Fam Relat. 1999;48(3):273–5.

35. Edwards N, Peterson WE, Davies BL. Evaluation of a multiple component intervention to support the implementation of a "therapeutic relationships" best practice guideline on nurses' communication skills. Patient Educ Couns. 2006;63(1–2):3–11.

36. Jalongo MR. Promoting active listening in the classroom. Childhood Education. 1995;72:13–27.

37. Sifton CB. Listening: the art of communication. Alzheimer's Care Quarterly. 2002;3:2–5.

38. Mishara BL, Chagnon F, Daigle M, Balan B, Raymond S, Marcoux I, et al. Which helper behaviors and intervention styles are related to better short-term outcomes in telephone crisis intervention? Results from a silent monitoring study of calls to the US 1–800-SUICIDE network. Suicide Life Threat Behav. 2007;37(3):308–21.

39. Adler RB, Rosenfeld LB, Proctor RF. Interplay: the process of interpersonal communication. Oxford: Oxford University Press; 2006.

40. Canary DJ, Cody MJ, Manusov VL. Interpersonal communication: a goals-based approach. New York: Bedford/St. Martin's; 2003.

41. Devito JA. The interpersonal communication book. New York: Pearson; 2007.

42. Trenholm S, Jensen A. Interpersonal communication. Oxford: Oxford University Press; 2004.

43. Verderber KS, Verderber RF. Inter-act: interpersonal communication concepts, skills, and contexts. Oxford: Oxford University Press; 2004.

44. Wood JT. Interpersonal communication: everyday encounters. New York: Wadsworth; 1998.

45. Levitt DH. Active listening and counselor self-efficacy: emphasis on one micro-skill in beginning counselor training. Clin Supervisor. 2001;20:101–15.

46. Simon C. The functions of active listening responses. Behav Processes. 2018;157:47–53.

47. Englar RE. Common clinical presentations in dogs and cats. Hoboken, NJ: Wiley/Blackwell; 2019.

48. Shaw JR, Adams CL, Bonnett BN, Larson S, Roter DL. Use of the roter interaction analysis system to analyse veterinarian-client-patient communication in companion animal practice. J Am Vet Med Assoc. 2004;225(2):222–9.

49. Murphy SA. Consumer health information for pet owners. J Med Libr Assoc. 2006;94(2):151–8.

Chapter 6

Defining Entry-Level Communication Skills

Empathy

Empathy is the "almost magical" emotion that persons or objects arouse in us as projections of our feelings. Empathy requires passion, more so than does equanimity, so long cherished by physicians. Medical students lose some of their empathy as they learn science and detachment, and hospital residents lose the remainder in the weariness of overwork and in the isolation of the intensive care units that modern hospitals have become. Conversations about experiences, discussions of patients and their human stories, more leisure and unstructured contemplation of the humanities help physicians to cherish empathy and to retain their passion. Physicians need rhetoric as much as knowledge, and they need stories as much as journals if they are to be more empathetic than computers.(1)

The capacity to demonstrate empathy is an essential skill for the development and maintenance of interpersonal relationships.(1–4)

Empathy is often defined as putting yourself in someone else's shoes.(5–7) That being said, there is no universal definition of empathy.(5, 8–14) Empathy carries a variety of meanings for a variety of people. There are also different types of empathy.(2, 15, 16)

6.1 Cognitive Empathy

So-called *cognitive* empathy can be thought of as:(2)

- identifying with another individual
- developing a conscious awareness for how someone else experiences the world
- embracing someone else's perspective to obtain a different vantage point
- demonstrating understanding of another person's experience
- showing sensitivity towards another person's situation
- recognizing that someone else feels a certain way and making the effort to understand why.

Being empathetic at a *cognitive* level simply means that you can identify with the individual with whom you are engaging.(13) You may or may not agree with this person's perspective or insight, but you can appreciate his or her thought process. You get why she or he thinks the way she or he does about certain scenarios or events.(2) This form of empathy is purely cerebral.

Veterinarians require cognitive empathy in order to understand their client's point of view.(13)

Consider the following clinical vignettes and appreciate how the client in each scenario could benefit from receiving this form of empathy.

- A geriatric, toy-breed dog has developed an acute, wet cough. The client is concerned that the dog has developed congestive heart failure.
- A hunting dog has developed acute non-weight-bearing lameness on his left pelvic limb. The client worries that the underlying condition is osteosarcoma.
- A cat presents for evaluation of a persistent and enlarging, post-vaccinal integumentary mass. The client fears that the lump is an injection site sarcoma.
- A cat presents for evaluation of dyspnea. The client associates this presentation with a recent visit to the human emergency room with his asthmatic son.

Cognitive empathy allows the veterinary team to see each clinical scenario from the perspective of the client, whether or not the client's perspective is accurate. This recognition paves the way for the veterinarian to acknowledge and address the client's concerns so that there is mutual understanding. It is only by addressing these concerns that both parties move forward with diagnostic and/or treatment options.

Note that being empathetic does not mean that you necessarily agree with the individual for whom you are exhibiting empathy.(6)

In other words:

- that geriatric, toy-breed dog with an acute, wet cough may not be in congestive heart failure
- that hunting dog with lameness of the left pelvic limb may not have osteosarcoma
- that cat with a post-vaccinal integumentary mass may not have injection site sarcoma
- that dyspneic cat may not have asthma.

That is okay. Being empathetic is not about agreeing with the client. It is about viewing the case from the client's perspective. To do so requires you to set aside your own core benefits to accept the client's position as a starting point for how she or he feels about the present situation.

6.2 Missed Opportunities for Empathetic Displays in Healthcare

Have you ever been placed in a situation where you felt uncomfortable and did not know how to respond?

Envision yourself at a family gathering or high school reunion. Maybe you are approached by someone who says something that catches you off-guard. Maybe you were not expecting to hear this from him or her, or maybe you do not even know the person all that well. Perhaps they are an estranged family member, or someone that you have not talked to since grade school.

At best, the situation is awkward.

Thinking back on those times, consider how our own discomfort with these situations handicaps our ability to respond. We may be unsure what constitutes an appropriate response. We may not even know where to begin, in terms of what to say or do.

In situations where we feel uncomfortable, we default to what we know. We may change the subject to a content area that is neutral or deemed safe, such as the weather or sporting events.

SPEAKER: I'm really worried about Uncle Joe.

YOU: Say, he had a great time at the ballgame last night. What did you think of that home run during the final innings?

We may interrupt the speaker or finish his thought, even if we complete it with something that is incorrect:

SPEAKER: I'm really worried about Uncle Joe. Does he seem …?

YOU: Old? Eh, who isn't starting to feel their age around here?

We may invalidate the speaker's concerns:

SPEAKER: I'm really worried about Uncle Joe. Does he seem more confused to you?

YOU: No, not at all. You just haven't seen him for a while. He's his same ol' self.

We may even terminate the conversation:

SPEAKER: I'm really worried about Uncle Joe. Does he seem more confused to you?

YOU: Oh, look, here comes Mary. Hi Mary, how's it going?

Any of our responses, above, lack empathy.

In the moment, our words are protective. They take us away from the feelings that we do not want to feel. They prevent us from connecting to another person at a time when we want to maintain our distance.

Maybe we do not want to think about Uncle Joe's health. Maybe we are scared about it, too. Maybe we do not want to accept what is happening to him. Maybe we do not even want to acknowledge it.

So, we either turtle ourselves – we tuck ourselves out of the way and into a shell, until the moment passes and it is safe to come out – or we push past it until the moment is a distant memory.

These moments happen all the time. Sometimes we are aware of them; many times we are not.

What is important to note is that these situations are not restricted to our personal lives. They often present themselves in clinical practice. As professionals, we strive to maintain certain standards. By our own education, we are often praised for being objective and for maintaining professional distance from our patients/clients. This is intended to be protective.

Yet, the process of building walls is obstructive, particularly when the principles of relationship-centered care tell us that walls should be torn down. We have become so good at building walls that we often do not even know that they are there. When we are busy or otherwise stressed – physically, mentally, or emotionally – those walls feel even more constricting as if they are closing in on all sides. It makes it hard to catch our breath.

This leads to missed opportunities in clinical practice to connect to our clients through empathy. We may not hear the words that our clients/patients use. Or we may hear them, but choose to skip over them. Consider the following clinical vignette, taken from veterinary practice.

> VETERINARIAN: After we amputate Pasta's leg, he will stay in the hospital until Friday. Then we'll discharge him home to your care. The hospital is closed over that three-day holiday weekend, so you will need to be prepared to provide for his needs, including helping him to get in and out of the house to eliminate.

> CLIENT: I'm not sure how that is going to work. I live alone and he's too heavy for me to lift.

> VETERINARIAN: Now let's talk about what the surgery is going to involve.

In this clinical vignette, the client is worried about patient aftercare. The client expresses concern about her ability to care for the patient postoperatively, particularly knowing that the clinic will be closed. The client provided clues that indicated her desire to discuss these concerns in greater detail.

What did the veterinarian do? How did the veterinarian respond? Instead of taking a moment to acknowledge the client's reservations, the veterinarian hit the fast-forward button and skipped over the client's expression of concern. The veterinarian defaulted back to what was comfortable: focusing on procedural logistics.

This happens all the time in clinical practice. Empathy is apt to break down during difficult or distressing conversations.(17)

Healthcare providers often miss out on opportunities to express empathy.(2, 18–22) Recent studies in human medicine by Morse et al., Bylund and Makoul, and Levinson et al. demonstrate that these missed opportunities are not few and far between: they represent the majority (70–90%).(18–20)

Sometimes physicians are unaware when opportunities for empathetic displays present themselves. They may be so focused on a case or on a specific line of questioning that they have tunnel vision. This is restrictive. Tunnel vision causes doctors to miss out on key features or facts of the case because they are so caught up with paying attention to what they think is most important. They proceed with cases with only one goal in mind: to get to the finish line, the diagnosis.

Other times, physicians may recognize opportunities as they arise, but fail to take the time to explore feelings that are beneath the surface.(20) Physicians may mistakenly believe that they should mind their own business so as not to come across as prying, when in fact the patient is opening the door to the discussion that she or he wants to have.

On other occasions, physicians may intentionally ignore cues. For example, they may terminate discussions when consultations become emotional.(20) Alternatively, they may invalidate a patient's concerns ("Of course you don't have cancer! Don't be ridiculous!") or use humor inappropriately ("All you need to do is sign up for The Biggest Loser") to deflect discussions when emotional threads become uncomfortable for the physician.(20)

Human medical doctors are not the only members of the healthcare industry to skip out on opportunities to exhibit empathy. Veterinarians are equally apt to miss or ignore client cues in 59–93% of clinical scenarios.(21, 22)

Some veterinarians acknowledge a fear of getting "stuck" in a conversation that is uncomfortable.(23) Other veterinarians believe that clients benefit from objectivity rather than empathy.(13, 21, 24) Because veterinarians do not always know how to cope with client's intense emotions, they make an intentional decision not to go there.(13) Fear of the unknown provokes anxiety.(25)

To reduce discomfort, many veterinarians deflect empathy toward the patient rather than the veterinary client.(2, 21, 26) How this is perceived by the client varies.(13, 21, 27)

Veterinarians may also resort to labelling the client as being "difficult" rather than acknowledging their own personal discomfort with the situation.(13, 25) In today's day and age of social media groups that are closed to veterinary professionals only, it is tempting to trade anecdotes, about clients and their reactions – or perceived overreactions.(13, 25) However, this is counterproductive. It does not make us any more likely to develop or demostrate empathy.(13, 25) Instead, it stirs the pot by reinforcing judgmental tendencies instead of focusing on ways that empathy can impact the practice and its bottom line.

If veterinarians lack cognitive empathy, then they miss out on the opportunity to connect to their clients. At the same time, they run the risk that they will misidentify, misunderstand, or misconstrue the emotional undercurrent of each situation.

If the client's perspective is not addressed, then he or she may not buy into recommendations for patient care. The client may also not feel heard or valued as a member of the patient's healthcare team. This goes against the grain of relationship-centered care.

Client satisfaction with the veterinary team is largely based upon perceptions of the veterinary–client–patient relationship.(5, 27–32) Clients who do not feel valued are less likely to return for follow-up or refer others to the practice.(32, 33)

6.3 Emotional Empathy

Cognitive empathy is an important starting point for the veterinary team. *Emotional* empathy takes it a step further. Emotional empathy is the capacity to feel as another, instead of feeling for him or her.(2, 8) This figure of speech implies that, through empathy, we can become one with another person. We can connect to that individual through emotion. We can feel what they feel.

Emotional empathy is raw. It connects us to our client on the deepest level possible as we work hard to not only identify with, but experience another person's emotional state as much as we can in order to appreciate what that individual is going through.(5–7, 13, 14)

Emotional empathy can be immensely rewarding for the human healthcare provider and patient, veterinarian and client alike.

Like active listening, empathy humanizes medicine. It strengthens the bond between healthcare provider and client because it conveys the following unspoken messages.

- "I get you."
- "I feel for you."
- "I am there for you."
- "I can relate to you."
- "Your pain is my pain."

6.4 The Impact of Empathy on Case Outcomes

Because of its ability to reinforce interpersonal connectivity, empathy is associated with several positive outcomes in human healthcare:(13, 16, 22, 34–45)

- improved rapport between doctor and patient
- increased accuracy of data gathering, for instance, during history taking
  - patients are more likely to share complete histories
  - patients are likely to engage in full disclosure
- increased accuracy of diagnosis
- increased adherence of patients to treatment recommendations
- increased patient satisfaction
- reduced malpractice risk
- increased physician satisfaction
- improved physician health and wellbeing.

Empathy yields similar outcomes in veterinary practice:(16, 21, 34, 46)

- increased satisfaction among clients
- improved client adherence to treatment recommendations
- increased satisfaction among veterinarians.

What is it about empathy that makes it such a positive skill for healthcare providers to possess?

Empathy builds relationships. It connects two individuals through one person's attempt to experience another person's reality so that she or he may more easily relate to, accept, and understand that individual's perspective.(5, 6, 47)

Teh intent behind empathy is to be helpful. It paves the way for *empathetic concern*. Healthcare team members who exhibit empathetic concern not only relate to and connect with the patient's plight; they also want to effect change to help the patient work through it.(2)

6.5 Empathy versus Sympathy

Empathy is often mistaken for sympathy.(13, 48) Sympathy is an emotional response that is involuntary.(13, 21, 49, 50) In particular, sympathy typically involves responding to someone else's misfortune with sadness or pity.

For example, you may be sympathetic to someone's plight. You may sympathize with someone else's situation. You may express sympathy for another person's loss. In other words, you may feel for the person who is experiencing the emotion, be it sadness, sorrow, intense grief, or pain.

Sympathy cards are perhaps society's best example of expressing condolences.

- "I'm sorry for your loss."
- "Keeping you close in thought, with sincere sympathy"
- "Thinking of you, with sympathy, during this difficult time."

These statements are intended to provide support to the bereaved. However, the feelings of sorrow that such condolences express are kept at arm's length, meaning that they originate from outside of the supporter's frame of reference. They are external. They are not an attempt to experience grief as one's own in order to appreciate more fully the bereaved's experience.

Unlike sympathy, empathy is not an immediate or involuntary response to another person's experience.(13, 22, 51) Empathy is not innate, although some people's temperaments cause them to be more easily suited to empathetic displays. Empathy is a skill that is cultivated over time.(13, 22, 51)

Empathy can also be modified by the following factors:(4, 47, 52–55)

- genetics
- gender:
  - women have historically had higher human–human empathy scores than men(55–60)
  - women have historically had higher human–animal empathy scores than men(56, 57, 61–63)
- diet:
  - vegetarians and vegans reportedly have higher human–human empathy scores than omnivores(4, 58, 64)
  - vegetarians and vegans reportedly have higher human–animal empathy scores than omnivores(58)
- familiarity
- prior experiences
- professional aspirations:
  - veterinary students who prefer conservation medicine or small animal medicine have, on the whole, higher human–animal empathy scores than those who pursue production medicine.(65)

Note that human–human empathy and human–animal empathy are related, but not necessarily equivalent between groups of people and even within individuals.(4, 66–69)

Empathy takes time to develop because it requires:(13, 19, 22, 34, 50, 51, 70, 71)

- the ability to identify the non-verbal cues that another person is displaying
- the emotional intelligence to recognize how another person is feeling
- the ability to reflect upon our initial perceptions, confirm their accuracy, and/or modify them if they were incorrect
- the ability to communicate mutual understanding to the affected individual
- the ability to act on that level of understanding in a supportive manner.

Empathy requires you to tap into another person's perspective.

The best distinction that I have found to share with my students is credited to Rebecca O'Donnell: "Empathy is walking a mile in someone else's moccasins. Sympathy is being sorry their feet hurt."

6.6 The Human–Animal Bond Creates Opportunities for Empathy in Veterinary Practice

Opportunities to demonstrate empathy are plentiful in veterinary practice. Patients and patient outcomes are often tied to client emotions. Client emotions may vary tremendously depending upon the role in which they view themselves and their pets.

Clients may consider themselves to be pet "parents."(72) As such, they may feel responsible for meeting their "child's" needs and making informed decisions about healthcare.(72) When financial constraints hinder or prevent decision making, they may feel guilty that they could not do "everything" despite wanting to.

Clients that are dating, engaged, or married, may especially see themselves in the role of parents. It is not uncommon for couples to experience their first cat or dog together before they experience their first child.

Beyond the obvious link to pediatric medicine, veterinary patients may also act as surrogates for other human relationships. Veterinary patients may represent links to the deceased. The cat may be the only living tie to a deceased parent or grandparent, spouse or sibling.

Alternatively, veterinary patients may represent links to relationships that are no longer in existence; for instance, the dog may have been retained by the ex-wife following a divorce, and as such, represents the accumulation of memories from her past, failed chapter of marriage.

Some clients recognize the extent to which these links bind them to their pets; others are unconscious of this until something catastrophic happens and forces them into the realization of why so much emotion comes bubbling up to the surface.

6.7 The Dangers of Making Assumptions about Client Emotions

As veterinarians, we cannot and should not make assumptions about how a client feels or why she or he might feel that way. The human–animal bond means something different to every pet owner. No two clients are identical, just as no two pets are identical. No two relationships are equivalent.

For that reason, we should not express how difficult it is to see a client lose her "son" or "baby" unless we know for certain that is how she views their relationship. We should listen closely to how our clients describe their pets and reflect back the same language that they share with us.

We may be able to predict when and why some clients become emotional about their pets; for others, emotion may come as a surprise. It is not up to us to decide when and where emotion surfaces. We can only listen and relate and do our best to understand.

6.8 When Might Clients Become Emotional?

In veterinary practice, clients are more likely to become emotional during discussions about:(13)

- trauma and other aspects of emergency medicine
- unexpected death
- quality of life
- anticipatory grief
- euthanasia

- acute illness
- chronic disease
- terminal disease
- injury or disease that could have been prevented
- financial constraints.

There is no "right" or "wrong" emotion for a client to feel. Sadness, resentment, guilt, and blame may all play roles in the way a case unfolds.

Although veterinarians are not trained psychologists and there are certain boundaries that we should not cross, we do owe it to our clients to do what we can to understand. We may not be able to move forward with patient care until we get to the bottom of these emotions and/or provide a safe space for client emotions to be articulated.

Empathy is one communication tool that we can use to connect with our client, particularly during emotional and/or otherwise distressing times.

6.9 The Challenges Associated with Empathetic Displays in Clinical Practice

Despite plentiful opportunities for displays of empathy in veterinary practice, empathetic statements are expressed in the minority of appointments.(5, 13, 21, 22, 31)

Empathy is also one of several communication-based reasons why formal complaints by veterinary clients are lodged against practitioners through licensing boards.(73)

If empathy is so essential to the successful practice of veterinary medicine, then why is it so challenging to demonstrate? Empathy is difficult to define and describe. A statement may be inherently empathetic or not, but it is not always easy to articulate how or why that is so. Likewise, it is difficult for students who do not feel particularly empathetic to act empathetic towards a given situation or individual.

Students and practitioners alike may struggle with empathy when client emotions make them uncomfortable. Sometimes when we are uncomfortable, we may want to change the subject. Changing the subject when we are uncomfortable is tempting, however, doing so is not particularly empathetic.

Students may struggle with empathy because it is difficult to fake. When empathy is forced, clients can tell, and students come across as being insincere. Students may also struggle with this skill because it is difficult to set aside judgment. For instance, a student once expressed to me that it was difficult to display empathy to a client that had administered acetaminophen to her cat because it was the wrong thing to do.

Recognize that being empathetic does not necessarily mean that you agree with a client's actions; it means that you understand why they did what they did.

Even experienced clinicians may struggle with expressing empathy. We may miss out on opportunities for us to be empathetic in the consultation room.(13, 21, 22) Clients are not always direct about their feelings, though they may provide hints.(6, 13, 70, 74) If we are not on the lookout for indirect statements or nonverbal cues, then we lose the chance to explore how our client is experiencing life in the moment.(13)

In the process of trying to check in with our clients and clarify their perspective, we need to be cautious about how we phrase our questions. Our goal is not to interrogate or to convey judgment.(13)

Avoid questions that begin with, "Why?"(13, 24)

- "Why do you think that?" may come across as being judgmental, even when it was not intended to be.
- "Why do you think that?" may incite defensiveness when in fact all we were trying to do was gather information.

"What makes you say that?" is a gentler approach to the same question.

Gentler approaches are more likely to instill trust in our clients, who, as a result, may be more likely to share their perspective, including their concerns with us. If we are too direct, we may create discomfort that mutes conversation.(13)

Consider, for example, the common clinical scenario in which a veterinarian advises a client to pursue dental prophylaxis under general anesthesia for a geriatric cat. Despite making this recommendation, the veterinarian senses pushback from the client. It is important that the veterinarian pick up on this resistance and address it. However, the way in which it is handled can have different results.

If the veterinarian is well intentioned, but too direct, and asks, "What makes you uncomfortable about placing your cat under anesthesia?", the client may be reluctant to share.

The client may be more likely to share if the veterinarian phrases the inquiry using the third person.(13) For example: "A lot of clients are uncomfortable with anesthetizing their senior pets …", which provides an opening in the conversation that allows a more hesitant client to speak up.(13) Alternatively, the veterinarian can lead with, "Some of my clients are concerned about anesthesia in an older pet. Can we talk about that?"(13)

These strategies can facilitate clinical conversations, particularly those in which it is essential to create connections between healthcare provider and client.

Even so, empathizing with clients day in, day out, is demanding. Not all clinicians feel empathetic towards every client at every appointment, every day.

In truth, a clinician's empathy depends upon a number of circumstances including:

- the clinical scenario and associated circumstances
- the client's comfort
- the client's emotions
- the physician's comfort
- the physician's stress level
- the timing of the appointment.

External factors play a major role. What else may be going on, behind the scenes, in the clinician's life, matters greatly in terms of whether or not the clinician is capable of expressing empathy in the moment.

If I have had to euthanize 25 patients before coming into my 26th exam room of the day to discuss quality of life, then I may be emotionally exhausted. For self-preservation, I may not want to put myself in my client's shoes. In that case, I need to lean on other communication tools to ensure that I still fully invest in the relationship.

6.10 Displaying Empathy through Actions in Clinical Practice

Empathy may take the form of words or actions.(6, 13, 21, 23, 74) For the novice, empathetic actions are usually easier to demonstrate sincerely than empathetic words.
   Empathetic actions include:

*   making eye contact(6, 13)
*   maintaining eye contact when a client is expressing an emotion(6, 13)
*   mirroring the client's posture, that is, if the client is seated, seat yourself(6, 13, 14, 23)
*   angling your body at a 5–10 degree angle from the horizontal line between you and the client(14)
*   avoiding towering above the client, if you are standing
*   sitting on the floor, with your eye level below the client's, to put the patient at ease and to reduce feelings of vulnerability that the client may have(23, 75)
*   decreasing the distance between you and the client, that is, bringing one's chair nearer to the client or sitting beside the client on an examination room bench
*   talking slowly to allow the client to process details(6)
*   using a moment of silence(6)
*   using touch appropriately at one of the following locations: the client's shoulder, upper arm, forearm, or top of the hand to console(25)
*   touching the patient, particularly if the clinician is uncomfortable with touching the client(75)
*   offering a box of tissues to a grieving or crying client.

Note that offering tissues gets mixed reviews. Some clients feel comforted. Others feel like it's a gesture that says "stop crying" or "I'm uncomfortable with tears, so here, let's dry them up."

6.11 Displaying Empathy through Words in Clinical Practice

Empathy can also be demonstrated through the use of words or phrases.
   Note that not every clinician will make use of the same words or phrases to convey similar intentions.(13) Not every client will respond to the veterinarian's chosen words or phrases in the same way.(13) There is a great deal that is beyond the clinician's control.
   What is within the clinician's power is to select words and phrases that are sincere.
   Empathetic phrases include statements of acknowledgement.

- "I see that you care very deeply about Juniper."
- "I can see how hard it is for you to make this decision."
- "I can tell that Sam's battle with cancer is really weighing on your mind."
- "I know that you would do anything in your power to take away Simba's pain."
- "I appreciate that you are putting her needs first and that you do not want Tigress to suffer."
- "You two have been through so much together. Saying goodbye to Darcy today must feel like losing family."

Sometimes these statements of acknowledgement mirror reflective listening.(13)

- "It sounds like your greatest concern is …"
- "It sounds like you aren't sure what we need to do next to figure out what's wrong with Tuxedo."
- "I hear that you are worried most about …"
- "I'm hearing you say that you cannot administer injections at home."
- "I'm hearing that quality of life is most important to you as we consider Fluffy's care."
- "What you're saying is that Rose acts like she's in pain and that is distressing to you."
- "What you're telling me is that you don't want Gina to suffer."

Refer to Chapter 5 for more information about reflective listening.
    Empathetic phrases also include statements that normalize and/or validate the client's expressed emotion.(13)

- "It must have been so difficult for you to discuss this with me."
- "It must have been so scary to see Fluffy in that condition."
- "It's absolutely frightening to have to witness Turnip seizing."
- "It's so overwhelming to consider all the ways that we need to adjust Tulip's lifestyle."
- "It's understandable that you would worry about Fiji's appetite being off: we both know that anorexic cats may develop liver disease if we don't intervene quickly."

Empathetic phrases include connectivity statements that express shared experiences.(13)

- "Your concern is my concern. I am worried about that, too."
- "When my own cat developed diabetes, I also wondered how I could make injections work with my current schedule."
- "I know what it's like to have a large-breed dog with arthritis: I cannot lift mine up or down the stairs either, so I understand how difficult it is going to be at home to manage Trolley's hip pain."

Empathetic phrases may also include statements of honesty and full disclosure that you have not ever experienced the same situation first hand.

- "I can only imagine what you are going through."
- "I can't begin to understand the depth of your pain."

6.12 The Potential Dangers of Empathy in Clinical Practice: the Client's Perspective

Empathy can be overused in clinical practice.(13) Empathy that is premature or empathy that lacks sincerity is hazardous to relationship-building.(13)

Clients value honesty.(5, 32, 76) In fact, when the general public ranks professionals in terms of character traits, veterinarians are consistently ranked above human physicians, accountants, and lawyers.(5)

Clients want their veterinarians to be kind and gentle.(5, 77) Being kind means being real. Clients know when empathetic responses are genuine. Clients know when they are not. Empathy cannot be faked well. There is only one thing worse than having no empathy: faking it.

We may fake empathy by saying what we think the clients want to hear. However, what clients will hear is that your words were forced.(13)

Clients will also see if our words are supported by the appropriate nonverbal cues. (13) When verbal and nonverbal cues are at odds, clients believe the latter.(5, 13, 23) For instance, if we say the right words, in the right tone, but convey the following nonverbal cues, then the client is likely to lose trust in us:

- acting uncomfortable by breaking eye contact and looking away
- acting disinterested or distracted, by looking at one's watch or smart phone
- crossing one's arms against one's chest
- leaning away.

Refer to Chapter 7 for additional information on nonverbal cues.

The bottom line is that whatever you say, make it true to you. Make it sound legitimate. Make it sound real, and true to the moment, rather than rehearsed. If you cannot say something empathetic; do something empathetic. If all you can do is provide attentive silence, then that is still better than faking empathy. Clients will appreciate your presence above all.

6.13 The Potential Dangers of Empathy in Clinical Practice: the Clinician's Perspective

There is a growing concern throughout the healthcare industry that both medical and veterinary providers are at increasing risk of compassion fatigue.(8, 78–80)

Compassion fatigue occurs when providers are overwhelmed by the physical and/or emotional distress of those under their care.(79, 81–84) Repeated exposure to challenging emotional threads creates anxiety for the provider, who may feel powerless to effect change for the patient.(79, 82, 85)

If a provider's capacity to give is exceeded by the burden of caring, particularly if she or he is spread too thin, then the provider may shut down as a means of self-protection. Empathy is replaced with numbness, and the provider may avoid any reminder that links him or her to the patient.(79, 82, 83)

Compassion fatigue that is not addressed may lead to burnout.(79, 81–84) Burnout occurs when the provider cannot continue in the role of caregiver due to exhaustion, frustration, or perceived loss of control.(79, 81–84) The path to burnout is accelerated by environmental factors, such as time constraints, increased workload, and inadequate social networks.(84, 86)

Burnout is significant in the veterinary profession.(79) Although more current studies are needed to evaluate its incidence in clinical practice today, two-thirds of female veterinarians in the United States demonstrated symptoms of burnout in a 1992 report.(87)

Because the provider is no longer able to perform the role that she or he was trained to do, she or he may become clinically depressed.(88–90) Fear of failure and fear of losing one's professional identify may prevent the provider from reaching out to others for support.(81, 91) Lack of support breeds isolation, and isolation is self-perpetuating. Thus, the cycle of dysfunctional coping continues.(81, 92)

The incidence of depression in veterinary professionals continues to be extensively studied. In 2012, 66% of Alabama veterinarians self-reported that they had at least once experienced "clinically significant depression."(93) In 2015, the Centers for Disease Control and Prevention (CDC) surveyed 10,254 veterinarians in the United States. Based upon their responses to standardized questions from the Kessler-6 psychological distress scale, almost 7% of male veterinarians and 11% of female veterinarians had evidence of active psychological distress.(88, 94) These values are twice that which have been recorded for the general population.(88, 94–96)

If appropriate coping mechanisms are not established, depression may result in suicidal ideation, suicide attempts, and/or suicide completion.(97–99) Veterinary professionals are more likely to commit suicide than members of the general population.(88, 93, 99–106) One-sixth of veterinarians in the United States have contemplated suicide. (88) In Australia, New Zealand, and the UK, suicide completion occurs by veterinarians at a rate of three to four times that of the general public.(100)

In the past, it was believed that detachment from patients was the key to physician survival.(8, 78, 107) Empathy was viewed as being too costly.(8, 78) Clinicians who were overly empathetic were considered to be overinvolved with their cases, and in danger of becoming overwhelmed by their patients' distress.(8, 78) It was assumed that the empathetic practitioner could not practice objectivity, and would be unable to provide adequate care.(8, 37, 78)

Subsequent studies have disproven the belief that empathy is an obstacle to clinical encounters.(8, 108, 109) Empathetic doctors are in fact less susceptible to compassion fatigue and burnout, provided that they develop appropriate coping mechanisms to shoulder the emotional burden.(8, 108, 109)

How can we adapt, both individually and as a profession, to better cope with our role as caregivers?

We need to find ways around the paralysis of overwhelming emotion through acknowledgement and self-care. These include:(79, 81, 110–112)

- preparing our students for the realities that they will face in clinical practice
- anticipating problems before they arise and devising practical solutions
- creating safe, supportive environments to discuss professional and personal struggles
- promoting resiliency
- developing positive professional identities
- providing ourselves and each other with strong support systems
- finding creative ways of restoring work-life balance
- reshaping attitudes about our role in patient care
- encouraging self-awareness
- accepting ourselves for who we are, including our limitations.

6.14 The Decline of Empathy?

There is concern that human–human empathy is on the decline, within the United States, as a society and as a nation.(17)

There is also growing concern that the training that students receive in medical school has the potential to reduce human–human empathy.(11, 113–122)

Equal concern exists that veterinary student training dampens human–animal empathy.

- First-year veterinary students score higher for human–animal empathy than fourth-year veterinary students.(4)
- Second-year veterinary students are more likely to propose pain management than fourth-year veterinary students.(123)

Whether these trends are due to a loss of idealism or the need to distance oneself from one's patients in order to survive remains unclear.(4, 124, 125) Stress and fatigue may also be contributing factors.(4)

In addition, third-year veterinary students are much more likely than first- or second-year veterinary students to report personal distress.(35) As Schoenfeld-Tacher et al. report:

> This is especially concerning because the enhanced unease in interpersonal interactions coincides with students entering clinical rotations in the third year – the very time when these traits are necessary for quality client and patient care.(35)

As veterinary educators, we do not yet know how to address changes in students' levels of empathy as they progress through veterinary training programs. As a profession, we do not yet know the best way to intervene to counteract these trends.

What we do know is this. Workplace learning can have a significant impact on student empathy as well as their perceptions of animal welfare.(65, 126) We need to do all that we can to keep empathy alive and well in clinical consultations. Empathy encourages connectivity. It bonds us to our clients and vice versa.

Empathy strengthens the veterinarian–client–patient relationship that we hope to make lifelong.

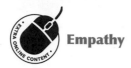 **Empathy**

References

1. Spiro H. What is empathy and can it be taught? Ann Intern Med. 1992;116(10):843–6.
2. Adams CL, Kurtz SM. Skills for communicating in veterinary medicine. Oxford: Otmoor Publishing and Dewpoint Publishing; 2017.
3. Garden R. Expanding clinical empathy: an activist perspective. J Gen Intern Med. 2009;24(1):122–5.
4. Calderon-Amor J, Luna-Fernandez D, Tadich T. Study of the levels of human–human and human–animal empathy in veterinary medical students from Chile. J Vet Med Educ. 2017;44(1):179–86.
5. Shaw JR. Four core communication skills of highly effective practitioners. Vet Clin North Am Small Anim Pract. 2006;36(2):385–96, vii.
6. Silverman J, Kurtz S, Draper J. Skills for communicating with patients. Oxford: Radcliffe Medical Press; 2008.
7. Kurtz SM, Silverman JD, Draper J. Teaching and learning communication skills in medicine. Grand Rapids, MI: Radcliffe; 2004.
8. Preusche I, Lamm C. Reflections on empathy in medical education: what can we learn from social neurosciences? Adv Health Sci Educ Theory Pract. 2016;21(1):235–49.
9. Halpern J. What is clinical empathy? J Gen Intern Med. 2003;18(8):670–4.
10. Hojat M. Empathy in patient care: antecedents, development, measurement, and outcomes. New York: Springer; 2007.
11. Pedersen R. Empirical research on empathy in medicine – a critical review. Patient Educ Couns. 2009;76(3):307–22.
12. Singer T, Lamm C. The social neuroscience of empathy. Ann N Y Acad Sci. 2009;1156:81–96.
13. McMurray J, Boysen S. Communicating empathy in veterinary practice. Vet Irel J. 2017;7(4):199–205.
14. Shea SC. Psychiatric interviewing: the art of understanding. Second ed. Philadelphia, PA: WB Saunders Company; 1998.
15. Panksepp J, Panksepp JB. Toward a cross-species understanding of empathy. Trends Neurosci. 2013;36(8):489–96.

16. Schoenfeld-Tacher RM, Shaw JR, Meyer-Parsons B, Kogan LR. Changes in affective and cognitive empathy among veterinary practitioners. J Vet Med Educ. 2017;44(1):63–71.
17. Schumann K, Zaki J, Dweck CS. Addressing the empathy deficit: beliefs about the malleability of empathy predict effortful responses when empathy is challenging. J Pers Soc Psychol. 2014;107(3):475–93.
18. Morse DS, Edwardsen EA, Gordon HS. Missed opportunities for interval empathy in lung cancer communication. Arch Intern Med. 2008;168(17):1853–8.
19. Bylund CL, Makoul G. Examining empathy in medical encounters: an observational study using the empathic communication coding system. Health Commun. 2005;18(2):123–40.
20. Levinson W, Gorawara-Bhat R, Lamb J. A study of patient clues and physician responses in primary care and surgical settings. JAMA. 2000;284(8):1021–7.
21. McArthur ML, Fitzgerald JR. Companion animal veterinarians' use of clinical communication skills. Aust Vet J. 2013;91(9):374–80.
22. Shaw JR, Adams CL, Bonnett BN, Larson S, Roter DL. Use of the Roter interaction analysis system to analyse veterinarian-client-patient communication in companion animal practice. J Am Vet Med Assoc. 2004;225(2):222–9.
23. Carson CA. Nonverbal communication in veterinary practice. Vet Clin North Am Small Anim Pract. 2007;37(1):49–63; abstract viii.
24. Cornell KK, Kopcha M. Client-veterinarian communication: skills for client centered dialogue and shared decision making. Vet Clin North Am Small Anim Pract. 2007;37(1):37–47; abstract vii.
25. Bateman SW. Communication in the veterinary emergency setting. Vet Clin North Am Small Anim Pract. 2007;37(1):109–21; abstract ix.
26. Roberts F. Speaking to and for animals in a veterinary clinic: a practice for managing interpersonal interaction. Res Lang Soc Interac. 2004;37(4):421–46.
27. Case DB. Survey of expectations among clients of three small animal clinics. J Am Vet Med Assoc. 1988;192(4):498–502.
28. Antelyes J. Client hopes, client expectations. J Am Vet Med Assoc. 1990;197(12):1596–7.
29. Antelyes J. Client retention. J Am Vet Med Assoc. 1990;197(4):461–3.
30. Antelyes J. Difficult clients in the next decade. J Am Vet Med Assoc. 1991;198(4):550–2.
31. Bylund CL, Makoul G. Empathic communication and gender in the physician–patient encounter. Patient Educ Couns. 2002;48(3):207–16.
32. Show A, Englar RE. Evaluating dog and cat owner preferences for Calgary–Cambridge communication skills: results of a questionnaire. J Vet Med Educ. 2018:1–10.
33. Hall MA, Dugan E, Zheng B, Mishra AK. Trust in physicians and medical institutions: what is it, can it be measured, and does it matter? Milbank Q. 2001;79(4):613–39, v.
34. Shaw JR, Adams CL, Bonnett BN, Larson S, Roter DL. Veterinarian satisfaction with companion animal visits. J Am Vet Med Assoc. 2012;240(7):832–41.
35. Schoenfeld-Tacher RM, Kogan LR, Meyer-Parsons B, Royal KD, Shaw JR. Educational research report: changes in students' levels of empathy during the didactic portion of a veterinary program. J Vet Med Educ. 2015;42(3):194–205.
36. Decety J, Fotopoulou A. Why empathy has a beneficial impact on others in medicine: unifying theories. Front Behav Neurosci. 2014;8:457.
37. Halpern J. Clinical Empathy in medical care. In: Decety J, editor. Empathy: from bench to bedside. Cambridge, MA: MIT Press; 2012. pp. 229–44.
38. Riess H, Kelley JM, Bailey RW, Dunn EJ, Phillips M. Empathy training for resident physicians: a randomized controlled trial of a neuroscience-informed curriculum. J Gen Intern Med.

2012;27(10):1280–6.

39. Maguire P, Faulkner A, Booth K, Elliott C, Hillier V. Helping cancer patients disclose their concerns. Eur J Cancer. 1996;32A(1):78–81.

40. Stewart MA. Effective physician–patient communication and health outcomes: a review. CMAJ. 1995;152(9):1423–33.

41. Bertakis KD, Roter D, Putnam SM. The relationship of physician medical interview style to patient satisfaction. J Fam Pract. 1991;32(2):175–81.

42. Goodchild CE, Skinner TC, Parkin T. The value of empathy in dietetic consultations. A pilot study to investigate its effect on satisfaction, autonomy and agreement. J Hum Nutr Diet. 2005;18(3):181–5.

43. Graugaard PK, Holgersen K, Finset A. Communicating with alexithymic and non-alexithymic patients: an experimental study of the effect of psychosocial communication and empathy on patient satisfaction. Psychother Psychosom. 2004;73(2):92–100.

44. Ong LM, Visser MR, Lammes FB, de Haes JC. Doctor–patient communication and cancer patients' quality of life and satisfaction. Patient Educ Couns. 2000;41(2):145–56.

45. Norfolk T, Birdi K, Walsh D. The role of empathy in establishing rapport in the consultation: a new model. Med Educ. 2007;41(7):690–7.

46. Kanji N, Coe JB, Adams CL, Shaw JR. Effect of veterinarian–client–patient interactions on client adherence to dentistry and surgery recommendations in companion-animal practice. J Am Vet Med Assoc. 2012;240(4):427–36.

47. Loffler-Stastka H, Datz F, Parth K, Preusche I, Bukowski X, Seidman C. Empathy in psychoanalysis and medical education – what can we learn from each other? BMC Med Educ. 2017;17(1):74.

48. Gelhaus P. The desired moral attitude of the physician: (I) empathy. Med Health Care Phil. 2012;15(2):103–13.

49. Davis MA. A perspective on cultivating clinical empathy. Comp Thera Clin Pract. 2009;15(2):76–9.

50. Neumann M, Bensing J, Mercer S, Ernstmann N, Ommen O, Pfaff H. Analysing the "nature" and "specific effectiveness" of clinical empathy: a theoretical overview and contribution towards a theory-based research agenda. Patient Educ Couns. 2009;74(3):339–46.

51. Berger DM. On the way to empathic understanding. Amer J Psychotherapy. 1984;38(1):111–20.

52. McDonald D, Messinger DS. The development of empathy: how, when, and why. In: Acerbi A, Lombo JA, Sanguineti JJ, editors. Free will, emotions and moral actions: Philosophy and neuroscience in dialogue: IF Press; 2011.

53. de Waal FB. Putting the altruism back into altruism: the evolution of empathy. Annu Rev Psychol. 2008;59:279–300.

54. Hegazi I, Wilson I. Maintaining empathy in medical school: it is possible. Med Teach. 2013;35(12):1002–8.

55. Williams B, Brown T, McKenna L, Boyle MJ, Palermo C, Nestel D, et al. Empathy levels among health professional students: a cross-sectional study at two universities in Australia. Adv Med Educ Pract. 2014;5:107–13.

56. Fernandez AM, Dufey M, Kramp U. Testing the psychometric properties of the interpersonal reactivity index (IRI) in Chile empathy in a different cultural context. Eur J Psychol Assess. 2011;27(3):179–85.

57. Paul ES. Empathy with animals and with humans: are they linked? Anthrozoos. 2000;13(4):194–202.

58. Preylo BD, Arikawa H. Comparison of vegetarians and non-vegetarians on pet attitude and

empathy. Anthrozoos. 2008;21(4):387–95.

59. Erlanger ACE, Tsytsarev SV. The Relationship between empathy and personality in undergraduate students' attitudes toward nonhuman animals. Soc Anim. 2012;20(1):21–38.

60. Austin EJ, Evans P, Magnus B, O'Hanlon K. A preliminary study of empathy, emotional intelligence and examination performance in MBChB students. Med Educ. 2007;41(7):684–9.

61. Mathews S, Herzog HA. Personality and attitudes toward the treatment of animals. Soc Anim. 1997;5(2):169–75.

62. Rothgerber H. Underlying differences between conscientious omnivores and vegetarians in the evaluation of meat and animals. Appetite. 2015;87:251–8.

63. Colombo ES, Pelosi A, Prato-Previde E. Empathy towards animals and belief in animal-human-continuity in Italian veterinary students. Anim Welfare. 2016;25(2):275–86.

64. Filippi M, Riccitelli G, Falini A, Di Salle F, Vuilleumier P, Comi G, et al. The brain functional networks associated to human and animal suffering differ among omnivores, vegetarians and vegans. PLoS One. 2010;5(5):e10847.

65. Hazel SJ, Signal TD, Taylor N. Can teaching veterinary and animal-science students about animal welfare affect their attitude toward animals and human-related empathy? J Vet Med Educ. 2011;38(1):74–83.

66. Ascione FR, Weber CV. Children's attitude about the humane treatment of animals and empathy: one-year follow up of a school-based intervention. Anthrozoos. 1996;9(4):188–95.

67. Sprinkle JE. Animals, empathy, and violence can animals be used to convey principles of prosocial behavior to children? Youth Violence Juv J. 2008;6(1):47–58.

68. Rothgerber H, Mican F. Childhood pet ownership, attachment to pets, and subsequent meat avoidance. The mediating role of empathy toward animals. Appetite. 2014;79:11–7.

69. Norring M, Wikman I, Hokkanen AH, Kujala MV, Hanninen L. Empathic veterinarians score cattle pain higher. Vet J. 2014;200(1):186–90.

70. Suchman AL, Markakis K, Beckman HB, Frankel R. A model of empathic communication in the medical interview. JAMA. 1997;277(8):678–82.

71. Shaw JR, Bonnett BN, Roter DL, Adams CL, Larson S. Gender differences in veterinarian–client–patient communication in companion animal practice. J Am Vet Med Assoc. 2012;241(1):81–8.

72. Murphy SA. Consumer health information for pet owners. J Med Libr Assoc. 2006;94(2):151–8.

73. Shaw JR, Adams CL, Bonnett BN. What can veterinarians learn from studies of physician-patient communication about veterinarian–client–patient communication? J Am Vet Med Assoc. 2004;224(5):676–84.

74. Adams CL, Frankel RM. It may be a dog's life but the relationship with her owners is also key to her health and well being: communication in veterinary medicine. Vet Clin North Am Small Anim Pract. 2007;37(1):1–17; abstract vii.

75. Morrisey JK, Voiland B. Difficult interactions with veterinary clients: working in the challenge zone. Vet Clin North Am Small Anim Pract. 2007;37(1):65–77; abstract viii.

76. Englar RE, Williams M, Weingand K. Applicability of the Calgary–Cambridge Guide to dog and cat owners for teaching veterinary clinical communications. J Vet Med Educ. 2016;43(2):143–69.

77. Brown JP, Silverman JD. The current and future market for veterinarians and veterinary medical services in the United States. J Am Vet Med Assoc. 1999;215(2):161–83.

78. Gleichgerrcht E, Decety J. The costs of empathy among health professionals. In: Decety J, editor. Empathy: from bench to bedside. Cambridge, MA: MIT Press; 2012. pp. 245–61.

79. Englar RE. Using a standardized client encounter to practice death notification after the unexpected death of a feline patient following routine ovariohysterectomy. J Vet Med Educ. 2019:1–17.

80. McArthur ML, Andrews JR, Brand C, Hazel SJ. The prevalence of compassion fatigue among veterinary students in australia and the associated psychological factors. J Vet Med Educ.44(1):9–21.

81. McArthur M, Mansfield C, Matthew S, Zaki S, Brand C, Andrews J, et al. Resilience in veterinary students and the predictive role of mindfulness and self-compassion. J Vet Med Educ.44(1):106–15.

82. Lloyd C, Campion DP. Occupational stress and the importance of self-care and resilience: focus on veterinary nursing. Ir Vet J. 2017;70:30.

83. Hunsaker S, Chen HC, Maughan D, Heaston S. Factors that influence the development of compassion fatigue, burnout, and compassion satisfaction in emergency department nurses. J Nurs Scholarsh. 2015;47(2):186–94.

84. Wu S, Singh-Carlson S, Odell A, Reynolds G, Su Y. Compassion fatigue, burnout, and compassion satisfaction among oncology nurses in the United States and Canada. Oncol Nurs Forum. 2016;43(4):E161–9.

85. Figley CR. Compassion fatigue: psychotherapists' chronic lack of self care. J Clin Psychol. 2002;58(11):1433–41.

86. Perry B, Toffner G, Merrick T, Dalton J. An exploration of the experience of compassion fatigue in clinical oncology nurses. Can Oncol Nurs J. 2011;21(2):91–105.

87. Elkins AD, Kearney M. Professional burnout among female veterinarians in the United States. J Amer Vet Med Assn. 1992;200(5):604–8.

88. Nett RJ, Witte TK, Holzbauer SM, Elchos BL, Campagnolo ER, Musgrave KJ, et al. Risk factors for suicide, attitudes toward mental illness, and practice-related stressors among US veterinarians. J Amer Vet Med Assn. 2015;247(8):945–55.

89. Maslach C, Schaufeli WB, Leiter MP. Job burnout. Annu Rev Psychol. 2001;52:397–422.

90. Maslach C. What have we learned about burnout and health? Psychol Health. 2001;16(5):607–11.

91. Griffith JL, Kohrt BA. Managing Stigma effectively: what social psychology and social neuroscience can teach us. Acad Psychiatry. 2016;40(2):339–47.

92. Siebert DC. Personal and occupational factors in burnout among practicing social workers: implications for researchers, practitioners, and managers. J Soc Serv Res. 2006;32(2):25–44.

93. Skipper GE, Williams JB. Failure to acknowledge high suicide risk among veterinarians. J Vet Med Educ. 2012;39(1):79–82.

94. Kessler RC, Barker PR, Colpe LJ, Epstein JF, Gfroerer JC, Hiripi E, et al. Screening for serious mental illness in the general population. Arch Gen Psychiatry. 2003;60(2):184–9.

95. Reeves WC, Strine TW, Pratt LA, Thompson W, Ahluwalia I, Dhingra SS, et al. Mental illness surveillance among adults in the United States. MMWR Suppl. 2011;60(3):1–29.

96. Baca-Garcia E, Perez-Rodriguez MM, Keyes KM, Oquendo MA, Hasin DS, Grant BF, et al. Suicidal ideation and suicide attempts in the United States: 1991–1992 and 2001–2002. Mol Psychiatry. 2010;15(3):250–9.

97. Conwell Y, Duberstein PR, Cox C, Herrmann JH, Forbes NT, Caine ED. Relationships of age and axis I diagnoses in victims of completed suicide: a psychological autopsy study. Am J Psychiatry. 1996;153(8):1001–8.

98. Lesage AD, Boyer R, Grunberg F, Vanier C, Morissette R, Menard-Buteau C, et al. Suicide and

mental disorders: a case-control study of young men. Am J Psychiatry. 1994;151(7):1063–8.

99. Bartram DJ, Baldwin DS. Veterinary surgeons and suicide: a structured review of possible influences on increased risk. Veterinary Record. 2010;166(13):388–97.

100. Veterinary mental health: an international issue. Veterinary Record. 2015;176(13):324.

101. Blair A, Hayes HM, Jr. Mortality patterns among US veterinarians, 1947–1977: an expanded study. Int J Epidemiol. 1982;11(4):391–7.

102. Jones-Fairnie H, Ferroni P, Silburn S, Lawrence D. Suicide in Australian veterinarians. Aust Vet J. 2008;86(4):114–6.

103. Miller JM, Beaumont JJ. Suicide, cancer, and other causes of death among California veterinarians, 1960–1992. Am J Ind Med. 1995;27(1):37–49.

104. Platt B, Hawton K, Simkin S, Mellanby RJ. Suicidal behaviour and psychosocial problems in veterinary surgeons: a systematic review. Soc Psychiatry Psychiatr Epidemiol. 2012;47(2):223–40.

105. Skegg K, Firth H, Gray A, Cox B. Suicide by occupation: does access to means increase the risk? Aust N Z J Psychiatry. 2010;44(5):429–34.

106. Mellanby RJ. Incidence of suicide in the veterinary profession in England and Wales. The Veterinary record. 2005;157(14):415–7.

107. MacLean PD. The brain in relation to empathy and medical education. J Nerv Ment Dis. 1967;144(5):374–82.

108. Brazeau CM, Schroeder R, Rovi S, Boyd L. Relationships between medical student burnout, empathy, and professionalism climate. Acad Med. 2010;85(10 Suppl):S33–6.

109. Gleichgerrcht E, Decety J. Empathy in clinical practice: how individual dispositions, gender, and experience moderate empathic concern, burnout, and emotional distress in physicians. PLoS One. 2013;8(4):e61526.

110. Kogan LR, McConnell SL, Schoenfeld-Tacher R. Veterinary students and non-academic stressors. J Vet Med Educ. 2005;32(2):193–200.

111. Bakker DJ, Lyons ST, Conlon PD. An exploration of the relationship between psychological capital and depression among first-year doctor of veterinary medicine students. J Vet Med Educ.44(1):50–62.

112. Meyer-Parsons B, Van Etten S, Shaw JR. The Healer's Art (HART): veterinary students connecting with self, peers, and the profession. J Vet Med Educ.44(1):187–97.

113. Chen D, Lew R, Hershman W, Orlander J. A cross-sectional measurement of medical student empathy. JGIM. 2007;22(10):1434–8.

114. Diseker RA, Michielutte R. An analysis of empathy in medical-students before and following clinical-experience. J Med Educ. 1981;56(12):1004–10.

115. Craig JL. Retention of interviewing skills learned by 1st-year medical-students – a longitudinal study. Med Educ. 1992;26(4):276–81.

116. Khajavi F, Hekmat H. Comparative study of empathy – effects of psychiatric training. Arch Gen Psychiat. 1971;25(6):490–3.

117. Newton BW, Barber L, Clardy J, Cleveland E, O'Sullivan P. Is there hardening of the heart during medical school? Academic Medicine. 2008;83(3):244–9.

118. Newton BW, Savidge MA, Barber L, Cleveland E, Clardy J, Beeman G, et al. Differences in medical students' empathy. J Acad Med. 2000;75(12):1215-.

119. Bellini LM, Shea JA. Mood change and empathy decline persist during three years of internal medicine training. J Acad Med. 2005;80(2):164–7.

120. Mangione S, Kane GC, Caruso JW, Gonnella JS, Nasca TJ, Hojat M. Assessment of empathy in different years of internal medicine training. Med Teach. 2002;24(4):370–3.

121. Stratton TD, Saunders JA, Elam CL. Changes in medical students' emotional intelligence: an

exploratory study. Teach Learn Med. 2008;20(3):279–84.

122. Khademalhosseini M, Khademalhosseini Z, Mahmoodian F. Comparison of empathy score among medical students in both basic and clinical levels. J Adv Med Educ Prof. 2014;2(2):88–91.

123. Hellyer PW, Frederick C, Lacy M, Salman MD, Wagner AE. Attitudes of veterinary medical students, house officers, clinical faculty, and staff toward pain management in animals. J Am Vet Med Assoc. 1999;214(2):238–44.

124. Batt-Rawden SA, Chisolm MS, Anton B, Flickinger TE. Teaching empathy to medical students: an updated, systematic review. Acad Med. 2013;88(8):1171–7.

125. Nunes P, Williams S, Sa B, Stevenson K. A study of empathy decline in students from five health disciplines during their first year of training. Intl J Medical Educ. 2011;2:12–7.

126. Pollard-Williams S, Doyle RE, Freire R. The influence of workplace learning on attitudes toward animal welfare in veterinary students. J Vet Med Educ. 2014;41(3):253–7.

Chapter 7

Defining Entry-Level Communication Skills

Nonverbal Cues

Think about the last time you were in a dispute with someone and you had to agree to disagree.

If you are a student, maybe you and your anatomy lab partner did not see eye-to-eye on the dissection guide. Evan wanted to bisect muscle "X" to appreciate the structures beneath, but you were not ready to cut. You were still trying to get your bearings regarding the muscle's origin and insertion. You may have ultimately agreed to Evan's plan. You may have even given in with an affirmative response, such as "okay, fine."

But were you fine? And was everything okay? More importantly, how did Evan know that it was not? Chances are that what you said and what you displayed by way of behavioral signals did not align.

Consider the following contributors to your conversation.

- Body language
  - Did you lose eye contact?
  - Which facial expressions did you exhibit?
    - Did you furrow your brow?
    - Did you roll your eyes at Evan?
  - Did you cross your arms?
  - Did your body tense?
  - Did you alter your posture?
- Spatial relationships
  - Did you move away from Evan?
  - Did you place a physical object, such as the dissection table or guide, between you?
- Paralanguage
  - What was your tone of voice?
  - What was your voice volume?
  - Which, if any, words did you accentuate?

- Autonomic response
  - Did you change your breathing pattern?
  - Did you flush or blanch?
  - Did you tear up?
  - Did you break into a sweat?

All of the above are ways that you may have conveyed a message of discontent to Evan. Some of these behavioral signals may have been intentional, such as an eye roll. Others, such as the autonomic responses, are outside of your control.

Either way, if Evan was receptive to your behavioral cues, he should have gotten the message loud and clear: what you were saying was not exactly an accurate representation of what it was that you were feeling.

These incongruences are daily occurrences in everyday conversations – not just in the anatomy lab.

Consider, for instance, the parent who gives a directive to a child that the child does not like: "Clean your room or else Suzy can't come over to play." Or "Eat your spinach if you want to have dessert." The child may provide a verbal agreement. The child may even do as she or he was told. However, the child is likely to give off behavioral cues that air his or her discontent with the plan.

Clinical practice also has its share of discrepancies between what is shared aloud and how the body responds physically. Consider the client who agrees to a treatment plan; however, their reluctance to follow through is plastered over their face. Or the veterinarian who responds, "It's fine," to the client who is 45 minutes late to his or her appointment, but then, by way of body language, demonstrates otherwise as the examination progresses.

Both veterinarians and clients demonstrate nonverbal communication during clinical conversations.(1, 2) This means that both parties have the opportunity to read each other's cues and respond accordingly.(1)

In the former scenario, if the veterinarian fails to pick up on the client's nonverbal cues that indicate reluctance to proceed with patient treatment, then she or he may miss the opportunity to effectively manage patient care. The veterinarian may discharge the client prematurely, assuming that she is going to follow through, only to find that she is lost to follow up.

In the latter scenario, if the client picks up on the veterinarian's nonverbal cues that suggest irritation over the client's tardiness, then the client is likely to feel uncomfortable. How likely is that client to engage the veterinarian in conversation? How likely is that client to share a comprehensive history with the veterinarian? How likely is that client to prolong the appointment by asking the appropriate follow-up questions? How likely is that client to return to the practice?

Nonverbal communication is a powerful conversational tool, yet it is often forgotten or pushed to the side as an "extra," to be considered only after spoken words are rehearsed and/or modified in clinical practice.

When we think about communication as a means of connecting two or more individuals, our brains automatically prioritize the spoken word as being central to mutual understanding. Oral communication is something that we focus on, as clinicians, because it is such a key component of our day-to-day work as doctors.

We rely upon speech to take a patient history, discuss physical examination findings with a client, review the diagnostic and/or therapeutic plan with a client, obtain consent, explain test results, and share patient prognosis.

In turn, we rely upon our client's speech to fill in the blanks, ask questions, clarify, share concerns, and consent to treatment.

However, as much as 80 to 90% of clinical communication is nonverbal.(1, 3–6) Nonverbal communication influences how the spoken word is perceived.(2, 7, 8)

In the ideal world, nonverbal communication complements the spoken word to reinforce a message.(2, 3) In reality, nonverbal communication may contradict what is said aloud.(2, 3, 9) The resultant mixed message is confusing to the receiver. At the end of the day, which message does the receiver believe?

Nonverbal communication is most likely to predict behavior.(3, 9) So it is that when nonverbal and verbal communication are not in alignment, the former is what most people believe to be true.(3, 9–11)

To reduce incongruent messages and the potential for miscommunication, clinicians would do well to address how they respond to clients, in terms of their nonverbal cues, as much as which specific words are said.(4, 8, 9, 12–22)

Student or new graduates may not be aware of their behavioral cues or how they impact a client's experience during the clinical consultation.(1) Successful clinicians devote time to the study of their behavioral cues as much as their speech in order to fine-tune their awareness. This maximizes the opportunities for mutual understanding between them and their clients.(3, 4, 13) Like any other skill, nonverbal communication can be practiced and refined.(1)

7.1 The History of Nonverbal Cues in Clinical Conversations

The ability of a physician to perceive and appropriately respond to nonverbal cues has long been valued in human healthcare.(23) The perception that nonverbal communication guides the success of a doctor in clinical practice dates back to the days of Hippocrates and Osler.(23–25) This belief persisted throughout the 20th century and was advanced by such physicians as George Engel of the University of Rochester Medical Center.(26, 27) Engel is credited with the development of the biopsychosocial model, the view that health and illness are intricately tied to the interplay of biological, psychological, and social factors.(27) Engel believed that case outcomes could be influenced by the doctor–patient relationship.(27) Positive outcomes required a patient-centered approach care and the humanization of medicine.(27, 28) This approach emphasized relationships and how communication between providers and patients could strengthen the bond between them in such a way as to improve health.

7.2 The Importance of Nonverbal Cues in Clinical Conversations

Nonverbal behavior is an essential part of communication because we each send out and receive signals all the time.(2) To do so is human. Humans are social.(5) As social creatures, we seek out messages from one another to establish, secure, and maintain bonds. Messages reinforce interpersonal relationships and help us to navigate our day-to-day interactions with one another.

Both doctors and patients, veterinarians and clients have emotional responses to people and situations.(2) The emotions are often displayed on our faces and throughout our body, based upon the way in which we carry ourselves, regardless of whether or not we try to mask them.(2)

As a species, we are surprisingly good at picking up on emotions from nonverbal cues.(1, 2) As early as 375 milliseconds after witnessing nonverbal communication, we are able to identify emotion and be fairly accurate with regards to our interpretation.(1, 29, 30)

Ambady et al. referred to these snippets of communication as "thin slices of behavior"(29) and found that predictive accuracy based upon 0.5 minute interactions was equal to observations that lasted 4-5 minutes.(29)

People judge others based upon brief observations, and these judgments are often spot-on, even when they are about virtual strangers.(2, 29, 31–36) A glimpse is all that is needed, concerning behavior, to make a fairly accurate assessment about mood, temperament or disposition, social status, and/or performance.(29, 37) Intuition may therefore be more reliable, in some cases, than reason when we are prompted to make decisions. (29, 38)

7.3 What Contributes to Accuracy in Judgment Making Based upon Fleeting Observations?

Gender is thought to contribute to the accuracy of judgment making. Females are better able than males to convey, identify, and interpret emotion via nonverbal cues.(2, 30, 39)

The role of the message recipient also appears to influence the accuracy of perceived judgments. Patients are more accurate than physicians in their assessment of each other's emotional states. As compared to self-ratings by patients, physicians are more likely to:(40)

- underrate patient satisfaction
- rate patients as being more negative than patients perceived themselves to be
- rate patients as being less positive than the patient perceived themselves to be
- rate patients as being worse in health than patients believed they were.

It is unclear why physicians are significantly less aware of their patients' emotional states. Proposed theories include the following.(40)

- Physicians are trained to look for disease, so perhaps they have a "low threshold for 'seeing' signs of emotional negativity."
- Physicians may make assumptions about how patients perceive their chronic disease states.

Physicians need to find a way to reduce these discrepancies so as to gain a more complete and accurate clinical picture.

If physicians overemphasize negative signals and at the same time underappreciate positive ones, then they are at risk of responding "in a way that contributes to a climate of negativity."(40)

7.4 What are Nonverbal Cues?

If judgments can be formed on the basis of observation alone, then it behooves us, both as individuals and collectively as a profession, to consider which signals we are giving off that allow others to infer information about ourselves.

A study of nonverbal communication is essential:

Clinical experience shows that until people are allowed to express their emotions, they are usually not ready to take steps towards solving their problem. Therefore, before veterinarians can help their clients to solve their animals' medical problems, they need to know how to attend to client emotions.(1)

Nonverbal communication is the primary way in which emotions are expressed.(1) Nonverbal cues are loosely defined as any form of communication without words.(2, 41) Four categories of nonverbal communication were introduced at the start of this chapter, using slightly different terminology. These categories are: (1)

- kinesics
- proxemics
- paralanguage
- autonomic shifts.

Each of these categories will be defined in the sections below (7.5–7.8) as they relate to clinical veterinary practice.

7.5 Kinesics

Kinesics is the study of gestures and body movements as a means of nonverbal communication. Simply put, kinesics is what most often comes to mind when we consider body language.(1)

As a whole, body language may reflect safety, fight, or flight.(1)

All people have a basic need to feel safe.(1) The drive to protect ourselves is ingrained.(1) This need for self-preservation extends into the consultation room. Clients need to feel secure in their ability to express what is on their minds within the context of a safe and supportive environment.(1) Clients who feel safe are more willing to be vulnerable, that is, they are more likely to share their concerns and fears with the veterinary team.(1)

Whether or not a client feels safe and secure can be conveyed through body language.(1)

Body language includes:(1–3, 5, 20, 42–46)

- body position and posture
  - open versus closed body posture
  - forward versus backwards lean
- whole body movement
- body part isolations and movements
- body tension
- eye contact
- facial expressions
- facial micro-expressions
- gestures
- touch.(5, 7, 47–50)

In general, clients who feel safe tend to present themselves with an open body posture. Arms and legs tend to be uncrossed or, at the very least, loose, rather than taut with tension.(1) Facial expressions tend to be relaxed, rather than tight or forced.(1) Clients will position themselves to face us as they engage in conversation.(1)

If the consultation room becomes less safe as difficult conversations arise, clients may go into "fight or flight" mode. Clients who are on the attack tend to demonstrate one or more of the following confrontational signs:(1)

- taut mouth
- tight jaw
- clenched fists
- narrowed palpebral fissures
- lowered brow
- forward lean
- reluctance to remain seated
- decreased personal space.

Other clients may retreat at the first indication of conflict. These individuals are experiencing the desire for flight. Although their bodies may respond with tension, as is true of those who are experiencing "fight," those exhibiting classic signs of flight tend to disengage from conversation.(1) They may:(1)

- lean away
- increase personal space
- place physical barriers in the way, for instance, retreating to the opposite side of the examination room table
- create a figurative wall around themselves by crossing their arms or legs
- break eye contact
- turn their heads and necks away
- clutch the patient tightly.

As clinicians, we need to be perceptive to these changes. It is important to recognize when clients have moved from a safe to non-safe mindset.

It is our responsibility to do everything in our power to recreate safety so that we can be as comprehensive as possible in our approach to patient care. A client who does not feel safe is unlikely to provide us with the level of detail that we need to effectively manage the patient's health.

7.5.1 Tips on Kinesics for the Clinician, from the Client's Perspective

Just as our clients are giving off signals for us to make inferences about their comfort or discomfort about a given situation, we, as clinicians, reciprocate. Whether we are aware of it or not, whether we mean to put our emotions on display or not, we do. Clients pick up on our cues as much as we pick up on theirs, if not more so. Clients are very in tune with what it is we are conveying, regardless of the words we choose to pair with our body actions. Let us take a look now at what some of our actions convey to clients.

7.5.1 Body Posture Basics

Body posture is how we hold ourselves in space, upright, against gravity.(51) There is good posture and there is bad posture.

When standing, good posture involves:(51)

- standing tall (rather than hunched)
- keeping your shoulders back and your head level
- maintaining your feet approximately a shoulder-width apart
- bearing weight primarily on the balls of your feet
- tucking your stomach in
- allowing your arms to hang naturally at your sides.

When sitting, good posture involves:(51)

- sitting tall with your back straight and your shoulders back

- keeping your elbows close to the body
- distributing your body weight evenly between hips
- not twisting at the waist
- allowing your buttocks to touch the back of your chair
- bending your knees at right angles and keeping them even with or slightly higher than hips
- not crossing your legs
- allowing your feet to touch the floor.

Good posture is essential for health.(51–53) Good posture allows us to maintain proper alignment between bones and joints and to use our muscles properly. Because muscles are being used more efficiently, the body is less likely to become fatigued.

Good posture also reduces the amount of wear and tear on the surfaces of joints, as well as reduces the stress on ligaments, which hold the joints together.

Sometimes we are physically limited by what we can do in terms of posture because of our own medical challenges. If, for example, you have scoliosis, you may not be able to stand straight and tall. For the purposes of this chapter, focus on what is within your ability to correct.

It is important for us to be aware of our body posture because our clients may make assumptions based on how we hold our bodies. From the client's vantage point, good posture is aesthetically pleasing. A tall, erect posture communicates engagement and professionalism.(3, 54–56) Those who stand tall convey confidence and attentiveness. It communicates to your client that you are focused and ready to work.

By contrast, a slumped or slouched posture suggests apathy. You appear to be less invested in the case at hand. Clients may feel that you are not committed or that you do not care.

7.5.3 Facing the Client

A study of body posture also includes the direction that we are facing. This is often referred to as body position. When we face our clients directly, we appear to be invested in what they have to say. When we do not face our clients, for instance, if we have our back to them as we are typing on the computer, it may appear that we are not interested in their perspective and/or that we do not value them as members of the healthcare team.

7.5.4 Open versus Closed Body Posture

Body posture may also be described as open or closed.

Clinicians who display open body posture face the client and keep their arms and hands apart. If they are standing, they will allow their arms to hang naturally at their sides. If they are seated, they might choose to place each hand on its respective arm rest.

An open body posture conveys that "I am listening."

On the other hand, clinicians who display a closed body posture may or may not face the client directly, and they are likely to fold their arms across their chest.

Note that clinicians who cross their arms may just be cold to the touch – I personally have a tendency to fold my arms across my chest when I am trying to warm up. However, to the client, it may appear that I am closed off to conversation or worse, that I am defensive.

7.5.5 Leaning into the Conversation

Clinicians may maintain good posture, yet lean forward as a means of reinforcing their engagement and attentiveness to the client.(5, 6, 57–59) Clinicians who lean into the conversation are considered to be warm, responsive, and involved.(60)

Clients are more likely to continue sharing what is on their mind when their clinicians demonstrate forward poise.(60)

7.5.6 Mirroring the Client's Body Posture

Sometimes, clinicians make a concerted effort to mirror our client's body posture. Another way to consider this is matching your posture to your client's to create a mirror image.

If your client is seated, it may be best to seat yourself so that you are speaking at their level, literally.(42) If, conversely, your client is standing, you may wish to stand with them so that you are at eye level.

If your client is standing up and angry, you may try to encourage them to sit down. You, in turn, can sit down. This gives the client the opportunity to mirror you. Doing so may or may not be effective, depending upon the client and the clinical scenario. However, it is worth the effort in an attempt to diffuse the tension.

7.5.7 Body Part Isolations and Movements

Section 7.5.6 considered the body as a whole. Now let's consider the body in parts. Body part isolations and movements include:

* affirmative head nodding
* head shaking
* finger tapping
* toe tapping
* hand wringing.

Head actions are a type of gesture, that is, the movement of one or more body parts to convey a particular action, either in combination with speech, or in place of it.

Another example of a head action is the affirmative head nod. This action is a means of demonstrating interest in the conversation.(5, 61, 62) An affirmative head nod may also encourage the speaker to continue to share his or her story with the audience by way of silent encouragement.(5) Heading nodding implies either agreement ("You're right") or mutual understanding ("I'm with you," "I am following you"). Those who nod their heads are often seen as being friendlier and more engaged in conversation.(5, 58)

Head shaking is another form of gesture that represents the opposite of affirmative head nodding. A horizontal head shake implies "no" or "I disagree." A horizontal head shake, paired with a gaping mouth and/or an audible gasp may even imply disbelief, as if to say, "no way!"

Finger tapping, toe tapping, and hand wringing are body isolations that have the potential to be distracting. These are often unconsciously done by the clinician. However, these actions may convey disinterest, disengagement or boredom. They may also communicate "Hurry up." Hand wringing may indicate of nervousness. Clients who witness this action may question whether or not the clinician has told them everything about a particular situation or is instead withholding information.

7.5.8 Eye Contact

Eye contact, sometimes referred to as eye gaze, is meeting someone's eyes with your own.(5)

In western cultures, eye contact is established between the provider and the client during the initial stage of the visit, when an appropriate greeting is made. Refer to Chapter 4 for more information on greeting the client. The degree to which eye contact is comfortably established and maintained is largely determined by the cultural norm. In western cultures, for instance, eye contact is established between the provider and the client during the initial stage of the visit, when an appropriate greeting is made. By contrast, the use of eye contact in many cultures, including eastern, may be interpreted as being disrespectful or even rude. In these cultures, lack of eye contact does not mean that the individual with whom you are speaking is not paying attention. This text emphasizes the use of eye contact in western cultures.

Once it has been established, eye contact between two individuals is most comfortable when it is intermittent. Intermittent eye contact means that you look the client directly in the eye from time to time, but not to the point that it becomes an uncomfortable hard stare.

Intermittent eye contact is the preferred form of eye gaze for clinical consultations. It conveys that "I am listening to you."(5) It tells the client that "I care about you and what you have to say." Intermittent eye contact denotes respect. Clients also interpret it as a positive sign that the clinician is competent, credible, and transparent. (5, 58, 63)

When paired with a pause, intermittent eye contact serves as a means to check in with the client, to be clear that the information received was understood.(5, 64)

In western cultures, eye contact avoidance during conversations is considered to be unusual and counterproductive to rapport building.(5, 58) When you do not meet the eyes of your client during a clinical consultation, your client may make one or more of the following assumptions about you.

- You are not confident.
- You are intimidated.
- You are disinterested.
- You do not like the client as a person.
- You do not respect the client as a person.
- You are finished listening to what the client has to say, regardless of whether or not the client has finished speaking.
- You are nervous.
- You are hiding something from the client.
- You are avoiding bad news delivery: in other words, there is something you need to tell them, but you are reluctant to do so for fear of their reaction.

Be aware of your use of eye contact in the consultation room. Also be aware of what else you may be paying attention to, instead of your client, during clinical conversations. For example, be cautious about making repeated eye contact with your watch. You may simply be looking at your watch to measure the patient's heart rate or respiratory rate, however, the client may assume that you are running out of time or that you are not invested in this appointment.

7.5.9 Facial Expressions

Facial expressions are another form of nonverbal communication. They require the movement of muscles beneath the skin of the face to convey a great variety of emotional states. Facial expressions may result in a change in the positioning of the brow or eyebrows, the openness of the eyelids, the shape of the mouth, and tension at and around the mouth and jaw.

Some facial expressions are universally recognized. Consider, for instance, those facial expressions that convey anger, fear, joy, sadness, and surprise.

Other facial expressions may not necessarily be universal, but may be easily interpreted.

- A raised brow may suggest skepticism or doubt. The client may feel that you do not believe him or her.
- A furrowed brow may suggest irritation, puzzlement, or confusion.
- A clenched jaw may suggest anger.
- A wrinkled nose, squinted eyes, and a scrunched face may convey disgust.

Facial expressions may be voluntarily or unconsciously conveyed. Consider, for instance, a smile, which could be either.

When it is a voluntary expression, a smile can be a great relationship builder.(5, 65) It conveys warmth and receptivity to what the client is sharing.(5, 42, 60, 62)

The power of a smile is something that we can all relate to. It is so universally understood that it permeates literature. Consider, for instance, the following quote, which appears in F. Scott Fitzgerald's *The Great Gatsby*:

> He smiled understandingly much more than understandingly. It was one of those rare smiles with a quality of eternal reassurance in it, that you may come across four or five times in life. It faced – or seemed to face – the whole eternal world for an instant, and then concentrated on you with an irresistible prejudice in your favor. It understood you just as far as you wanted to be understood, believed in you as you would like to believe in yourself, and assured you that it had precisely the impression of you that, at your best, you hoped to convey.(66)

Smiles put the recipient at ease when the smile is genuine and well intentioned. They denote respect and kindness, patience, and understanding. As such, smiles are a bridge to relationships. They open the door to mutual understanding by allowing two individuals to bond over a statement or content area. Simply put, a smile says, "I can relate to that, I can relate to you."

In that context, smiles are appropriate to set the tone for greetings, introductions, and small talk, particularly during general wellness visits or when the client and patient both appear to be in good health.

Smiles are less appropriate during difficult conversations or, for example, in the middle of triaging an emergency.

For some individuals, nervous energy forces an unconscious smile. These individuals need to find a way to dampen that tendency so as not to give the client the wrong impression that he or she is making light of the situation.

The same is true of a laugh. There are appropriate and inappropriate times to laugh.

7.5.10 Gestures

The affirmative head nod and the head shake were introduced in Section 7.5.7 as two types of gestures. Unlike facial expressions, gestures are not limited to the face. They often involve the hands and other parts of the body.

One example of a gesture is a handshake. There is no universal etiquette concerning a proper handshake. Whether or not to shake hands, for how long to shake hands, and whether or not you will pair the handshake with eye contact varies largely between countries. For example, in Thailand, handshakes are uncommon. Contrast that with western cultures, in which handshakes are an important part of the greeting process. This text emphasizes the proper use of a handshake as it pertains to western cultures. It is considered professional for clinicians to shake hands with clients, firmly and deliberately, when meeting them for the very first time.(13, 67–77) Subsequent visits may or may not involve a handshake, depending upon clinician and patient preference.

Recall from Chapter 4 that handshakes are preferred by roughly 78% of human medical patients. However, not all clients desire them.(67) In fact, older patients are less likely to expect or want to shake hands.(67)

In addition to the handshake, several other gestures are universal:(44)

- thumbs down
- shoulder shrug
- beckoning ("come here").

Other gestures exhibit regional, national, or cultural differences.(44) These are beyond the scope of this text. However, recognize that the potential for misinterpretation is high and that the need for cultural competence in the healthcare industry is growing.

7.5.11 Touch

Touch is a specific form of nonverbal communication that involves physical contact between two individuals.(7) Touch may be procedural or task oriented, that is, it is associated with and/or required for a task to be performed, or it may be spontaneous and expressive, to enhance interpersonal relationships.(7, 47–50, 78, 79)

Touch has been poorly studied in the veterinary profession and only superficially examined in the human medical literature, yet both human medical doctors and their patients believe that touch has the power to improve communication.(7)

As a fundamental demonstration of connectivity between people, touch humanizes medicine.(7) Touch conveys that "I care" and "I am here to comfort you."(5, 80, 81)

A 2013 study by Cocksedge et al. examined doctors' and patients' perceptions of touch and found that human medical patients in particular were receptive to its use in consultations. Patients self-reported that:

> [Being touched made me feel ...] that they understood ..., they weren't just going through the motions ...(7)

> Even if it's just putting a hand out ... can be very reassuring.(7)

Physicians agreed that touch could be a powerful statement about benevolence.(7) One doctor explained it best:

> A little frail, old lady who's had to lie down for me to examine her abdomen, I will just help her sit up and steady her or hold her stick out, help her put her coat back

on ... I think, first of all, you're a human being, the same as you would do helping somebody at home or cross the street ... Your first thing is that you're a human and not a machine.(7)

Despite both patients and physicians being in agreement that touch could be therapeutic and humanizing, the latter expressed reluctance to making use of expressive touch in the examination room. Several factors appear to influence how touch is used in clinical practice and by whom. These include: (7)

• the clinical scenario
• the patient's age
• the patient's sex
• the location on the recipient's body
• the physician's personality.

Clinical scenarios that are likely to inspire touch are at end of life and during those situations where physicians wish to comfort the bereaved.(7)

Older patients are more likely to be touched than younger patients, particularly if younger patients are female and the care provider is of the opposite sex.(7) Male patients are less likely to be touched by physicians of the same sex.(7)

When touch is used in clinical practice, it is often restricted to safe zones, such as the hand or forearm.(7) Other safe zones, although used less frequently, include the upper arm or shoulder.

Touch may also take the form of a hug, for instance, during an emotionally challenging time in veterinary practice, such as euthanasia.

Note that clinicians are often hesitant to make use of touch for fear of being wrongfully accused of being inappropriate:(7) "You have to be careful with it. You don't want it to be misconstrued." (7)

For this reason, many clinicians are selective about dispensing touch.(7) They may, for instance, only attempt touch when it is with someone that they have known for a long time.(7) There is security in having already established a solid working relationship.

Even then, when a relationship has been longstanding, touch may feel awkward or forced. To that end, touch is a very personal action that not everyone is comfortable with giving or receiving.

As with all gestures, we need to be culturally aware and sensitive.

You may even consider checking with your client before dispensing touch in the consultation room. It may sound awkward, but I often ask my long-term clients to share their needs with me. For instance, I may say, "You look like you could use a hug right now, is that okay?"

This gives clients the opportunity to say "yes" or "no." If ever a client displays signs of discomfort, then it is important to back off. It is your responsibility to respect the client's decision.

Likewise, you have the right to your own comfort and personal space. Just as a client can refuse touch that comes from a clinician, you have the right to set boundaries with a touchy-feely client. It's okay to say, "That makes me uncomfortable."

Both you and the client share that right.

7.6 Proxemics

Proxemics refers to the use of space, specifically, how space is created and shaped to fit the needs of those who are circulating through the usable space.(1)

In the veterinary practice, a consideration of proxemics includes:(1, 3, 82, 83)

- the physical distance between the client and veterinarian
- height differences between the client and the veterinarian
- any physical barriers that obstruct the view of and/or get in between the client and veterinarian
  - the medical record
  - the patient
  - the patient's carrier or crate
  - seating, including benches, that are built into consultation room walls and corners
  - the examination room table
  - consulting room computer(s) and/or television monitor(s)
  - watches, pagers, and/or cellular phones – the client's and/or the veterinarian's
  - the reception desk, within the waiting area.

7.6.1 Addressing Differences in Height

Height differences between the client and the veterinarian were addressed in Section 7.5.6 with regards to mirroring the client's body posture. The goals of mirroring the client's body posture are to:(42)

- build rapport
- improve eye contact by conversing at eye level
- reduce height differences between the client and the veterinarian.

If your client is standing, stand with him or her; if your client is seated, then join him in having a seat.(42)

7.6.2 Removing Physical Barriers

Where you place yourself in the examination room relative to the client also contributes to the conversational tone.(42) Standing across from one another, particularly if there is a physical obstacle between you and the client, such as the examination room table, may come across as either distancing or confrontational.(42)

Instead, position yourself at the end of the table.(42) This allows you to create an "L" shape with the client.(42) This shape is thought to facilitate conversation by leveling the playing field and reducing the spatially perceived position of authority.(42)

Alternatively, you may elect to stand side-by-side with your client, shoulder-to-shoulder.(42) This positioning demonstrates an active attempt to partner and collaborate with the client to devise a healthcare plan that will be best for the collective you.(42)

Eliminating physical barriers conveys an open approach to healthcare. It reinforces the trend towards relationship-centered care. It conveys to the client that you are a team, and you will not let anything stand in the way. More than that, you are open to navigating the healthcare journey with the client at your side.

7.6.3 Modern Day Physical Barriers: Computers

The patient's medical record and the examination room table used to be the primary physical barriers in the examination room. In today's modern world, the computer has taken their place as a potential obstacle to patient care.

The computer was first introduced to human healthcare in the western world in the 1980s.(84, 85) By 1999, more than 90% of Dutch, Canadian, British, and Swedish general practices were using computers to facilitate consultations.(84, 86, 87)

Physicians are now tasked with balancing history taking, data gathering, physical examinations, explanation, and planning with data entry into a computer.(85)

Veterinarians have an additional consideration to balance against computer use: the patient.

Computers are used in healthcare to:(84, 85, 88–90)

- improve physician preparation for the visit by reviewing past pertinent history
- allow for more efficient data entry by support staff
- facilitate data collection and storage
- allow for data mining for research, such as incidence and prevalence studies for diseases of interest
- improve efficiency of medical record keeping through the development of electronic medical records (EMRs)
- encourage multitasking in healthcare
- eliminate the potential for medical errors due to illegible handwriting
- reduce the potential for medical errors due to built-in drug interaction detection software

- improve compliance and adherence to preventative care guidelines
- share patient-specific data with patients and other healthcare providers
  - past appointment data
  - trends
  - diagnostic test results (labwork and imaging)
- offer diagnostic support for doctors
- facilitate record transfer
- process electronic requests for prescriptions and diagnostic tests
- improve billing and accounting.

Although physicians and patients both agree that computer use in the consultation room has the potential to enhance efficiency, it may also detract from clinical communication. (84, 85, 89, 91)

When computers were first introduced to the consultation room in human healthcare, many patients and clients feared that technology would lessen the personal touch of the healthcare industry.(90, 92, 93) These fears were not necessarily unsubstantiated.

Computer use has the following potentially deleterious effects on clinical communication:(12, 84, 92, 94–99)

- increased computer use makes appointments seem depersonalized
- increased computer use may cause clinicians to become more task oriented at the expense of building rapport
- increased computer use may create a distraction in the examination room
- clinicians are more likely to remain silent when using the computer, thereby shutting down doors of communication rather than opening them
- increased computer use may exacerbate inefficiency in the consultation, particularly if the provider has poor computer skills
- increased computer use may reduce eye contact between the provider and patient/client
- increased computer use creates a physical barrier that obscures nonverbal cues, such as body position and posture
- increased computer use may elevate the client's fears of loss of confidentiality, as through a privacy breach.(85, 89, 92, 97, 100–104)

Computers in the consultation room are here to stay. If anything, our reliance upon them may only increase as more veterinary practices switch to EMRs.

What, then, are some strategies that we can employ to improve client communication while maintaining efficiency of provider services?

We can remind clients that computers are not intended to replace the veterinarian–client–patient relationship. They are there to support it. Moreover, we can suggest that clients view computers through the following lens:

It is the attitude of doctors to patients that affects overall satisfaction. The attitude of doctor to computer is barely relevant. A computer is a tool. Would you ask if we were concerned about a doctor's attitude to his stethoscope?(89)

In other words, computers are physician assistants. They help doctors to get work done, but they are not a replacement for clinical conversation.

To reinforce that perspective, we may consider the following ways to improve customer service in the face of technology.(12, 105)*

- Review the EMR prior to entering the examination room to obtain past pertinent history.
- Allow the client to complete his or her opening statement without interruption before making an entry into the patient's the medical record.
- Explain to the client when and why referring to the EMR is necessary.
- Keep pauses when consulting notes to 5 seconds or less.

The consultation room computer has its place. However, as is summed up beautifully by Christopher Pearce, "computers can't listen." Pearce offers a reminder that:

In attempting to implement both clinical evidence and new technologies into practice, we must remind ourselves that [general practitioners] primarily use data contained in the stories our patients tell us, and the completeness of these stories depends upon a relationship that is intricately and delicately woven. While both computers and [evidence based medicine] clearly bring benefits to the consultation, they are merely tools to be used judiciously and not totems to be revered beyond their utility. We must be careful not to lose what we have recently gained. If we lose the narrative, we lose the plot.(99)

7.7 Paralanguage

Paralanguage is the category of nonverbal communication that describes the following characteristics of language:(1)
- volume
- rate of speech
- pausing
- pitch
- tone
- emphasis.

At its most basic, paralanguage refers to how we speak as opposed to the specific words that we use.

Every veterinarian and every client bring a unique mix of paralanguage to the consultation room.

Consider even just your closest circle of friends and family, and you'll see what I mean. We all speak at different volumes. We all make use of different tones and inflections. Our rate of speech is not identical. It also changes with level of excitement and engagement. I tend to speak *very fast the more animated I become!*

Being different is what sets us apart. It is what makes us stand out as individuals.

The purpose of paralanguage studies is not to get everyone to parrot each other. We do not all need to speak the same way to achieve the same end result with our clients.

That being said, your client *does* need to be able to hear you.

7.7.1 Volume of Speech

Volume, specifically the ability to modulate one's volume, plays an important role in the consultation experience.

Soft-spoken voices may be difficult to follow, particularly if the client is hard of hearing. Soft-spoken voices may also convey a lack of confidence to your client. At the other extreme, booming, loud voices may be jarring and disorienting. Aim for a happy medium. Use a comfortable, indoor voice to be conversational.

7.7.2 Pace of Speech

The pace of a clinical consultation is also important. Ideally, the pace of conversational flow should match the urgency of the situation. Consider, for example, if you are triaging a hit-by-car patient that is decompensating, and you need to obtain verbal permission for your team to initiate cardiopulmonary resuscitation (CPR). It would be inappropriate to speak slowly. The pace at which you speak must convey urgency. You need to know and you need to know now.

Conversely, consider the clinical scenario in which you must address quality of life concerns with the owner of a patient with chronic disease. The topic of euthanasia has been broached. The client is devastated. Your task is to help your client to make an informed decision. To do so, they must be able to process the situation as well as their anticipatory grief. Provided that the patient is stable, you can help the client best by cautiously pacing the conversation. Slow down your words and be articulate. Pair this sluggish rate of conversational flow with a calm, quiet voice so that the client does not feel rushed or forced into decision-making.

Pausing is an exceptionally profound tool to allow the client to process the information that you have shared. Pausing gives both you and the client time to collect yourselves and determine where to go from here.

Sometimes this is referred to as the power of the pause. This phraseology highlights how important it is for the pace of conversation to halt at critical momentsso that all contributors of the conversation can exist in the moment, without pressure to move forward until they are ready.

7.7.3 Tone of Speech

In addition to voice volume and rate of speech, you need to attend to your tone. Tone can convey irritation or disrespect in much the same way as eye rolling.

For instance, suppose a client asks you if Fifi's anal sacs can be expressed while she is in the treatment area for venipuncture. There's a difference between you saying "Sure" (nicely) and "Sure" (with annoyance). Clients can pick up on tension.

Not only might clients feel uncomfortable in the moment, they may be reluctant to reach out in the future with questions or concerns, for fear of being ignored, rejected, or lambasted.

If you find that you cannot manage your tone in a constructive manner and the patient is stable, then it is best that you take a time out. Time outs are essential, particularly when you find yourself carrying baggage from one consultation room into the next. Rather than punish the next client with an aggravated state of mind, take a breath. Stand outside, even for a moment, just to get some fresh air.

If it is too late and you're already inside of the consultation room, find an excuse to step out for just a moment.

It is tempting to say that you do not have the time to do so in a busy clinical practice. However, one moment of your time is time well spent so that you do not find yourself in the situation of having to apologize for an inappropriate tone.

7.8 Autonomic Shifts

Autonomic shifts comprise the one category of nonverbal communication that is largely outside of our control.(1) Autonomic shifts are directed responses by our nervous system to help our body respond to perceived threats.(1)

Each and every one of us has "triggers." These are emotional currents that run deep inside of us.

Some are large; some are small. All have the potential to be reactive.

Every now and then, a consultation sets off one or more of those "triggers."

Our body responds as if it has been catapulted into "fight or flight" mode. This may set off a chain reaction inside of us. Our body may respond with one or more of the following physical changes:(1)

- facial flushing or blanching
- sweaty palms
- glistening conjunctiva
- altered breathing
  - holding one's breath
  - increasing one's respiratory rate
  - reducing the depth of respiration such that breaths become more shallow.

Although we have little to no control over the development of these changes, we are still responsible for managing our emotions.

As professionals, it is up to us to lead by example and to recognize when we may need to step away from a case, patient, client, or situation so that it does not escalate.

It also behooves us to engage in self-reflection, after the fact, to consider what triggered the autonomic reaction in the first place. Sometimes we are acutely aware of the cause. Other occasions require dedicated introspection to establish the causative agent.

Although self-reflection does not erase what transpired or the physical and/or emotional aftermath, self-awareness does help you to recalibrate so that you may be able to approach a similar situation differently in the future. Perhaps you can diffuse future conversations before they reach the critical breaking point.

7.9 Revisiting the Impact of Nonverbal Cues on Clinical Conversations

Clinical conversations are the bread and butter of veterinary companion animal practice. If you met with one client every half-hour, for 8 hours each day, for 5 days each week, for 4 weeks each month, for 12 months each year, then you would average 3840 conversations annually. This number does not take into account after-hours telephone calls or electronic correspondence with clients.

Now expand that number out to encompass the number of client interactions that you have over your professional career. That number has been estimated to exceed 100,000 client encounters.(106)

Consider that all conversations have an impact on the following:

* your patient
* your client
* your health
* your license to practice medicine and, by default, your livelihood
* your colleagues
* your support staff
* your practice.

Think about how much time we spend in person, on the phone, or writing emails, trying to craft the perfect words to say, in the moment, to each client about every patient, in every clinical scenario. It is impossible.

There are no perfect words, just as there are no perfect people. Medicine is, by default, an imperfect science. We can only do our best and start each day, refreshed and renewed, hoping to make a difference to those who will walk through our doors. Putting forth our best effort requires us to acknowledge that communication is not always about what we say. In fact, it is quite the opposite.

As we've discovered through the course of this chapter, communication is more often than not about the nuances – that is, what we don't say, but what we imply, by way of nonverbal cues.

To summarize, nonverbal cues are an enormous aspect of client communication that we cannot take for granted.

Patient satisfaction in human healthcare is largely tied to the effective use of nonverbal cues by the physician.(7, 20) The following nonverbal cues are particularly valued by the human medical patient: (3, 54–56)

- open body posture
- eye contact
- gesturing, as through affirmative head nods
- using a caring tone of voice
- being expressive with emotion.

Body language is an integral part of how clients formulate opinions about us, including our perceived compassion, competence, and confidence.

In addition, nonverbal cues affect the:(2, 7, 20, 107)

- patient's level of anxiety
- patient's willingness to follow through with treatment recommendations
- patient's decision to persue follow-up
- patient's decision to make use of healthcare services in the future.

7.10 When Words and Nonverbal Cues Do Not Align: How to Handle Mixed Messages

Despite our best efforts, our words do not always align with our nonverbal cues. The latter may contradict the former, and vice versa.(2, 3, 9) The same can be said of our clients. They may tell us "yes," but through nonverbal communication, they may be screaming, "no!"

How do we handle this incongruence?

Ignoring the problem will not make it go away. Instead, we need to address it respectfully, but directly. You might start by acknowledging the discrepancy.(1)

- "I'm getting the feeling that you're not quite onboard with Champ's treatment plan."
- "I feel as though you're uncomfortable with the plan that we've discussed."
- "I sense you're not quite sure about proceeding with Champ's surgery."

Follow this up with a pause. Allow the client time to process, reflect, and answer.

If you are met with silence, press onward with one of the following approaches.

- "Am I correct in thinking that you're hesitant about starting this medication?"
- "Can you share with me what's going through your mind right now?"
- "Can we talk about any concerns that you might have?"
- "Is there anything further that I can share with you to help guide our decision making?"
- "What can I do to assist you in decision making?"

If you are sensing discomfort, yet the client is still unwilling or unable to share, consider a gentler tactic. Switch to the third person.(1) Respond using one of the following approaches.

- "Many of my clients aren't too sure how they feel about this new deworming protocol."
- "Cost is a significant concern for a number of my clients."
- "A lot my clients worry that …"

Again, pause after finishing your thought. Allow the client time to reflect and process.

If you have succeeded in creating a safe and supportive space, then your client is more likely to open up to you. This should allow him to speak what is on his mind, in which case, his words should more accurately match the nonverbal cues that gave you pause in the first place.

You may be able to reach mutual understanding with your client and find common ground in a plan that you feel strongly will benefit the patient.

7.11 Nonverbal Skills Development

Clients are perceptive and accurate when it comes to reading nonverbal cues. We must constantly work on ourselves and strive for self-awareness so that we know which cues we are giving off and what inferences they lead to.

Nonverbal cues may be more natural to some students than others, but they are not innate or just a "gift" or "nice to have."(1) Like any other skill, they can be learned.

Each of us has nonverbal strengths to fall back upon. Each of us has nonverbal weaknesses. We cannot "fix" everything about ourselves at once. There are certain habits that are deeply engrained that we cannot change, even if we may want to.

So rather than get overwhelmed, take a moment to consider what you can work on today.

Then think about tomorrow. And the day after that.

It is a process. Take it slowly.

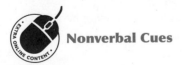 **Nonverbal Cues**

References

1. Carson CA. Nonverbal communication in veterinary practice. Vet Clin North Am Small Anim Pract. 2007;37(1):49–63; abstract viii.

2. Roter DL, Frankel RM, Hall JA, Sluyter D. The expression of emotion through nonverbal behavior in medical visits: mechanisms and outcomes. J Gen Intern Med. 2005;21(Suppl 1):S28–34.

3. Shaw JR. Four core communication skills of highly effective practitioners. Vet Clin North Am Small Anim Pract. 2006;36(2):385–96, vii.

4. Kurtz SM, Silverman JD, Draper J. Teaching and learning communication skills in medicine. Grand Rapids, MI: Radcliffe; 2004.

5. Caris-Verhallen WM, Kerkstra A, Bensing JM. Nonverbal behaviour in nurse-elderly patient communication. J Adv Nurs. 1999;29(4):808–18.

6. Gross D. Communication and the elderly. POTG. 1990;9(1):49–64.

7. Cocksedge S, George B, Renwick S, Chew-Graham CA. Touch in primary care consultations: qualitative investigation of doctors' and patients' perceptions. Br J Gen Pract. 2013;63(609):e283–90.

8. Hall JA, Harrigan JA, Rosenthal R. Nonverbal behavior in clinician patient interaction. Appl Prev Psychol. 1995;4(1):21–37.

9. Adams CL, Kurtz SM. Skills for communicating in veterinary medicine. Oxford: Otmoor Publishing and Dewpoint Publishing; 2017.

10. Koch R. The teacher and nonverbal communication. Theory Pract. 1971;10(4):231–42.

11. McCroskey JC, Larson CE, Knapp ML. An introduction to interpersonal communication. Englewood Cliffs, N.J.: Prentice Hall; 1971.

12. Silverman J. Doctors' non-verbal behaviour in consultations: look at the patient before you look at the computer. Brit J Gen Pract. 2010(February):76–8.

13. Silverman J, Kurtz S, Draper J. Skills for communicating with patients. Oxford: Radcliffe Medical Press; 2008.

14. McArthur ML, Fitzgerald JR. Companion animal veterinarians' use of clinical communication skills. Aust Vet J. 2013;91(9):374–80.

15. Friedman HS. Nonverbal-communication between patients and medical practitioners. J Soc Issues. 1979;35(1):82–99.

16. Kanji N, Coe JB, Adams CL, Shaw JR. Effect of veterinarian–client–patient interactions on client adherence to dentistry and surgery recommendations in companion-animal practice. J Am Vet Med Assoc. 2012;240(4):427–36.

17. MacDonald K. Patient–clinician eye contact: social neuroscience and art of clinical engagement. Postgrad Med. 2009;121(4):136–44.

18. Roter DL, Hall JA. Doctors talking with patients/patients talking with doctors: improving communication in medical visits. Westport, CT: Auburn House; 2006.

19. Shaw JR, Adams CL, Bonnett BN, Larson S, Roter DL. Veterinarian–client–patient communication during wellness appointments versus appointments related to a health problem in companion animal practice. J Am Vet Med Assoc. 2008;233(10):1576–86.

20. Marcinowicz L, Konstantynowicz J, Godlewski C. Patients' perceptions of GP non-verbal communication: a qualitative study. Br J Gen Pract. 2010;60(571):83–7.

21. Larsen KM, Smith CK. Assessment of nonverbal-communication in the patient-physician interview. J Fam Practice. 1981;12(3):481–8.

22. Mehrabian A. Communication without words. Psychol Today. 1968;2(4):53–5.

23. DiMatteo MR, Taranta A, Friedman HS, Prince LM. predicting patient satisfaaction from physicians' nonverbal communication skills. Medical Care. 1980;18(4):376–87.

24. Hippocrates. On decorum and the physician. English translation by E.H.S. Jones. London: William Heinemann Ltd.; 1923.

25. Osler W. The master-word in medicine. Aequanimitas with other addresses to medical students, nurses, and practitioners of medicine. Philadelphia, PA: Blakiston; 1904. p. 369.

26. Engel GL. The care of the patient: art or science? Johns Hopkins Med J. 1977;140(5):222–32.

27. Borrell-Carrio F, Suchman AL, Epstein RM. The biopsychosocial model 25 years later: principles, practice, and scientific inquiry. Ann Fam Med. 2004;2(6):576–82.

28. Smith RC. The biopsychosocial revolution – interviewing and provider-patient relationships becoming key issues for primary care. JGIM. 2002;17(4):309–10.

29. Ambady N, Rosenthal R. Thin slices of expressive behavior as predictors of interpersonal consequences – a metaanalysis. Psychol Bull. 1992;111(2):256–74.

30. Rosenthal R, Hall JA, DiMatteo MR, Rogers PL, Archer D. Sensitivity to nonverbal communication: the PONS test. Baltimore, MD: Johns Hopkins University Press; 1979.

31. Hall JA, Bernieri FJ. Interpersonal sensitivity: theory and measurement. Mahwah, NJ: Erlbaum; 2001.

32. Albright L, Kenny DA, Malloy TE. Consensus in personality judgments at zero acquaintance. J Pers Soc Psychol. 1988;55(3):387–95.

33. Babad E, Bernieri F, Rosenthal R. Nonverbal-communication and leakage in the behavior of biased and unbiased teachers. J Personality Soc Psych. 1989;56(1):89–94.

34. Babad E, Bernieri F, Rosenthal R. When less information is more informative – diagnosing teacher expectations from brief samples of behavior. Brit J Educ Psychol. 1989;59:281–95.

35. O'Sullivan M, Ekman P, Friesen WV. The effect of comparisons on detecting deceit. J Nonverbal Behav. 1988;12(3):203–15.

36. Watson D. Strangers ratings of the 5 robust personality-factors – evidence of a surprising convergence with self-report. J Personality Soc Psych. 1989;57(1):120–8.

37. Goffman E. Gender advertisements. New York: Harper & Rowe; 1979.

38. Wilson TD, Schooler JW. Thinking too much: introspection can reduce the quality of preferences and decisions. J Pers Soc Psychol. 1991;60(2):181–92.

39. Hall JA. How big are nonverbal sex differences? The case of smiling and sensitivity to nonverbal cues. In: Canary DJ, Dindia K, editors. Sex differences and similarities in communication: critical essays and empirical investigations of sex and gender in interaction. Mahwah, NJ: Erlbaum; 1998. pp. 155–7.

40. Hall JA, Stein TS, Roter DL, Rieser N. Inaccuracies in physicians' perceptions of their patients. Med Care. 1999;37(11):1164–8.

41. Knapp ML, Hall JA. Nonverbal communication in human interaction. Sixth edn. Belmont, CA: Wadsworth; 2005.

42. Myers WS. Nonverbal communication speaks volumes: building better client relationships. Exceptional Veterinary Team. 2009(November):3–5.

43. Verderber RF, Verderber KS. Inter-Act: using interpersonal communication skills. Belmont, CA: Wadsworth; 1980.

44. Gabbott M, Hogg G. The role of nonverbal communication in service encounters: a conceptual framework. JMM. 2001;17:5–26.

45. Duggan AP, Parrott RL. Physicians' nonverbal rapport building and patients' talk about the subjective component of illness. Human Communication Research. 2001;27(2):299–311.

46. Endres J, Laidlaw A. Micro-expression recognition training in medical students: a pilot study. BMC Med Educ. 2009;9:47.

47. Peloquin SM. Helping through touch: the embodiment of caring. J Relig Health. 1989;28(4):299–322.

48. Edwards SC. An anthropological interpretation of nurses' and patients' perceptions of the use of space and touch. J Advanced Nursing. 1998;28(4):809–17.

49. Estabrooks CA, Morse JM. Toward a theory of touch – the touching process and acquiring a touching style. J Advanced Nursing. 1992;17(4):448–56.

50. Connor A, Howett M. A conceptual model of intentional comfort touch. J Holist Nurs. 2009;27(2):127–35.

51. Grandjean E, Hunting W. Ergonomics of posture – review of various problems of standing and sitting posture. Appl Ergon. 1977;8(3):135–40.

52. Hansson KG. Body mechanics and posture. Jama-J Am Med Assoc. 1945;128(13):947–53.

53. Watson AW, Mac Donncha C. A reliable technique for the assessment of posture: assessment criteria for aspects of posture. J Sports Med Phys Fitness. 2000;40(3):260–70.

54. Hall JA, Roter DL, Katz NR. Task versus socioemotional behaviors in physicians. Med Care. 1987;25(5):399–412.

55. Hall JA, Roter DL, Rand CS. Communication of affect between patient and physician. J Health Soc Behav. 1981;22(1):18–30.

56. Weinberger M, Greene JY, Mamlin JJ. The impact of clinical encounter events on patient and physician satisfaction. Soc Sci Med E. 1981;15(3):239–44.

57. Von Cranach M. The role of orienting behaviour in human interaction. In: Esser AH, editor. Behaviour and environment. New York: Plenum Press; 1971. pp.217–37.

58. Heintzman M, Leathers DG, Parrott RL, Cairns I. Nonverbal rapport-building behaviors' effect on perceptions of a supervisor. MCQ. 1993;7(2):181–208.

59. Rosenfeld HM. Conversational control functions of nonverbal behaviour. In: Siegman AW, Feldstein S, editors. Nonverbal behaviour and communication. New York: Wiley; 1978. pp. 291–328.

60. Reece MM, Whitman RN. Expressive movements, warmth, and verbal reinforcement. J Abnorm Soc Psychol. 1962;64:234–6.

61. Anderson PA. Nonverbal immediacy in interpersonal communication. In: Siegman AW, Feldstein S, editors. Multichannel integrations of nonverbal behavior. London Erlbaum Associates; 1985. pp. 1–36.

62. Mehrabian A. Nonverbal communication. Chicago, IL: Aldine Atherton; 1972.

63. Burgoon K. Handbook of interpersonal communication. Nonverbal signals. Thousand Oaks, CA: SAGE Publications; 1994. pp. 229–71.

64. Collier G. Emotional expressions. Hillsdale, NJ: Erlbaum; 1985.

65. Herzmark G, Brownbridge G, Fitter M, Evans A. Consultation use of a computer by general practitioners. J R Coll Gen Pract. 1984;34(269):649–54.

66. Fitzgerald FS. The great gatsby. New York: Scribner; 1961.

67. Makoul G, Zick A, Green M. An evidence-based perspective on greetings in medical encounters. Arch Intern Med. 2007;167(11):1172–6.

68. Thompson TL. The initial interaction between the patient and the health professional: communication for health professionals. Lanham, MD: Harper & Row Publishers, Inc.; 1986.

69. Zeldow PB, Makoul G. Communicating with patients. In: Wedding D, Stuber ML, editors. Behavior & medicine. Cambridge, MA: Hogrefe & Huber Publishers; 2006. pp. 201–18.

70. Lipkin M, Frankel RM. Performing the interview. In: Lipkin M, Putnam SM, Lazare A, editors. The medical interview: clinical care, education, and research. New York: Springer-Verlag NY Inc.; 1995. pp. 65–82.

71. Coulehan JL, Block MR. The medical interview: mastering skills for clinical practice. Philadelphia, PA: FA Davis Co Publishers; 1997.

72. Makoul G. The SEGUE Framework for teaching and assessing communication skills. Patient Educ Couns. 2001;45:23–34.

73. Billings JA, Stoeckle JD. The clinical encounter: a guide to the medical interview and case presentation. St. Louis, MO: Mosby Year Book Inc.; 1999.

74. Lloyd M, Bor R. Communication skills for medicine. New York: Churchill Livingstone, Inc.; 1996.

75. Smith RC. The patient's story: integrated patient–doctor interviewing. Boston, MA: Little Brown & Co, Inc.; 1996.

76. Ranjan P. How can doctors improve their communication skills? JCDR. 2015;9(3):1–4.

77. Frankel RM, Stein T. Getting the most out of the clinical encounter: the four habits model. The Permanente Journal. 1999;3(3):79–88.

78. Jourard S. Disclosing man to himself. New York: Van Nostrand Reinhold Company; 1968.

79. Watson WH. Meanings of touch – geriatric nursing. J Commun. 1975;25(3):104–12.

80. McCann K, Mckenna HP. an examination of touch between nurses and elderly patients in a continuing care setting in Northern Ireland. J Advanced Nursing. 1993;18(5):838–46.

81. De Wever MK. Nursing-home patients perception of nurses affective touching. J Psychol. 1977;96(2):163–71.

82. Argyle M. Spatial behavior. In Englar M, editor. Bodily communication. Second edn. Madison, CT: International Universities Press; 1988. pp. 168–87.

83. Hall E. Space speaks. The silent language. Garden City, NY: Anchor Press; 1973. pp. 162–85.

84. Noordman J, Verhaak P, van Beljouw I, van Dulmen S. Consulting room computers and their effect on general practitioner-patient communication. Fam Pract. 2010;27(6):644–51.

85. Ridsdale L, Hudd S. Computers in the consultation – the patients view. BJGP. 1994;44(385):367–9.

86. Stroppe J, J. DM, Cennaeme R. A picture of primary health care in Europe. In: De Maeseneer J, Beolchi L, editors. Telematics in primary care in europe. Amsterdam: IOS Press; 1995. pp. 1–30.

87. Martin S. Computer use by Canada's physicians approaches 90% mark. Can Med Assoc J. 2001;165(5):632-.

88. Pearce C, Dwan K, Arnold M, Phillips C, Trumble S. Doctor, patient and computer – a framework for the new consultation. Int J Med Inform. 2009;78(1):32–8.

89. Lelievre S, Schultz K. Does computer use in patient-physician encounters influence patient satisfaction? Can Fam Physician. 2010;56(1):e6–12.

90. Pringle M. Using computers to take patient histories. BMJ. 1988;297(6650):697–8.

91. Als AB. The desk-top computer as a magic box: patterns of behaviour connected with the desk-top computer; GPs' and patients' perceptions. Fam Pract. 1997;14(1):17–23.

92. Rethans JJ, Hoppener P, Wolfs G, Diederiks J. Do personal computers make doctors less personal? Br Med J (Clin Res Ed). 1988;296(6634):1446–8.

93. Cruickshank PJ. Computers in medicine: patients' attitudes. J R Coll Gen Pract. 1984;34(259):77–80.

94. Frankel R, Altschuler A, George S, Kinsman J, Jimison H, Robertson NR, et al. Effects of exam-

room computing on clinician–patient communication: a longitudinal qualitative study. J Gen Intern Med. 2005;20(8):677–82.

95. Rouf E, Whittle J, Lu N, Schwartz MD. Computers in the exam room: differences in physician-patient interaction may be due to physician experience. J Gen Intern Med. 2007;22(1):43–8.

96. Bensing JM, Tromp F, van Dulmen S, van den Brink-Muinen A, Verheul W, Schellevis FG. Shifts in doctor–patient communication between 1986 and 2002: a study of videotaped general practice consultations with hypertension patients. BMC Fam Pract. 2006;7:62.

97. Strayer SM, Semler MW, Kington ML, Tanabe KO. Patient attitudes toward physician use of tablet computers in the exam room. Fam Med. 2010;42(9):643–7.

98. Booth N, Robinson P, Kohannejad J. Identification of high-quality consultation practice in primary care: the effects of computer use on doctor–patient rapport. Inform Prim Care. 2004;12(2):75–83.

99. Pearce C, Trumble S. Computers can't listen – algorithmic logic meets patient centredness. Aust Fam Physician. 2006;35(6):439–42.

100. Solomon GL, Dechter M. Are patients pleased with computer use in the examination room? J Fam Pract. 1995;41(3):241–4.

101. Sullivan F, Mitchell E. Has general practitioner computing made a difference to patient care? A systematic review of published reports. BMJ. 1995;311(7009):848–52.

102. Garrison GM, Bernard ME, Rasmussen NH. 21st-century health care: the effect of computer use by physicians on patient satisfaction at a family medicine clinic. Fam Med. 2002;34(5):362–8.

103. Hsu J, Huang J, Fung V, Robertson N, Jimison H, Frankel R. Health information technology and physician-patient interactions: impact of computers on communication during outpatient primary care visits. J Am Med Inform Assoc. 2005;12(4):474–80.

104. Brownbridge G, Herzmark GA, Wall TD. Patient reactions to doctors' computer use in general practice consultations. Soc Sci Med. 1985;20(1):47–52.

105. Newman W, Button G, Cairns P. Pauses in doctor–patient conversation during computer use: The design significance of their durations and accompanying topic changes. Int J Hum-Comput St. 2010;68(6):398–409.

106. Morrizey JK, Voiland B. Difficult interactions with veterinary clients: working in the challenge zone. Vet Clin N Am-Small. 2007;37(1):65-+.

107. Bensing J, Verheul W, van Dulmen A. Patient anxiety in the medical encounter: a study of verbal and non-verbal communication in general practice. Health Educ. 2008;108(5):373–83.

Chapter 8

Defining Entry-Level Communication Skills

Open-Ended Questions and Statements

As veterinarians, we spend a significant amount of time in the consultation room gathering information from clients about our patients and what ails them. History taking is an essential component of clinical practice for the following reasons.

- It demonstrates respect for the client as part of the healthcare team:
  - you may be an expert in veterinary medicine, however, your client is an expert about the patient and its day-to-day care.
- It invites the client to share his or her perspective:
  - history taking is the first opportunity to establish the client's full agenda for the consultation(1–3)
  - history taking allows the client the freedom to describe what has been going on, why it is of concern, and what the client would like to pursue at today's visit.(4–8)
- It provides insight into the patient's presentation.
  - What happened? (Or, what does the client *think* happened?)
  - When did it happen? (Or, when does the client *think* it happened?)
  - How did it happen? (Or, how does the client *assume* the issue came to be?)
  - Why did it happen? (Or, why does the client *suppose* the issue has arisen?)
- It provides key details that are essential to making the diagnosis.(9–13)
  - The diagnostic value of history taking cannot be understated.(14)
  - Sixty-to-eighty percent of diagnoses in human healthcare can be made based upon data was obtained from history taking alone.(15–20)

8.1 The Comprehensive Patient History

History taking may seem overwhelming to the student doctor, when she or he considers all the data that must be gathered to paint a complete portrait of our patient and its lifestyle. Even something as simple, on the surface, as a new kitten or puppy wellness visit requires attention to detail.

A comprehensive anamnesis includes:(21–25)

- the patient's demographic data (collectively, this information is referred to as the patient's signalment)
  - age
  - sex
  - sexual status
  - breed
  - species
- patient acquisition history
  - purchased
  - adopted (from shelter or a private owner)
  - rescued stray
- the client's expectations for the visit
- the client's expectations for the patient
  - for instance, is the patient intended to be a companion
  - or is the patient:
    - a service dog (guide, mobility, hearing, medical alert, autism service, and psychiatric service dogs)
    - a therapy dog
    - a working dog (search and rescue, explosives detection, narcotics and agriculture detection, allergy alert dog, cancer detection, and bed bug sniffing)
- the patient's primary concern, that is, its presenting or chief complaint – a concise summary statement that identifies the reason for the veterinary medical consultation
- the client's secondary concerns:
  - in human healthcare, the majority of patients have more than one concern that needs to be addressed during the current visit(26–30)
  - these concerns may be late breaking, that is, if they are not elicited early on in the appointment, then they are likely to emerge at the end of the consultation, when the clinician is attempting to wrap up the case(1, 26, 31–34)
- the patient's lifestyle:
  - whether the patient is indoor-only, such as a housecat
  - whether the patient is outdoor-only, such as a barn cat
  - whether the patient is indoor–outdoor:
    - is the patient outdoors only when supervised or does the patient experience outdoor living unsupervised?
    - does the patient come and go as it likes, for instance, by way of a pet door?
    - is the patient reliant upon the client to let it in or out?
- activity level
  - whether the patient is sedentary
  - whether the patient goes for walks, hikes, or runs
  - whether the patient performs agility, herding, or hunting
- travel history

- - no travel outside of the home
  - travel within the region
  - travel within the country
  - international travel
- serological status
  - cats: feline leukemia (FeLV) and feline immunodeficiency virus (FIV)
  - dogs:
    - heartworm (HW)
    - Lyme disease
    - *Ehrlichia*
    - *Anaplasma*
  - other:
    - fungal infections, such as coccidioidomycosis (valley fever)
    - protozoal infections, such as toxoplasmosis
- diet history
  - home-made or commercial diet
  - volume fed
  - frequency of feeding (ad libitum or meal fed)
  - treats and table scraps
- current medications
  - over-the-counter products
  - prescriptions
  - vitamins
  - supplements
- history of preventative care, including vaccinations
- past familial, medical, surgical, and reproductive history
- past pertinent diagnostic tests and test results, including laboratory and imaging
- past pertinent therapeutic trials and outcomes.

It is easy to see how copious data collection can become, yet it is essential.

The history is our window into the home life, environment, and experience of the patient. Short of making a home visit, it is the closest that we come to fully appreciating what it is like to be that individual.

Background information is not extraneous. Clues are often hidden in the details that clients may not recognize as being important. The successful veterinarian is a detective. She or he learns the *right* questions to ask and in which order, in order to accumulate a substantial database about the patient and its needs.

At the same time, the successful veterinarian makes use of history taking as a means of building rapport with the client. History taking is our opportunity to connect with clients by inviting them to share, acknowledging what they say, and addressing their concerns.

8.2 Why is it Critical to Elicit the Patient's Concerns? The Human Medical Perspective

Consumers of all healthcare industries have undergone a dramatic shift. Today's veterinary clients are much less concerned about what their provider knows. It matters more to them that their provider cares.(35, 36) This is consistent with the movement away from medical paternalism and the trend towards relationship-centered care.(35, 37)

A patient-centered approach in human healthcare drives consumer satisfaction.(38)

- Patients that are invited to share their story are more satisfied with the healthcare team.
- Patients appreciate the opportunity to voice their questions.(39)
- Patients want to have their concerns acknowledged and addressed.(39–42)
- Patients feel heard when they feel connected to providers through nonverbal cues. (43–46) Please also refer to Chapter 7.

Patients that are satisfied with their healthcare team have better clinical outcomes.(47)

- Patients are more likely to exhibit compliance with healthcare recommendations when providers invite them to share their knowledge base, core beliefs, and concerns.(48, 49)
- Patients are more likely to exhibit adherence to treatment plans when they participate in decision making.(50)
- Patients are more likely to report shorter durations of illness and faster recovery periods when they contribute to treatment plans.(51, 52)

Patients that are satisfied with their healthcare team are less likely to sue.(53, 54)

8.3 Why is it Critical to Elicit the Client's Concerns? The Veterinary Perspective

The veterinary profession has been slower to investigate the impact of veterinarian–client interactions on patient outcomes than the human healthcare industry.(37) However, we now know that relationship building and connectivity are valued by the veterinary client.

The veterinary client's experience is contingent upon their perception of effective communication. When breakdowns in communication occur, clients may:(37, 55–62)

- feel judged
- feel ignored
- not feel heard
- feel misinformed
- misunderstand

- feel rushed
- not feel as if they have choices
- feel pressured into making a decision
- feel that they have not been given all the options
- fail to understand why recommendations have been made
- fail to see why a particular treatment is important
- not follow through with treatment recommendations
- not return for follow-up care.

8.4 Noncompliance in Healthcare

Noncompliance is a huge problem in both human and veterinary healthcare industries. Recent research has demonstrated that, contrary to popular thought, noncompliance is often not because cost is an obstacle to care.(58) Rather, non-compliance often stems from misinformation, misunderstanding, confusion, or uncertainty.(58) According to a 2008 study by Lue et al., 30% of owners do not follow recommendations from the veterinary team because they do not understand their value or why they are necessary.(58)

As part of the customer service, the veterinary profession needs to do a better job of conveying the value of care, that is, the "why?" or the "so what?" factor.

We need to do a better job of asking the right questions. We need to do a better job of listening to our clients' answers. Asking the right questions, in the right way, begins with history taking and ends with hearing our clients' response, without interrupting.

8.5 The Art of Listening and the Dangers of Interrupting during History Taking

Clients want us to invite them to share, and listen for the answer that they provide. Listening is a challenge for many clinicians. Clinicians may think that they are listening; however, what they think they hear may not be an accurate reflection of what it is that the client is trying to share. (Refer to Chapter 5 for additional insight into the communication skill of reflective listening.)

Listening incorrectly is problematic to patient outcomes for several reasons, not the least of which is that acquiring incorrect information may lead to incorrect diagnostic or therapeutic recommendations. However, even worse is when human healthcare providers do not listen at all.

In fact, clinicians frequently interrupt patients within seconds of asking them to share. In 1984, Beckman and Frankel published that 69% of physicians interrupt patients' opening statements within the first 18 seconds.(5) Only 23% of patients were allowed to complete their statement.(5)

The study concluded that:

> There is little doubt that the physician response and, in particular, early termination or interruption of patients during their initial expression of concerns at a time of the visit specifically reserved for such discourse, inhibits further patient identification of additional concerns. (5)

Fifteen years later, in 1999, Marvel et al. demonstrated minimal improvement, with interruptions occurring, on average, within the first 23.1 seconds.(63)

A decade later, a 2019 study by Ospina et al. documented that the human healthcare industry has backtracked, rather than advanced, when it comes to eliciting the patient's agenda: 67% of physicians interrupt after a median of 11 seconds.(64) Less than one-half, 49% of patients, were able to fully share their agenda with the attending physician in primary care visits as compared to 20% of patients in specialty care.(64)

Imagine how an interruption might be viewed from the client's perspective.

- Would you feel connected to your provider?
- Would you feel heard?
- Would you feel respected?
- Would you feel understood?
- Would you feel valued?
- Would you feel like a member of the healthcare team?
- Would you feel like your contributions were being taken seriously?
- Would you feel welcome to expand upon your story?
- How likely are you to answer subsequent questions with detailed responses?

If I were interrupted by my healthcare provider, I might make one or more of the following assumptions about him or her.

- She or he is in a hurry.
- She or he is running behind schedule.
- She or he does not have the time to hear me out.
- She or he does not welcome my involvement in decision making.
- She or he thinks that I do not know what I am talking about.
- She or he does not value what I have to say.
- What I have to say does not matter.

These assumptions may or may not be true. It could be that the clinician:

- is in a hurry that day
- does not agree with my perception of the problem
- is preoccupied – maybe there is another, more urgent case that is weighing heavily on his or her mind.

As the client, I will never know which of the these precipitated the interruption.

All I know, as the client, and what I will walk away from this appointment feeling, is that I was not heard. As a result, how likely am I to follow through with healthcare recommendations that were given to me at this visit?

There is a high probability that I will leave this practice with unmet concerns.

There are a variety of reasons why physicians interrupt their patients. Many worry that if their patients are granted the floor to speak, they will never stop talking. Physicians fear a runaway train of lengthy narratives that will distract and/or detract from the efficiency of care.

In truth, a handful of patients will take the reins and fail to give them back. However, the majority will not. When uninterrupted by general practitioners, most patients speak for less than 30 seconds.(5) Patients rarely speak for more than 90 seconds when consulting with specialists.(65)

Less than 2 minutes of our time is insignificant. Even in the busiest practice, barring an unexpected walk-in emergency, this is reasonable and should be sufficient for 80% of patients, even among those with complicated histories.(65)

Why is preserving this time so valuable to the clinical consultation?

An investment of time upfront breeds efficiency later. Patients are less likely to postpone voicing concerns until the visit's end, when they are granted the time for sharing upfront.

Patients are also more likely to invest in the conversation and hear what the doctor has to say when they are not preoccupied with remembering their concerns until the end of the consultation.

It is worth risking the runaway train narrative by granting patients (and veterinary clients) the floor to speak. Chances are, if we open the consultation with the right question and give them the opportunity to answer, they will provide precisely the information that we need without us having to inefficiently go fish for it.

8.6 The Art of History Taking: Introducing Two Styles of Questioning

History taking is an art as much as a science.

The poor history taker is robotic and tiresome as she or he fires away a laundry list of questions. The exceptional history taker knows how to craft seemingly disparate questions into a unified conversation.

How we, as clinicians, initiate that conversation makes a difference as to how the rest of it will flow. Initiating the consultation can be done via one of two styles of questioning:

- closed-ended questions
- open-ended questions or statements.

The words that we use to phrase our questions, and how it is that we ask our questions, matter.(4, 5, 8, 63, 66–70)

Word choice impacts information gathering because it directs the client to respond in a particular way. In fact, a single word difference has the power to alter what a client shares with his healthcare provider.(9) Consider, for instance, findings from a 2006 study by Robinson.(9, 71) Robinson reported that the following two questions solicited distinct answers from patients.(71)

- "How are you?"
- "How are you feeling?"

Clients who are asked the former question take it as an open-ended social opportunity. They may choose to share virtually anything about themselves – for instance, "Life's going great, the grandkids are coming over to visit this weekend, and work hasn't been so bad."

Clients who are asked, "How are you feeling?" tend to respond in a narrower manner that is biomedically focused.

Similarly, a 2007 study by Heritage et al. showed that patients responded very differently to the following two questions.(9, 28)

- "Is there something else you want to address in the visit today?"
- "Is there anything else you want to address in the visit today?"

Clients who were asked the former question identified fewer concerns than those who were asked the latter question.(9, 28)

According to Heritage et al.:

> This finding suggests that patient responses are often designed to meet the expectations set by physician questions and that patient answers can display sensitivity to the implications such questions inherently impose. (28)

We would do well to consider what information we are hoping to obtain from data gathering. That may guide us to phrase our question in such a way as to increase the likelihood of getting the answer that we want or need.

Closed- and open-ended questions are two distinct styles of inquiry that serve a purpose in the medical interview.

8.7 Closed-Ended Questions, Defined

Closed-ended questions are direct, short, and to the point. They direct clients to respond in an abbreviated manner.(66) The answer to a closed-ended question is often "yes" or "no."(66)

Consider the following examples of closed-ended questions that direct clients to respond with a definitive *yes* or *no*.

- Has Mychael coughed today?
- Has Mychael vomited?
- Has Mychael been his usual self?
- Has Mychael's attitude been off?
- Did Justin eat breakfast?
- Did he eat dinner last night?
- Did he sleep through the night?
- Did he keep you up all night?
- Did he walk normally after he got up from his nap?
- Did he limp on his left front leg?
- Have you seen Lowell squinting?
- Have you seen Lowell pawing at his eyes?
- Have you seen him act sensitive to light?
- Have you seen Lowell sneeze?
- Are his sneezes productive?
- Are his eyes goopy?
- Are his breaths rapid?
- Are they shallow?
- Are his breathing sounds raspy?
- Does he have a snotty nose?
- Is he wheezing?
- Is he choking?
- Is he open-mouth breathing?
- Has he developed ocular discharge?
- Has he developed nasal discharge?
- Has he been drinking?
- Has he been eating?
- Is Chewy eating?
- Is Chewy drinking?
- Is Bailey producing solid bowel movements?
- Is Nina urinating outside of the litter box?
- Do you plan on travelling outside of the state with Turnip?
- Do you want to proceed with the dental cleaning?
- Do you want an estimate?
- Do you want to discuss cost of care?
- Did you see blood in Jesse's vomit?
- Did you see diarrhea?
- Did you see straining to have a bowel movement?
- Did you see blood in his stool?

Note that not all closed-ended questions ask for a definitive yes or no. Some closed-ended questions ask the client to respond with a number.

- How many times did Bailey eat yesterday?
- How many times a day does Nina void?
- How many times did Timothy vomit overnight?
- How many times has Bentley been obstructed in the past?

Some closed-ended questions do not fit the descriptions above, yet still ask the question in such a way as to invite only an abbreviated answer from the client. For instance:

- How often does Squash vomit?
  - Possible answer: "three times a day."
- When did Buttercup stop eating?
  - Possible answer: "last night."
- What do you feed Pumpkin?
  - Possible answer: "canned Friskies."
- How frequently is Denver's house-soiling a problem for you?
  - Possible answer: "every two or three days."

8.7.1 The Value of Closed-Ended Questions in the Clinical Consultation

Closed-ended questions play an important part in the veterinary consultation: there are times when we need a definite, abbreviated answer.

Consider, for instance, if a patient is being dropped off at the clinic for surgery under general anesthesia. We have to ask our client, "When did you last feed Ginger?"

We need an exact answer. The answer determines whether or not the patient can undergo general anesthesia.

Similarly, in the unfortunate event that a patient arrests, the veterinarian needs an immediate answer to the question, "Do you want us to perform CPR on Pillsbury?"

8.7.2 The Limitations of Closed-Ended Questions in the Clinical Consultation

On other occasions, we benefit from having our clients share additional details with us. During these circumstances, closed-ended questions are inappropriate because there are limits to the amount of detail that can be obtained by asking them.

For instance, if a patient presents to us with a history of seizing, we need a description of what the client witnessed. A "yes" or "no" answer is inadequate.

We would have to ask a LOT of closed-ended questions to get the type of data that we need. For example, we might ask.

- Was Finn acting strange before this episode?
- Did Finn appear to be weak in his hind limbs before the episode?
- Did Finn seem wobbly just before a incident?
- How long did the event last?
- Did it take a while for Finn to recover?
- How long did it take for Finn to recover?
- Did Finn paddle his limbs during the event?
- Did he lose control of his bladder?
- Did he lose control of his bowels?
- Did Finn seem confused after the episode?
- Did Finn run into walls or otherwise appear to be blind after the incident?
- How long did this abnormal behavior persist?

This is not time efficient.

The client may also become frustrated by the assembly line of questions that are being fired at him or her.

To improve efficiency of history taking and to allow the client the freedom to share his or her perspective, we need to consider a different style of questioning, the open-ended question or statement.

8.8 The Open-Ended Question or Statement

Robinson and Heritage capture the distinction between closed- and open-ended questions best:

> Open-ended general inquiries claim a lack of knowledge of patient's problems, encourage their *de-novo* presentation, and frame patients (at least initially) as being active authorities over their own health information. Closed-ended requests claim prior knowledge of patients' problems (e.g., gathered from charted notes), encourage Yes–No confirmation-type answers, and frame patients as, at best, passive authorities. (4)

Unlike closed-ended questions, open-ended questions and statements invite clients to expand upon an answer. Rather than eliciting a yes, no, or one-word answer, open-ended questions and statements invite clients to share their story in greater detail.(72) In this regard, they are relationship builders. They help us to get to know our clients better. They open up doors so that we know more fully what it is that may be weighing on clients' minds.

Open-ended questions and statements let clients know that you value what they have to say and that you are interested in their thoughts. Open-ended questions and statements help clients to feel heard.

Clients that have the opportunity to expand upon their answers may also be more likely to share questions or concerns because this questioning style opens up the opportunity for dialogue.

Clients are able to respond to open-ended questions and statements with their own unique perspective. This allows them to share their thoughts, ideas, concerns, and emotions using words that are their own.

8.8.1 Examples of Open-Ended Questions or Statements

Open-ended statements often begin with:(66, 73–75)

- tell me
- help me
- show me
- share with me
- describe
- paint a picture for me.

For example:

- Tell me more about that.
- Tell me what the vomit looked like.
- Tell me more about what is concerning you most.
- Tell me how that makes you feel.
- Tell me what's going through your mind right now.
- Help me to better understand where you are coming from.
- Help me to see this through your eyes.
- Show me what you read online that has you so worried about the medication that I prescribed.
- Show me what the specialist's report said about Billy's hip dysplasia.
- Show me how Beau postured when he vomited.
- Share with me what you witnessed when Darling was attacked by the neighbor's dog.
- Share with me what your greatest concern is.
- Share with me what is most important for me to know about your cat while he will be staying with us in the hospital.
- Describe what you're seeing at home when you say that Johnny shakes.
- Describe how Justine's gait is off.
- Describe how Carolyn is acting painful.
- Paint a picture for me as to what a normal day is for Juniper.

Open-ended questions could theoretically begin with "Why."

- "Why do you think that Johnny's appetite is off?"
- "Why are you so worried about getting Figment spayed?"
- "Why are you reluctant to vaccinate Dobby against rabies?"

- "Why don't you want to pursue a dental cleaning?"
- "Why are you concerned about anesthesia?"

These are reasonable questions to ask, and they all do attempt to elicit the client's perspective.

However, questions that begin with "why" have the potential to stir up defensiveness. (66) Clients may feel that you are questioning them or their motives. Clients may feel wrongly judged, even if that is not your intent.

It would be better to lead off an open-ended question with the word, "How." Consider, for example, the following.

- "How do you feel about getting Figment spayed?"
- "How does the thought of vaccinating Dobby against rabies make you feel?"
- "How does a dental cleaning sound to you?"
- "How concerned are you about anesthesia?"

"How" questions also provide the opportunity for relationship building, by fostering rapport.

- "How did you come up with your dog's name?"
- "How did you decide upon this breed of cat?"
- "How is it that this little one came to be a part of your life?"

"How" questions also allow the opportunity for you to check in with the client about changes in the household and address potential problems before they escalate.

- "Your new pup is super sweet, but tell me, how is your cat handling this new addition to the household?"
- "How is housetraining going?"
- "How is the new puppy adjusting to his new home?
- "How is the new puppy settling into his new routine?"

Leading open-ended questions with the word, "What," may achieve similar effects as leading off with the word, "How."

- "What are your thoughts about getting Figment spayed?"
- "What is your gut reaction to getting Dobby vaccinated against rabies?"
- "What is your reluctance to vaccinate?"
- "What makes you reluctant to pursue a dental cleaning?"
- "What about anesthesia concerns you most?"

"What" is also a good way to open-up the consultation because it offers a broad solicitation.(76, 77)

- "What brings you in today?"
- "What may I do for you today?"
- "What's going on with Little John?"
- "What seems to be the trouble?"
- "What concerns would you like to discuss today?"

Note that "how" and "what" help form open-ended questions that invite the client to share.

Unlike "why" questions, they do not give the impression that you are finger-pointing or calling them out for not wanting to proceed with one or more recommendations for care.

They are therefore safer for use in the clinical consultation, particularly in the face of difficult conversations.

8.8.2 Ways to Soften Open-Ended Statements

Sometimes young clinicians are hesitant to ask open-ended questions because they fear that they might come across as seeming demanding or authoritative. *Tell me* may seem more like an order than a friendly invitation to share.

In truth, tone has much to do with it. If you say, tell me, in a respectful tone, then it is unlikely that the client will become defensive. That being said, there are ways to soften how you phrase your open-ended question. Instead of "tell me", you may say, "Please, can you tell me ..." Instead of "show me", you may say, "Please, can you show me ..."

8.8.3 Efficiency and Open-Ended Statements

Veterinarians share many of the same fears as human physicians. Like human doctors, veterinarians, too, are often afraid to ask open-ended questions because they worry that clients will take over the conversation.

Remember that open-ended questions, when spaced appropriately, are time-savers, not time-wasters. The descriptions that they provide are diverse and, without prompting, clients may share precisely what the veterinarian needed to ask.

Let's return to the case of the seizing patient in Section 8.7.2.

Twelve closed-ended questions were provided in the hopes of obtaining a complete history from the client. This would have been time-consuming.

What if instead of asking closed-ended questions, we invited the owner to share his story using one open-ended statement: "Tell me what you noticed with Finn."

This single open-ended statement might prompt the following response:

It was so strange, Doc. Finn woke up fine, he ate breakfast, we went for his morning run. Nothing was wrong. We came home. I got a telephone call. I turned my back for maybe five minutes. That's when I heard a sound. It sounded like a crash. I thought he'd knocked something over. I turned around to scold him. That's when I saw him lying on the floor. He was paddling all of his legs like he was going bicycling and he seemed really out of it – panting and whining and whimpering up a storm. I called out to him, but he didn't respond. The lights were on, but nobody was home. It felt like forever. He finally settled down a minute or two later. When he got up, he was soaked in pee. He seemed a bit off and shaky. He kind of walked into a wall like he couldn't see. But he worked his way out of it. By the time I got him here – an hour or so later – you wouldn't know anything had happened. He seems perfectly fine now.

Note how much information the client was able to provide. Note how many details we were able to obtain without having to pry them out of the client.

Just one open-ended statement yielded data about:

- the timeline of event
- what may have precipitated the event
- what the client witnessed:
  - the patient was laterally recumbent and paddling
  - the patient was disoriented
  - the patient was nonresponsive
  - the patient lost control of his urinary bladder during the event
- duration of event
- post-ictal period:
  - disorientation persisted
  - patient seemed wobbly
  - patient appeared to be blind
  - this phase lasted about 1 hour.

Can you appreciate the value that this style of questioning offers the clinician?

A single open-ended question allowed the client to paint a picture for us that described most of, if not all of, what we needed to understand just what had happened to the patient.

You can appreciate how much time this question saved, and also how it gave the client the freedom to share the experience, from his perspective, without the constant interruption of his line of thought that would have occurred with closed-ended questioning.

True, we may still need to ask a follow-up question here or there, but we got the bulk of what we needed to know in order to develop a diagnostic and/or treatment plan.

8.9 Is there a Place for Both Open- and Closed-Ended Questions?

Absolutely, there is a place in the consultation for both open- and closed-ended questions. One type is not "right" and one type is not "wrong." An experienced clinician knows how to ask a mix of questions that includes both varieties.

So how do you know which type to ask and when to ask it?

Most veterinarians are heavily reliant upon closed-ended questions out of habit.(59, 66) They may even use them exclusively to gather data. However, open-ended questions offer the following advantages:(66, 78)

- increased client satisfaction
- increased opportunity for mutual understanding
- increased opportunity to clarify the client's perspective
- increased likelihood of client 'buy-in' to the treatment plan and prescribed follow-up.

How, then, can we balance our default style of questioning against the need to broaden our approach to data gathering for the benefit of patient outcomes?

It is advisable to consider the veterinary consultation as a funnel, in which both open-ended and closed-ended questions have their place.(66, 73, 75) Open-ended questions are a good starting point for the consultation because they provide clients with the opportunity to share what is on their minds. Veterinarians may then clarify what has been shared or fill in the gaps by asking appropriate closed-ended questions as follow-up.

8.10 Client Preferences for Open-Ended Questions Based upon Species

My 2018 study with Alyssa Show evaluated dog- and cat-owner preferences for Calgary–Cambridge communication skills, including open-ended questions.(70) Based upon 215 submissions from canine owners and 166 submissions from feline owners, we established that the communication preferences of dog and cat owners overlap.(70)

Owners of both species prioritize reflective listening as the most important skill of the four that are discussed in Chapters 5–8.(70) However, open-ended questions were valued by dog-owners more so than cat-owners.(70)

In the words of a respondent for the canine survey:

Open-ended questions allow me to more completely fill in what my pets are doing or not doing and why I think there is a problem.(70)

It became apparent from our study that:

Dog owners tend to see themselves as experts when it comes to their dogs, and they worry that limiting themselves to a simple yes/no response may lead to an inaccurate diagnosis.(70)

Additional research is necessary to follow-up on these subtle distinctions between dog and cat owners. However, it does give us pause as veterinary educators. It may be that a "one size fits all" approach to clinical communication could benefit from revision as we further tailor communication skills based upon the species for whom we are providing care.

Taking a Patient History
Open-Ended Questions
Closed-Ended Questions

References

1. Tsai MH, Lu FH, Frankel RM. Learning to listen: effects of using conversational transcripts to help medical students improve their use of open questions in soliciting patient problems. Patient Educ Couns. 2013;93(1):48–55.
2. McWhinney I. The need for a transformed clinical method. In: Stewart M, Roter DL, editors. Communicating with medical patients. Newbury Park, CA: SAGE Publications; 1989. pp. 25–40.
3. Roter D. Three blind men and an elephant: reflections on meeting the challenges of patient diversity in primary care practice. Fam Med. 2002;34(5):390–3.
4. Robinson JD, Heritage J. Physicians' opening questions and patients' satisfaction. Patient Educ Couns. 2006;60(3):279–85.
5. Beckman HB, Frankel RM. The effect of physician behavior on the collection of data. Ann Intern Med. 1984;101(5):692–6.
6. Robinson JD. Closing medical encounters: two physician practices and their implications for the expression of patients' unstated concerns. Soc Sci Med. 2001;53(5):639–56.
7. Robinson JD. An interactional structure of medical activities during acute visits and its implications for patients' participation. Health Commun. 2003;15(1):27–57.
8. Heritage J, Robinson JD. The structure of patients' presenting concerns: physicians' opening questions. Health Commun. 2006;19(2):89–102.
9. MacMartin C, Wheat HC, Coe JB, Adams CL. Effect of question design on dietary information solicited during veterinarian-client interactions in companion animal practice in Ontario, Canada. J Am Vet Med Assoc. 2015;246(11):1203–14.
10. Cole SA, Bird J. The medical interview: the three-function approach. St. Louis, MO: Mosby; 2000.
11. Cassell E. Talking with patients. Second edn. New York: Oxford University Press; 1997.
12. Bates B, Bickley LS, Hoekelman RA. Physical examination and history taking. Sixth edn. Philadelphia, PA: Lippincott; 1995.
13. Stoeckle JD, Billings JA. A history of history-taking: the medical interview. J Gen Intern Med. 1987;2(2):119–27.
14. Rich EC, Crowson TW, Harris IB. The diagnostic value of the medical history. Perceptions of internal medicine physicians. Arch Intern Med. 1987;147(11):1957–60.
15. Lichstein PR. The medical interview. In: Walker HK, Hall WD, Hurst JW, editors. Clinical methods: the history, physical, and laboratory examinations. Boston, MA: Butterworths; 1990.
16. Takemura Y, Atsumi R, Tsuda T. Identifying medical interview behaviors that best elicit information from patients in clinical practice. Tohoku J Exp Med. 2007;213(2):121–7.
17. Hampton JR, Harrison MJ, Mitchell JR, Prichard JS, Seymour C. Relative contributions of history-taking, physical examination, and laboratory investigation to diagnosis and management of medical outpatients. Br Med J. 1975;2(5969):486–9.

18. Kassirer JP. Teaching clinical medicine by iterative hypothesis testing. Let's preach what we practice. N Engl J Med. 1983;309(15):921–3.

19. Peterson MC, Holbrook JH, Von Hales D, Smith NL, Staker LV. Contributions of the history, physical examination, and laboratory investigation in making medical diagnoses. West J Med. 1992;156(2):163–5.

20. Sandler G. The importance of the history in the medical clinic and the cost of unnecessary tests. Am Heart J. 1980;100(6 Pt 1):928–31.

21. Cameron S, Turtle-song I. Learning to write case notes using the SOAP format. J Couns Dev. 2002;80(3):286–92.

22. Rockett J, Lattanzio C, Christensen C. The veterinary technician's guide to writing SOAPS: a workbook for critical thinking. Heyburn, ID: Rockett House Publishing LLC; 2013.

23. Borcherding S. Documentation manual for writing SOAP notes in occupational therapy. Second edn. Thorofare, NJ: SLACK Incorporated; 2005.

24. Kettenbach G, Kettenbach G. Writing patient/client notes: ensuring accuracy in documentation. 4th edn. Philadelphia, PA: F.A. Davis; 2004.

25. Kettenbach G. Writing SOAP notes: with patient/client management formats. 3rd edn. Philadelphia, PA: F.A. Davis Company; 2004.

26. Robinson JD, Tate A, Heritage J. Agenda-setting revisited: when and how do primary-care physicians solicit patients' additional concerns? Patient Educ Couns. 2016;99(5):718–23.

27. Braddock CH, 3rd, Edwards KA, Hasenberg NM, Laidley TL, Levinson W. Informed decision making in outpatient practice: time to get back to basics. JAMA. 1999;282(24):2313–20.

28. Heritage J, Robinson JD, Elliott MN, Beckett M, Wilkes M. Reducing patients' unmet concerns in primary care: the difference one word can make. J Gen Intern Med. 2007;22(10):1429–33.

29. Middleton JF, McKinley RK, Gillies CL. Effect of patient completed agenda forms and doctors' education about the agenda on the outcome of consultations: randomized controlled trial. BMJ. 2006;332(7552):1238–42.

30. Rost K, Frankel R. The introduction of the older patient's problems in the medical visit. J Aging Health. 1993;5(3):387–401.

31. White J, Levinson W, Roter D. "Oh, by the way … ": the closing moments of the medical visit. J Gen Intern Med. 1994;9(1):24–8.

32. White JC, Rosson C, Christensen J, Hart R, Levinson W. Wrapping things up: a qualitative analysis of the closing moments of the medical visit. Patient Educ Couns. 1997;30(2):155–65.

33. Roter D, Hall JA. Doctors talking with patients / patients talking with doctors: improving communication in medical visits. Westport, CO: Auburn House; 1992.

34. Barsky AJ, 3rd. Hidden reasons some patients visit doctors. Ann Intern Med. 1981;94(4 pt 1):492–8.

35. Frankel RM. Pets, vets, and frets: what relationship-centered care research has to offer veterinary medicine. J Vet Med Educ. 2006;33(1):20–7.

36. Stein TS, Nagy VT, Jacobs L. Caring for patients one conversation at a time: musings from the interregional clinician patient communication leadership group. Permanente J. 1998;2(4):62–8.

37. Kanji N, Coe JB, Adams CL, Shaw JR. Effect of veterinarian–client–patient interactions on client adherence to dentistry and surgery recommendations in companion-animal practice. J Am Vet Med Assoc. 2012;240(4):427–36.

38. Arborelius E, Bremberg S. What can doctors do to achieve a successful consultation? Videotaped interviews analysed by the 'consultation map' method. Fam Pract. 1992;9(1):61–6.

39. Shilling V, Jenkins V, Fallowfield L. Factors affecting patient and clinician satisfaction with the clinical consultation: can communication skills training for clinicians improve satisfaction?

Psychooncology. 2003;12(6):599–611.

40. Eisenthal S, Lazare A. Evaluation of the initial interview in a walk-in clinic. The patient's perspective on a "customer approach". J Nerv Ment Dis. 1976;162(3):169–76.

41. Eisenthal S, Koopman C, Stoeckle JD. The nature of patients' requests for physicians' help. Acad Med. 1990;65(6):401–5.

42. Korsch BM, Gozzi EK, Francis V. Gaps in doctor–patient communication. 1. Doctor–patient interaction and patient satisfaction. Pediatrics. 1968;42(5):855–71.

43. Larsen KM, Smith CK. Assessment of nonverbal communication in the patient–physician interview. J Fam Pract. 1981;12(3):481–8.

44. DiMatteo MR, Hays RD, Prince LM. Relationship of physicians' nonverbal communication skill to patient satisfaction, appointment noncompliance, and physician workload. Health Psychol. 1986;5(6):581–94.

45. Weinberger M, Greene JY, Mamlin JJ. The impact of clinical encounter events on patient and physician satisfaction. Soc Sci Med E. 1981;15(3):239–44.

46. Griffith CH, 3rd, Wilson JF, Langer S, Haist SA. House staff nonverbal communication skills and standardized patient satisfaction. J Gen Intern Med. 2003;18(3):170–4.

47. Kurtz SM, Silverman J, Draper J, Silverman J. Teaching and learning communication skills in medicine. Second edn. Abingdon: Radcliffe Medical Press; 2005.

48. Inui TS, Yourtee EL, Williamson JW. Improved outcomes in hypertension after physician tutorials. A controlled trial. Ann Intern Med. 1976;84(6):646–51.

49. Maiman LA, Becker MH, Liptak GS, Nazarian LF, Rounds KA. Improving pediatricians' compliance-enhancing practices. A randomized trial. Am J Dis Child. 1988;142(7):773–9.

50. Schulman BA. Active patient orientation and outcomes in hypertensive treatment: application of a socio-organizational perspective. Med Care. 1979;17(3):267–80.

51. Little P, Williamson I, Warner G, Gould C, Gantley M, Kinmonth AL. Open randomized trial of prescribing strategies in managing sore throat. BMJ. 1997;314(7082):722–7.

52. Stewart M, Brown JB, Donner A, McWhinney IR, Oates J, Weston WW, et al. The impact of patient-centered care on outcomes. J Fam Pract. 2000;49(9):796–804.

53. Adamson TE, Bunch WH, Baldwin DC, Jr., Oppenberg A. The virtuous orthopaedist has fewer malpractice suits. Clin Orthop Relat Res. 2000(378):104–9.

54. Levinson W, Roter DL, Mullooly JP, Dull VT, Frankel RM. Physician–patient communication. The relationship with malpractice claims among primary care physicians and surgeons. JAMA. 1997;277(7):553–9.

55. Six steps to higher-quality patient care. In: Association AAH, editor. Lakewood, CO2009.

56. The path to high-quality care. Practical tips for improving compliance. In: Association AAH, editor. Lakewood, CO2003.

57. Coe JB, Adams CL, Bonnett BN. Prevalence and nature of cost discussions during clinical appointments in companion animal practice. J Am Vet Med Assoc. 2009;234(11):1418–24.

58. Lue TW, Pantenburg DP, Crawford PM. Impact of the owner–pet and client–veterinarian bond on the care that pets receive. J Am Vet Med Assoc. 2008;232(4):531–40.

59. Shaw JR, Adams CL, Bonnett BN, Larson S, Roter DL. Use of the Roter interaction analysis system to analyse veterinarian-client-patient communication in companion animal practice. J Am Vet Med Assoc. 2004;225(2):222–9.

60. Shaw JR, Adams CL, Bonnett BN, Larson S, Roter DL. Veterinarian–client–patient communication during wellness appointments versus appointments related to a health problem in companion animal practice. J Am Vet Med Assoc. 2008;233(10):1576–86.

61. Shaw JR, Bonnett BN, Adams CL, Roter DL. Veterinarian–client–patient communication patterns used during clinical appointments in companion animal practice. J Am Vet Med Assoc. 2006;228(5):714–21.

62. Coe JB, Adams CL, Bonnett BN. A focus group study of veterinarians' and pet owners' perceptions of veterinarian–client communication in companion animal practice. J Am Vet Med Assoc. 2008;233(7):1072–80.

63. Marvel MK, Epstein RM, Flowers K, Beckman HB. Soliciting the patient's agenda: have we improved? JAMA. 1999;281(3):283–7.

64. Ospina NS, Phillips KA, Rodriguez-Gutierrez R, Castaneda-Guarderas A, Gionfriddo MR, Branda ME, et al. Eliciting the patient's agenda – secondary analysis of recorded clinical encounters. JGIM. 2019;34(1):36–40.

65. Langewitz W, Denz M, Keller A, Kiss A, Ruttimann S, Wossmer B. Spontaneous talking time at start of consultation in outpatient clinic: cohort study. BMJ. 2002;325(7366):682–3.

66. Shaw JR. Four core communication skills of highly effective practitioners. Vet Clin North Am Small Anim Pract. 2006;36(2):385–96, vii.

67. Boyd EA. Bureaucratic authority in the "company of equals": the interactional management of medical peer. Am Sociol Rev. 1998;63(2):200–24.

68. Chester EC, Robinson NC, Roberts LC. Opening clinical encounters in an adult musculoskeletal setting. Manual Ther. 2014;19(4):306–10.

69. Zandbelt LC, Smets EMA, Oort FJ, de Haes HCJM. Coding patient-centred behaviour in the medical encounter. Soc Sci Med. 2005;61(3):661–71.

70. Show A, Englar RE. Evaluating dog and cat owner preferences for Calgary–Cambridge communication skills: results of a questionnaire. J Vet Med Educ. 2018:1–10.

71. Robinson JD. Soliciting patients' presenting concerns. In: Heritage J, Maynard D, editors. Communication in medical care: interactions between primary care physicians and patients. New York: Cambridge University Press; 2006. pp. 23–47.

72. Englar RE, Williams M, Weingand K. Applicability of the Calgary–Cambridge Guide to dog and cat owners for teaching veterinary clinical communications. J Vet Med Educ. 2016;43(2):143–69.

73. Kurtz SM, Silverman JD, Draper J. Teaching and learning communication skills in medicine. Grand Rapids, MI: Radcliffe; 2004.

74. Adams CL, Kurtz SM. Skills for communicating in veterinary medicine. Oxford: Otmoor Publishing and Dewpoint Publishing; 2017.

75. Silverman J, Kurtz S, Draper J. Skills for communicating with patients. Oxford: Radcliffe Medical Press; 2008.

76. Dysart LM, Coe JB, Adams CL. Analysis of solicitation of client concerns in companion animal practice. J Am Vet Med Assoc. 2011;238(12):1609–15.

77. Hunter L, Shaw JR. What's in your communication toolbox? Exceptional Veterinary Team. 2012(November/December):12–7.

78. Roter DL, Hall JA. Physician's interviewing styles and medical information obtained from patients. J Gen Intern Med. 1987;2(5):325–9.

Chapter 9

Defining Supplemental Communication Skills

Reducing Medical Jargon

Both inside and outside of the lecture hall, student doctors invest a significant portion of their time in learning how to communicate with other members of the healthcare team. Their introduction and orientation to medical jargon begins in foundational science coursework, such as anatomy and physiology, and continues well into clinical rotations.

So, it is that the student doctor who misidentifies a patient's diagnostic test as an *X-ray* in lieu of the proper term, *radiograph*, is called out in front of his classmates. The student doctor quickly learns that to fit in – to walk the walk – you must talk the talk in so-called doctor-speak.

This intense concentration on medical terminology presents an obstacle to the student doctor when he or she transitions into clinical practice. He or she should, but does not always consider, that which he or she needs to convey to the client and how to translate it into more relatable terms:

> As final year medical students we often fall into the trap of absorbing medical lingo without fully appreciating the effects of such phrases on patients.(1)

Throughout their training, student doctors are warned about the use of jargon in the wards.(2) They are specifically instructed to limit their use of medical terms with patients so as to avoid misunderstandings and misinterpretations.(2)

However, the message to use easy-to-understand language with clientele often falls upon deaf ears. Student doctors are likely to forget that patients may not always understand medical vocabulary. Some unintentionally reference medical terminology without even recognizing that its use may lead to confusion. Others use medical jargon intentionally, overestimating how much of it their patients comprehend.(3)

In addition to doctors-in-training, residents, and new graduates are likely to rely upon medical jargon to convey information to their patients.(4) Medical terminology is frequently employed in conversations with patients about healthcare, yet such terms are often poorly understood by those without a medical background.(4, 5)

Comprehension deficits are a significant concern in the healthcare industry because they complicate patient care and case outcomes.(6) Effective clinical communication correlates with patient understanding, satisfaction, recall, compliance, and adherence to physician-directed instructions.(6–14) To be successful, communication must be derived from shared vocabulary and common experiences.(6, 15–18)

When shared vocabulary is absent from conversation, patients are forced to interpret physician statements and directives based upon past experiences and prior knowledge. Patients who lack these are more likely to misunderstand the information that has been presented to them and/or misinterpret results. These patients are more likely to experience anxiety, confusion, or fear.(3, 19)

9.1 Defining Medical Jargon

Medical language is a form of jargon, that is, vocabulary that is unique to and shared by a particular group or profession, in this case, healthcare providers.(2, 3, 6, 19, 20) Mechanics have their own lingo, as do plumbers and electricians and any other group of individuals that collectively comes together to learn and practice a trade. Is it any surprise that doctors share their own language? This language is an attempt to standardize terms within the context of healthcare so that there is universal understanding among providers.(21)

Medical jargon includes key terms and phrases, including abbreviations, in order to communicate information about the following:(4)

- diagnostic testing – for example, EKG or ECG (electrocardiogram)
- diagnosis – for example, apnea, GERD (gastroesophageal reflux disease)
- patient-specific instructions – for example, NPO (nothing per os)
- prognosis – for example, terminal, cure, remission
- procedural actions – for example, intubate, extubate, catheterize
- recommendations for medical interventions – for example, Rx (prescription)
- recommendations for surgical intervention and discussion of surgical anatomy – for example, tonsillectomy, turbinates.

The purpose of medical jargon is to promote shared understanding among those who are familiar with it.(20) In that sense, it may be considered as a type of professional short-hand that, in theory, improves efficiency of correspondence between healthcare teams while reducing redundancy.(20)

9.2 The Limitations of Medical Jargon: the Provider's Perspective

Although its use may be viewed as professional by team members, medical jargon can become a barrier to communication for doctors and patients alike.

Consider potential limitations from the perspective of the healthcare provider. Most doctors have a poor understanding of the Latin language, from which much of medical jargon is derived.(4, 22) New generations of physicians are no longer expected to be trained in Latin.(4, 22) This has the potential to complicate interprofessional communication in healthcare.

9.2.1 The Challenges Associated with Medical Abbreviations

Shorthand terms that were developed to promote patient safety may in fact jeopardize patient health. Consider, for example, the abbreviations QD and QOD.

- QD stems from the Latin, *quaque die*, and is translated to mean each or every day, as in: take this medication daily.
- QOD stems from the Latin, *quaque altera die*, and is translated to mean every other day, as in: take this medication every other day.

There are many variations on instructions for prescription taking, including SID, BID, TID, and QID.

- SID stems from the Latin, *semil in die*, and is translated to mean once a day, as in: take this medication once daily.
- BID stems from the Latin, *bis in die*, and is translated to mean two times a day, as in: take this medication twice daily, or every 12 hours.
- TID stems from the Latin, *ter in die*, and is translated to mean three times a day, as in: take this medication three times a day, or every 8 hours.
- QID stems from the Latin, *quater in die*, and is translated to mean four times a day, as in: take this medication four times a day, or every 6 hours.

Abbreviations for anatomic regions have also historically been used to document clinical findings in the medical record or to provide detailed instructions for the topical administration of a prescribed medication.(23) Consider, for instance, the following.(23)

- AD stems from the Latin, *auris dextra* or *auris dexter*, and is translated to mean the right ear.
- AS stems from the Latin, *auris sinistra* or *auris sinister*, and is translated to mean the left ear.
- AU stems from the Latin, *auris uterque*, and is translated to mean both ears.
- OD stems from the Latin, *oculus dextra* or *oculus dexter*, and is translated to mean the right eye.
- OS stems from the Latin, *oculus sinistra* or *oculus sinister*, and is translated to mean the left eye.
- OU stems from the Latin, *oculus uterque*, and is translated to mean both eyes.

When these Latin terms are understood as they were intended, instructions for prescription taking are clear and concise. Their use has also been promoted as being both space saving (on the medical record) and time efficient.(22, 24, 25)

However, lack of familiarity with terms and their intended meanings makes these abbreviations error prone.(24) This is concerning because misinterpretations of written prescriptions all too easily may result in medication errors, both in terms of pharmacy dispensing and patient administering.(24)

The prevalence of error-prone abbreviations in medical charting for human healthcare has been reported to range from 8.4% (in Australia) to 30–33% (in the United States). (24, 26–28)

When they occur, errors may be minor or catastrophic.(24) For example, if the 'u' for unit is mistaken for a zero, then patients are at risk of experiencing a 10-fold overdose of a medication such as insulin.(24, 29)

9.2.2 The Changing Face of Healthcare

In addition to the challenges that are posed by medical abbreviations, the face of healthcare is changing.(21) Worldwide, there is increased emphasis in interprofessional collaboration. Moreover, there is an increase in multilingual healthcare environments in which medical language proficiency is assumed, but not always realized.(21) Proficiency with language implies that the speaker is articulate, that is, she or he is able to express opinions and ideas readily, without first having to translate it in writing or speech.(21)

Safe practice of medicine assumes that team members are linguistically competent; however, the team is constantly challenged by accents, dialects, idioms, and euphemisms.(21) Emphasis on the incorrect syllable can alter the meaning of a word or phrase significantly.(21) For example, the common word for excrement, *feces*, could sound much like *facies*, the word for facial expression, were it spoken with a thick accent. (21) When used in dialogue, in context, miscommunication between team members is less likely to occur.(21) However, communication may be jeopardized during critical situations when timely understanding is essential.(21) There is great potential for misunderstanding verbal orders.(21) When listeners are confused by what they hear, they are subject to errors in interpretation.(21, 30) Such errors could adversely impact case outcomes and patient health.(21, 30)

There are also regional differences in medical jargon that can compound the challenges associated with language comprehension. For example, a Canadian physician might not recognize the American term, *sonogram*. However, the Canadian physician is familiar with the synonymous term, *ultrasound*.(21)

In the UK, there is no talk of frequenting the *ER* – the emergency room – among human medical patients. Instead, patients discuss going to *A&E* – accident and emergency.(21) Likewise, the British equate *surgery* with a doctor's office.(21) Yet when an American says that she or he is going to *surgery*, they are referring a surgical procedure or operation.(21)

In the accounting office, NKA refers to no known address, whereas among healthcare providers, NKA refers to no known allergies.(21)

Jargon may be particularly confusing in the emergency room. In the United States, *call a code* is standard for announcing an emergency so that the healthcare team expedites care stat.(21) Specifically, *code blue* refers to either cardiac or respiratory arrest. (21) That terminology may hold little meaning for physicians of non-English speaking backgrounds.(21)

Similarly, Canadian and American medical and nursing associations routinely make use of terms such as *adverse events* or *near misses* when describing medical errors. An *adverse event* is a situation in which harm is caused to a patient unintentionally, whereas a *near miss* is a situation in which the patient would have been harmed had the risk not been identified and mitigated.(21) Both terms may hold little meaning for non-native speakers of the English language.(21)

9.3 The Limitations of Medical Jargon: the Patient's Perspective

If speaking with one another may be sufficiently challenging for healthcare providers, is it any surprise that patients might equally be at a loss to understand medical jargon? Consultations are subject to miscommunication and misinterpretation.(3) In fact, communication failures between doctors and patients may be more common than we think.

Communication failures are concerning because they adversely impact patient health, patient safety, and case outcomes.(3) If patients do not have a working knowledge of their medical predicaments, then they are unlikely to understand medical or surgical interventions.(3, 31) If they do not understand medical or surgical interventions, then they will exhibit decreased compliance and adherence to prescribed treatments.(3, 9, 13, 32–35)

9.3.1 Poor Working Knowledge of Anatomy

Providers often make erroneous assumptions about their patients' working knowledge of health and disease. They may incorrectly assume that patients understand basic human anatomy.(36) Studies from the 1960s through 1980s demonstrate poor understanding of body architecture among the general public, including the location of key body organs. (36–38)

In 1961, Samora et al. evaluated hospital patient understanding – and misinterpretation – of medical vocabulary. It became evident from their research that patients often did not comprehend anatomical terms. Consider, for instance, the question that a physician might ask of an inpatient: "Do you have a pain in the abdomen?" (39) Respondents indicated in the affirmative, but proceeded to describe pain in the following locations:(39)

- back
- buttocks

- heart
- sides
- urinary bladder
- uterus.

Others indicated, by their responses, that they believed the abdomen to be any portion of the body below the waist.(39)

When the same participants were asked to consider an appendectomy, it became clear that there was marked confusion about the term itself.(39) Definitions for appendectomy ranged from broad ("sickness" or "pain") to specific, yet inaccurate, and often pertaining to the wrong organ:(39)

- cut rectum
- the stomach
- something to do with the bowels
- something contagious
- something like an epidemic
- taking off an arm or leg.

Participants were equally at a loss to define the word, *nerve*. Definitions that they provided included:(39)

- arteries
- blood vessels
- something that feeds the blood
- something that goes to the heart
- something like a pink worm
- something like tissue in the body
- nervousness.

The process of *digestion* was equally difficult to define. Participants were unclear which aspect digestion referred to when they were asked by physicians, "How is your digestion?" Digestion was interpreted as meaning very different processes, including:(39)

- deglutition
- eructation
- food settling in the stomach
- normal passage of bowels
- constipation.

Participants answered the question based upon their interpretation of the question, which may or may not have been what the physician was intending to query.

Just over two decades later, in 1982, anatomy and anatomical processes remained a mystery to the general public. For example, only 12% of patients with gastrointestinal disease could correctly identify the location of the affected organ(s).(38)

A more recent study was conducted in 2014 to evaluate if baseline knowledge of anatomy among the general public had changed.(36) Ramanayake et al. provided questionnaire participants with a line diagram of the human body. Participants were asked to mark the location of the following organs:

- brain
- heart
- kidney
- liver
- lungs
- ovaries
- stomach
- thyroid gland
- urinary bladder
- uterus.

As compared to previous studies, these results were encouraging: 90% of participants could accurately locate half of the organs listed, and 50% could identify eight or more. (36) This performance is encouraging. It is thought to reflect curricular changes, namely the teaching of health science in grade school, as well as more widespread patient access to media, particularly the internet.(36)

However, it is important to recognize that not all patients share this foundation of scientific knowledge. The liver, kidney, and thyroid are the least identifiable organs by the general public, particularly among those with limited education.(36) Doctors should not assume that patients understand organs, organ locations, or organ functions.(36)

9.3.2 Poor Working Knowledge of Medical Pairs

Doctors should also not assume that patients understand medical pairs of words as being synonymous.(4, 40) A 2000 study by Lerner et al. evaluated patient understanding in an emergency setting and established that:(40)

- 79% of patients did not recognize that bleeding and hemorrhage were equivalent
- 78% of patients did not recognize that broken bone and fracture were equivalent
- 74% of patients did not recognize that heart attack and myocardial infarction were equivalent
- 38% of patients did not recognize that stitches and suture were equivalent
- 37% of patients did not recognize that loose stools and diarrhea were equivalent.

It is possible that the emergency nature of these clinical consultations impaired patient understanding. That is, it is possible that patients' emotional states altered their ability to comprehend that which is considered basic working knowledge of health and disease by physicians.

However, there are plenty of other examples in non-emergency settings that suggest otherwise. Consider, for instance, that oncology patients are frequently confused about the following terms:(3, 41–43)

- benign
- malignant
- metastasis
- palliative care
- remission
- tumor.

9.3.3 Poor Understanding of Basic Principles of Oncology

Oncology patients may be confused about the roles of various healthcare providers in their care, including the oncologist, pathologist, radiologist, and surgeon.(43)

Cancer patients may not grasp the various types of imaging that are essential for diagnosis and monitoring of treatment progress. For example, they may balk at terms such as mammogram, ultrasound scan, and magnetic resonance imaging (MRI).(43) They may not understand the advantages and/or the limitations of each technique, or why one modality is preferred over another.

It is equally challenging for many patients to understand the differences in treatment options, such as chemotherapy versus radiation.(43)

Radiation therapy (RT) patients are especially challenged to comprehend the following key terms that relate to their treatment modality:(19)

- beam
- dose
- electrons
- episode
- radiation
- seeds.

RT patients may have poor understanding of adverse side effects. They may not know what fatigue, nausea, and/or voiding means.(19)

9.3.4 Poor Understanding of Other Medical Disciplines

Cancer patients are not the only ones who struggle to comprehend medical jargon. In orthopedics, there is confusion over cast versus splint.(4, 40)

Other medical disciplines that have been shown to experience comprehension deficits include:(6, 44)

- anesthesiology – examples of challenging jargon: intubation, paresthesia, pulse oximetry (pulse ox), NPO
- cardiology – example of challenging jargon: myocardial infarction (MI)
- dentistry – examples of challenging jargon: fracture, mandible, occlusion, impacted tooth, temporomandibular joint (TMJ)
- gastroenterology – example of challenging jargon: GERD
- internal medicine – examples of challenging jargon: dialysis, hypertension.

Medical jargon challenges patient understanding of diagnoses, diagnostic procedures, and procedural actions. What patients do not comprehend, they often fear.(3, 19)

9.3.5 Poor Interpretation of Physician Recommendations

Patients are also likely to misinterpret therapeutic instructions.(45) Although more current studies are needed, a 1966 questionnaire by Riley highlighted key areas of disagreement between what physicians recommended and what patients heard. For example, the survey asked the following questions of patients:(45)

- "If the doctor told you to *avoid starch and sugar*, which of the following foods would you avoid?" – 38% of participants would not avoid crackers or prunes
- "If told to cut down your intake of salt as much as possible, would you …" – only 19% of participants would stop adding salt in food preparation
- "If told to *avoid solid foods* for 48 hours, would you …" – 37% of participants would eat semi-solid foods like egg or custard
- "If told to *avoid fatty foods*, which of the following foods would you avoid?" – 73% of participants would continue to eat sirloin, even knowing that it is estimated to contain 20% fat.

9.3.6 Poor Understanding of Symptom Management

Medical jargon may also lead to difficulties with symptom management.(46) If patients do not understand what medications they are taking, then what is their interest in taking them correctly or taking them at all? (46) This is particularly of concern in patients with chronic disease and/or concurrent conditions:

Patients and family members must coordinate medications among multiple providers, across inpatient and outpatient settings, and manage the integration of new prescriptions among existing regimens when new symptoms arise. (46)

This coordination of healthcare requires effective communication by the entire team. When communication flounders, the patient and his or her family are unable to make educated decisions about regimens.(46, 47) When regimens involve pain management, analgesic needs are unlikely to be met.(46, 48, 49) Medication errors are also more likely.(46, 50)

Compounding this issue is that many medication names are not explained in combination with the symptom for which they are intended to manage.(46, 51) Patients need to be told not only what medications they are taking, but why each is essential.(46) For example, patients should be told that senna is for management of constipation; amitriptyline is for management of nerve pain; and lorazepam is for management of anxiety. (46) Pairing each drug's name with its function, in plain language, should facilitate compliance, adherence, and high-quality symptom management.(46)

Providing written documentation may also facilitate patient comprehension. Physicians overestimate how much patients are able to recall following a consultation. Physicians also tend to overestimate just how much jargon patients can absorb and understand.(52) This is particularly concerning because when patients do not understand the content of clinical conversations, they may be reluctant to ask for clarification.(14) They may fear being judged by the medical team.(14) They may also want to save face so as not to appear ignorant.(14)

9.4 Easy-to-Understand Language Implies Transparency

Patients desire easy-to-understand language.(52–54) When language is complicated by jargon, patients question the veracity of information that is shared with them by providers.(52) In particular, parents of pediatric patients equate jargon with avoidance: they perceive that pediatricians use jargon to prevent parents from asking too many questions about topics that they would rather not discuss.(52, 54, 55) When parents do not feel that their concerns are being addressed or when they do not understand the situation for which their child presents, they may even go so far as to believe that the healthcare team is hiding something.(52)

Transparency is an essential part of trust, and trust is the building block of an effective doctor–patient relationship. When trust in the relationship breaks down, the relationship may be difficult to repair or rebuild. To prevent this issue of corrosion, patients want their doctors to "speak in terms that I can understand." (56) The physician that successfully acknowledges and validates patient concerns while using easy-to-understand language is seen as both compassionate and professional.(56)

9.5 Implications for the Veterinary Medical Profession

Human healthcare is leading the charge in medical literature when it comes to investigating and reporting the consequences of jargon in clinical consultations. Veterinary-specific studies are desperately needed to answer the following questions that are relevant to the comprehension and satisfaction of our clientele.

- What is considered plain language versus jargon?
  - What is commonly understood by the general public?
  - Which terms do we think are easy to understand, but in actuality are not?
  - Which explanations require additional clarification?
- How does the use of jargon impact the doctor–client–patient relationship?
- How does the use of jargon impact patient care?

It is likely that many of the same issues that face human healthcare providers also impact us as veterinarians. Consider, for example, the following surgical procedures that are routinely performed in companion animal practice:

- anastomosis
- castration ("neuter")
- cystotomy
- dental extraction
- enterotomy
- foreign body removal
- gastropexy
- gastrotomy
- laparotomy
- onychectomy ("declaw")
- ovariectomy
- ovariohysterectomy ("spay").

These terms are part of our everyday working knowledge, but are they clear to our clientele? If these terms appear on estimates, do our clients truly understand their meaning?

I would argue that, more often than not, clients are not fully made aware of key details that may impact the way in which they view a particular procedure. Consider, for instance, onychectomy, a surgical procedure that is still being performed in parts of the United States. This procedure is often referred to as "declawing." Few clients appreciate this procedure for what it is: surgical amputation of the most distal digit, the third phalanx. If our clients were better informed, would they still request it? Some would; some would not.

9.5.1 The Impact of Phraseology

The way we package medical terms – and our euphemisms for them – impacts our clients' response and acceptance of them as commonplace.

We have a tendency in practice to soften procedural names so that they do not appear to be too "clinical." We prefer to say "put to sleep" instead of "euthanize." Yet, while "put to sleep" is easy-to-understand language that sounds gentle and kind, it can be misconstrued.(14) Young children who hear this phrase may erroneously believe that the "put-to-sleep" patient can one day wake up.(14) Alternatively, they may develop a fear of bedtime, for fear that they, too, may be "put to sleep."

How do we know when language is easy to understand and clear, or concise, but not guarded or cold? How do we know when our meaning has been correctly conveyed and understood? How do we know when miscommunication or misinterpretation happens? How often does either occur? What is their impact on our patients and clinical outcomes?

The burden falls upon us as a profession to establish a working vocabulary that is both reasonable and consistent.

9.5.2 Easy-to-Understand Language is Not About "Dumbing it Down"

Sometimes, veterinary students wrongly equate the use of easy-to-understand language with "dumbing it down," as if our clients are uneducated and/or cannot handle the level of language proficiency that we expect of ourselves. Be cautious about taking on this view of the consultation.

It is critical to our success as a profession that we recognize our clients are not dumb. Even if they do not understand medical vocabulary, that does not mean they are uneducated. We have to put ourselves in their shoes. After all, we were in their shoes not all that long ago.

It is therefore our responsibility to make consultations clear and easy to follow. I would expect the same if I were the client of a mechanic. I don't know "car talk," so I need a clear explanation each time, every time that I am having auto trouble.

Our clients deserve the same from us.

9.5.3 Easy-to-Understand Language is Not About "Baby Talk"

Replacing medical jargon with easy to understand language represents a fine balance between respect and condescension. Our clients do not want us to talk over their heads. At the same time, our clients do not want to be talked at like toddlers; they want to be talked to as adults.

In order not to sound juvenile, avoid using the following words in the consultation:

- tummy – as in, "Your dog's tummy hurts"
- ouchy – as in, "Your dog's leg seems ouchy today."

Instead, ask if his stomach hurts, or comment that his leg seems painful.

Remember: you are the professional in the examination room. So, aim to be conversational, not condescending.

9.6 Strategies for Overcoming the Use of Medical Jargon

Using medical jargon is the default mode for veterinarians because it is how we talk to one another. However, the only way that we can accomplish care for our patient is to reach out and connect with the client.

Clients rely upon us to simplify medical details so that they are on the same page as us. Easy to understand language is an essential communication tool because it ensures mutual understanding.

If we fail to make use of this tool, then we run the risk of losing our client. The client may not know what we are saying. The client may even consent to something that she or he does not fully understand. Even worse, the client may decline treatment because of lack of understanding.

To avoid these failures of patient care, consider the way in which we speak to our clients.

9.6.1 Engage in Conversation, Not Dictation

Replace jargon with a conversational approach to the consult.

Do not think about the consultation as being a conversation between a veterinarian (the expert) and a client (the novice). Think about this as a consult between two people, on equal footing. Meet the client at his or her level; don't ask the client to rise to meet you at yours.

Aim to speak at a 5th grade (10–11 year old) reading level. Use words that you would find in the newspaper, such as *USA Today* or the *Daily Mail*, or any comparable chronicle. Doing so will assist with the flow of conversation and the likelihood that you and the client will be on the same page.

9.6.2 Convert Medical Jargon into Plain Language When Possible

Medical jargon is not always necessary. Consider the following scenario.

> You are an associate veterinarian in clinical practice. A 3-month-old unvaccinated puppy presents to you for evaluation of acute onset of bloody diarrhea.

After examining the patient, you are concerned that the dog has contracted parvovirus. When you mention the name of this infectious disease, your client asks an appropriate follow-up question: "What is that?"

There are several ways to answer this question. The least appropriate answer would be to launch into a textbook definition, such as:

Parvovirus is a non-enveloped, single-stranded DNA virus that affects dogs, wolves, and foxes. It can even affect cats. Pups that are not protected by maternal antibodies and dogs that are not protected by vaccination are exposed when they ingest infected feces or soil. We can also act as fomites if we handle infected material and then come into contact with a naïve dog. Once the virus is ingested, it replicates in lymphoid tissue before travelling in the bloodstream to the intestinal crypts. Here, it prevents absorption of food. Diarrhea results. Secondary bacterial infection is common and sepsis can result. There is a high mortality rate if we do not treat the infection.

Student doctors are often trained to memorize this level of detail and regurgitate it for examinations. However, this amount of detail is inappropriate for the average client. Although it may showcase our knowledge, it does very little to answer the client's question. The client likely is most interested in how the disease will affect the patient's health and longevity. The client may wonder how the dog acquired the infection; however, the exact circumstances surrounding viral pathophysiology are likely inconsequential. The client needs to know why the dog is sick, how the virus will affect the dog, and how you propose to medically manage the patient.

Instead of spitting out facts for the sake of sharing facts, be selective with what you share. Consider how you might substitute jargon for plain language.(42) You might begin to answer the client's query with the following statement:

Parvo is a virus that attacks the intestines. The intestines are made up of cells that absorb food once it is broken down into very tiny pieces. Parvo makes those cells sick so that they can't do their job. Now food isn't absorbed and comes out the other end as diarrhea. Are you with me so far?

This is more appropriate as a clinical conversation because it addresses the presumptive diagnosis without losing the client in jargon. Parvovirus is explained to the client using a simplistic approach that correlates the clinical sign of diarrhea with how the virus impacts the body.

The veterinarian even goes a step further and checks in with the client: is there mutual understanding or did the client get lost in the explanation? The check-in gives the client the opportunity to ask for clarification in the event that what the veterinarian shared was not understood.

Additional information about the communication skill of checking in will be covered in Chapter 15.

Other circumstances in which jargon is not necessary include conversations about clinical signs. Unless the client is in the medical field, a description of clinical signs using jargon is obstructive to the flow of conversation. For instance, you would not ask the client, "Is your dog exhibiting hematuria?" Instead, you'd ask if the client had noticed bloody urine.

Similarly, trade out the following medical terms for more ordinary descriptors:

- dyschezia
  - difficulty with bowel movements
  - difficulty passing stool
- dysuria
  - difficulty with urination
- epistaxis
  - nose bleed
- hematochezia
  - bloody stool
  - blood in feces
- hematemesis
  - bloody vomit
- stranguria
  - straining to urinate
- tenesmus
  - straining to defecate
  - straining to have a bowel movement
- voiding
  - urinating or defecating
  - peeing or pooping.

9.6.3 Explain Jargon When Used

Sometimes, medical jargon is essential and cannot be trimmed. Consider, for instance, the following diagnostic tests:

- complete blood count (CBC)
- chemistry panel
- computed tomography (CT) scan
- echocardiogram
- EKG or ECG
- fecal analysis
- MRI
- urinalysis (UA).

It is important that you be clear about which kind of test(s) are outlined in your recommendations.

However, in these situations, it is your responsibility to follow up with an easy-to-understand explanation so that any jargon that has been used is made clear. For example, you might suggest that you run a CBC to look for concerning changes in the patient's red or white blood cell count. You may go on to explain that white blood cells are often increased in number in the face of an infection.

Being clear about why a test is needed helps clients to understand the value of the diagnostic procedure. For example, if an estimate just lists UA without any explanation as to why this diagnostic test is deemed necessary, then the client may be inclined to decline this test if that is an option. Instead, share your reasoning with the client as to why each diagnostic test is essential. In a patient that is undergoing preanesthetic screening, you might explain that the UA is going to detect any changes in kidney function before they are detectable on bloodwork. Kidney function is essential because the drugs that you are planning to use to anesthetize the patient must be broken down by the kidneys in order for the patient to recover from anesthesia.

9.6.4 Assess the Client's Knowledge

Not all clients come to us with the same background information. Clients' past experiences shape their worldview. Some clients may be more experienced than others when it comes to routine healthcare, wellness, and preventive medicine by virtue of having had cats and dogs as pets before. These clients may already be familiar with heartworm disease (HWD) or vaccination protocols, so they need less introductory material. Instead, they may need refreshers or reminders about key take-away messages.

Some clients may have never owned a cat or dog before. These clients benefit from starting at the very beginning of patient care. What may seem obvious to me or you may not be so obvious to them. For example, clients that have previously owned outdoor-only cats may not have any concept of environmental enrichment for indoor-only cats.

Other clients may be well versed in certain disease states because they have personal experience managing that particular disease. Maybe a previous pet had diabetes mellitus, so they are familiar with blood glucose regulation and insulin injections. Maybe they themselves are diabetic and can extrapolate from their own health how being diabetic may impact the quality of their pet's life. In either case, these clients are unique in that they do not require an elementary lesson on diabetic lifestyle and disease management. We benefit instead by assessing their knowledge base so that we know what an appropriate starting point is for us to begin our clinical conversation.

It is appropriate to assess your client's knowledge every time that a diagnosis is made. Consider the following phrases that assist us with this communication skill.

- "Are you familiar with [insert disease name]?"
- "Did you know that cats could get [insert disease name]?"
- "What do you know about [insert disease name]?"
- "What is your experience managing [insert disease name] in cats?"

In addition to providing us with a starting point for clinical conversations, assessing out client's knowledge also allows us to check our client's knowledge against our own.

Maybe the client thinks that she or he is aware of something, but is not. Maybe the client thinks she or he knows more about something than she or he actually does. Maybe the client has incorrect or misguided information that requires correction.

Assessing our client's knowledge is an important communication skill that will be discussed at length in Chapter 13 of this text.

9.6.5 Translating Medical Documents

Student doctors of human healthcare can improve their communication skills by being asked to translate medical documents into plain language.(57) Veterinary students can benefit from the same tasks. Veterinary educators might consider asking students to review laboratory data, surgical notes, or radiographic reports and consider how they might relay the contents to their client. Role play may be of benefit so that students gain practice with word choice and the particular phrasing of their explanations.

In one teaching hospital, student doctors of human healthcare were asked to formulate letters to patients.(58) Patients were subsequently asked to review the letters and to underline any portion that they did not understand.(58) These portions included:(58)

- offensive statements
- medical jargon
- vague recommendations
- grammatical and/or spelling errors
- incorrect statements
- displays of obsequiousness.

Family medicine experts were also asked to perform the same evaluation of student letters.

Patients underlined phrases in 86 of 108 (79.6%) letters.(58) On average, 7.1% of text per letter was underlined.(58) Patients primarily underlined portions that were unclear because the phraseology was deemed too technical.(58) Family medicine experts underlined three times as many words and phrases as patients.(58)

The experience of letter-writing was thought to sensitize students to the need to improve clarity doctor-patient dialogue.(57) By having the patient weigh in on the student's use of jargon, the student could experience first hand what the patient felt like to be on the receiving end of his or her report. In this way, feedback was both relevant and personal. In theory, students could learn how to more effectively approach partnership with patients through the use of easy-to-understand language. At the same time, students could learn how the use of certain words or phrases impacted their patients for better or worse.

To the author's knowledge, this educational tool has not yet been studied in American colleges of veterinary medicine. However, any correspondence between students and clients that grants the opportunity for feedback in a safe, supportive environment has the potential to benefit learning. Students need assistance in discovering which words and phrases are unclear, and how to modify them to improve clarity of doctor–client dialogue.

Students may also be encouraged to invite feedback from their clients directly, through check-ins. However, clients may not be as willing, face-to-face, to acknowledge that they did not understand something. Therefore, students should be encouraged to engage with clients whenever and wherever possible. The more they practice clinical conversations, the more likely they will be to come across as relatable and knowledgeable, without sounding like a medical encyclopedia.

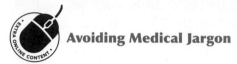 **Avoiding Medical Jargon**

References

1. Taylor A, Cantlay A, Patel S, Braithwaite B. Type two "endoleak": medical jargon that causes significant anxiety in patients. Eur J Vasc Endovasc Surg. 2011;42:851–2.
2. Fields AM, Freiberg CS, Fickenscher A, Shelley KH. Patients and jargon: are we speaking the same language? J Clin Anesth. 2008;20(5):343–6.
3. LeBlanc TW, Hesson A, Williams A, Feudtner C, Holmes-Rovner M, Williamson LD, et al. Patient understanding of medical jargon: a survey study of U.S. medical students. Patient Educ Couns. 2014;95(2):238–42.
4. Sevinc A, Buyukberber S, Camci C. Medical jargon: obstacle to effective communication between physicians and patients. Med Princ Pract. 2005;14(4):292.
5. Nikumb VB, Banerjee A, Kaur G, Chaudhury S. Impact of doctor–patient communication on pre-operative anxiety: Study at industrial township, Pimpri, Pune. Ind Psychiatry J. 2009;18(1):19–21.
6. Castro CM, Wilson C, Wang F, Schillinger D. Babel babble: physicians' use of unclarified medical jargon with patients. Am J Health Behav. 2007;31 Suppl 1:S85–95.
7. Hadlow J, Pitts M. The understanding of common health terms by doctors, nurses and patients. Soc Sci Med. 1991;32(2):193–6.
8. Heisler M, Bouknight RR, Hayward RA, Smith DM, Kerr EA. The relative importance of physician communication, participatory decision making, and patient understanding in diabetes self-management. J Gen Intern Med. 2002;17(4):243–52.
9. Ong LM, Visser MR, Lammes FB, de Haes JC. Doctor–patient communication and cancer patients' quality of life and satisfaction. Patient Educ Couns. 2000;41(2):145–56.
10. Piette JD, Schillinger D, Potter MB, Heisler M. Dimensions of patient–provider communication and diabetes self-care in an ethnically diverse population. J Gen Intern Med. 2003;18(8):624–33.
11. Silverman J, Kurtz S, Draper J. Skills for communicating with patients. Oxford: Radcliffe Medical Press; 2008.
12. Stewart M, Brown JB, Boon H, Galajda J, Meredith L, Sangster M. Evidence on patient–doctor communication. Cancer Prev Control. 1999;3(1):25–30.
13. Stewart MA. Effective physician–patient communication and health outcomes: a review. CMAJ. 1995;152(9):1423–33.

14. Adams CL, Kurtz SM. Skills for communicating in veterinary medicine. Oxford: Otmoor Publishing and Dewpoint Publishing; 2017.

15. Chapple A, Campion P, May C. Clinical terminology: anxiety and confusion among families undergoing genetic counseling. Patient Educ Couns. 1997;32(1–2):81–91.

16. Doak CC, Doak LG, Friedell GH, Meade CD. Improving comprehension for cancer patients with low literacy skills: strategies for clinicians. CA Cancer J Clin. 1998;48(3):151–62.

17. Doak CC, Doak LG, Root JH. Teaching patients with low literacy skills. Philadelphia, PA: Lippincott; 1996.

18. Weiner MF, Lovitt R. An examination of patients' understanding of information from health care providers. Hosp Community Psychiatry. 1984;35(6):619–20.

19. Schnitzler L, Smith SK, Shepherd HL, Shaw J, Dong S, Carpenter DM, et al. Communication during radiation therapy education sessions: the role of medical jargon and emotional support in clarifying patient confusion. Patient Educ Couns. 2017;100(1):112–20.

20. Subramaniam R, Sanjeev R, Kuruvilla S, Joy MT, Muralikrishnan B, Paul J. Jargon: a barrier in case history taking? A cross-sectional survey among dental students and staff. Dent Res J (Isfahan). 2017;14(3):203–8.

21. Hull M. Medical language proficiency: a discussion of interprofessional language competencies and potential for patient risk. Int J Nurs Stud. 2016;54:158–72.

22. Dunn EB, Wolfe JJ. Let go of Latin! Vet Hum Toxicol. 2001;43(4):235–6.

23. Englar RE. Writing skills for veterinarians. Sheffield: 5M Publishing; 2019.

24. Dooley MJ, Wiseman M, Gu G. Prevalence of error-prone abbreviations used in medication prescribing for hospitalized patients: multi-hospital evaluation. Intern Med J. 2012;42(3):e19–22.

25. Kuhn IF. Abbreviations and acronyms in healthcare: when shorter isn't sweeter. Pediatr Nurs. 2007;33(5):392–8.

26. Traynor K. Enforcement outdoes education at eliminating unsafe abbreviations. Am J Health-Syst Ph. 2004;61(13):1314-+.

27. Garbutt J, Milligan PE, McNaughton C, Waterman BM, Dunagan WC, Fraser VJ. A practical approach to measure the quality of handwritten medication orders. J Patient Saf. 2005;1:195–200.

28. Taylor S, Tak-Yan CM, Haack L, McGrath A. An intervention to reduce the use of error prone prescribing abbreviations in the emergency department. J Pharm Pract Res. 2007;37:214–6.

29. Aronson JK. Medication errors: what they are, how they happen, and how to avoid them. Qjm-Int J Med. 2009;102(8):513–21.

30. Robinson FP, Gorman G, Slimmer LW, Yudkowsky R. Perceptions of effective and ineffective nurse–physician communication in hospitals. Nurs Forum. 2010;45(July/September):206–16.

31. Ley P. Communicating with patients: improving communication, satisfaction, and compliance. London: Croom Helm; 1988.

32. Pendleton D, Hasler J. Doctor-Patient Communication. London: Academic Press; 1983.

33. Beck RS, Daughtridge R, Sloane PD. Physician–patient communication in the primary care office: a systematic review. J Am Board Fam Pract. 2002;15(1):25–38.

34. Street RL, Jr., Makoul G, Arora NK, Epstein RM. How does communication heal? Pathways linking clinician–patient communication to health outcomes. Patient Educ Couns. 2009;74(3):295–301.

35. Siminoff LA. Improving communication with cancer patients. Oncology (Williston Park). 1992;6(10):83–7; discussion 7–9.

36. Ramanayake BS, Liyanogoda NE, Dahananyake PK, Hemachandra MAD. Do patients understand medical communication? Scientific Res J. 2014;2(6):12–6.

37. Boyle CM. Difference between patients' and doctors' interpretation of some common medical terms. Br Med J. 1970;2(5704):286–9.
38. Pearson J, Dudley HA. Bodily perceptions in surgical patients. Br Med J (Clin Res Ed). 1982;284(6328):1545–6.
39. Samora J, Saunders L, Larson RF. Medical vocabulary knowledge among hospital patients. J Health Hum Behav. 1961;2(2):83–92.
40. Lerner EB, Jehle DV, Janicke DM, Moscati RM. Medical communication: do our patients understand? Am J Emerg Med. 2000;18(7):764–6.
41. Chapman K, Abraham C, Jenkins V, Fallowfield L. Lay understanding of terms used in cancer consultations. Psychooncology. 2003;12(6):557–66.
42. Pieterse AH, Jager NA, Smets EMA, Henselmans I. Lay understanding of common medical terminology in oncology. Psycho-Oncology. 2013;22(5):1186–91.
43. O'Connell RL, Hartridge-Lambert SK, Din N, St John ER, Hitchins C, Johnson T. Patients' understanding of medical terminology used in the breast clinic. Breast. 2013;22(5):836–8.
44. Dua R, Vassiliou L, Fan K. Common maxillofacial terminology: do our patients understand what we say? Surgeon. 2015;13(1):1–4.
45. Riley CS. Patients understanding of doctors instructions. Med Care. 1966;4(1):34–7.
46. Wittenberg E, Goldsmith J, Ferrell B, Platt CS. Enhancing communication related to symptom management through plain language. J Pain Symptom Manag. 2015;50(5):707–11.
47. Mayahara M, Foreman MD, Wilbur J, Paice JA, Fogg LF. Effect of hospice nonprofessional caregiver barriers to pain management on adherence to analgesic administration recommendations and patient outcomes. Pain Manag Nurs. 2015;16(3):249–56.
48. Schumacher KL, Plano Clark VL, West CM, Dodd MJ, Rabow MW, Miaskowski C. Pain medication management processes used by oncology outpatients and family caregivers part II: home and lifestyle contexts. J Pain Symptom Manage. 2014;48(5):784–96.
49. Schumacher KL, Plano Clark VL, West CM, Dodd MJ, Rabow MW, Miaskowski C. Pain medication management processes used by oncology outpatients and family caregivers part I: health systems contexts. J Pain Symptom Manage. 2014;48(5):770–83.
50. Mayahara M, Paice J, Wilbur J, Fogg L, Foreman M. Common errors in using analgesics by home-based nonprofessional hospice caregivers. J Hosp Palliat Nurs. 2014;16(3):134–40.
51. Wittenberg-Lyles E, Goldsmith J, Oliver DP, Demiris G, Kruse RL, Van Stee S. Using medical words with family caregivers. J Palliat Med. 2013;16(9):1135–9.
52. Links AR, Callon W, Wasserman C, Walsh J, Beach MC, Boss EF. Surgeon use of medical jargon with parents in the outpatient setting. Patient Educ Couns. 2019;102(6):1111–8.
53. Howe CJ, Cipher DJ, LeFlore J, Lipman TH. Parent health literacy and communication with diabetes educators in a pediatric diabetes clinic: a mixed methods approach. J Health Commun. 2015;20 Suppl 2:50–9.
54. Wiener RS, Gould MK, Woloshin S, Schwartz LM, Clark JA. What do you mean, a spot? A qualitative analysis of patients' reactions to discussions with their physicians about pulmonary nodules. Chest. 2013;143(3):672–7.
55. Konstantynowicz J, Marcinowicz L, Abramowicz P, Abramowicz M. What do children with chronic diseases and their parents think about pediatricians? A qualitative interview study. Matern Child Health J. 2016;20(8):1745–52.
56. Wiggins MN, Coker K, Hicks EK. Patient perceptions of professionalism: implications for residency education. Med Educ. 2009;43(1):28–33.
57. Bittner A, Jonietz A, Bittner J, Beickert L, Harendza S. Translating medical documents into

plain language enhances communication skills in medical students – a pilot study. Patient Educ Couns. 2015;98(9):1137–41.

58. Mrduljas Dujic N, Zitnik E, Pavelin L, Bacic D, Boljat M, Vrdoljak D, et al. Writing letters to patients as an educational tool for medical students. BMC Med Educ. 2013;13:114.

Chapter 10

Enhancing Relationship-Centered Care through Partnership

Although each veterinary client–patient relationship is unique, the human–animal bond, as a whole, has strengthened over the course of the past two decades, both within the United States and abroad.(1) In western society, the status of companion animals within the household has reached an all-time high.(2) Eighty-five percent of American clients currently regard pets as an integral part of the family structure.(1–6) Many even go so far as to consider dogs and cats to be their children.(1–5)

This elevation in social status for companion animals has changed the way that we practice veterinary medicine. Some clinics reflect this shift in philosophy by defining their workspace as a "veterinary family practice."(3, 7)

As pets have increased their value as members of the family, clients have begun to expect more from the veterinary team concerning patient care.(1, 5) Practices that cater to clients as "pet parents" are more likely to be successful and to experience better outcomes for their patients.(1, 5)

As "caregivers" for their "children, "pet parents" are driven by an increased sense of responsibility.(6) Today's veterinary clients are more invested in case outcomes. They may be more willing to commit to caring for patients with chronic disease, particularly if they are assured that quality of life for the patient can remain high.

"Pet parents" have benefited from the Information Age and the plethora of resources that are available online to guide decision making. Although their sources may be questionable, they enter into consultations as educated partners in the delivery of healthcare.(1)

"Pet parents" expect healthcare to be a joint effort. This implies an investment by the veterinary team in a collaborative approach to the practice of medicine. Collaboration requires effective communication that often involves more than one member of the patient's family. Patient's families are increasingly diverse and may include:

- children
- parents
- adult (grown) "children"
- grandparents
- spouses
- extended family.

Support networks may also include, in some cases, friends of the family, particularly if these members have a medical background; cat and/or dog breeders; or pet sitters, particularly in those cases when "pet parents" travel and authorize others to make decisions in their absence.

This network of support is increasingly valuable to "pet parents," who can lean on others for financial and emotional advice. However, it creates a web of communication for the veterinary team to navigate.

It is rare that everyone in the network will have the same communication style or needs. Yet the veterinary team must be able to connect to and communicate with them all. Communication between members of the family must be consistent.

When breakdowns in communication occur, "pet parents" are more likely to vocalize their concerns and seek retribution.(1, 4, 8–13) Today's veterinary clients are also more emotionally invested in the life and death of their pet.(6, 14, 15) Seventy percent of clients report that the death of a companion animal is emotionally challenging, and nearly one-third of clients acknowledge severe grief or devastation at end-of-life for their pet.(14, 16) For those who are faced with the decision to euthanize their dog or cat, it is common to feel guilt.(14, 16)

A client's grief can be lessened or exacerbated by the veterinary team.(14) The perception by clients that the veterinary team cares, acknowledges, and validates their grief is valued immensely.(14) However, emotional support is not merely appreciated; it is expected.(14)

10.1 The Shift towards Partnership

Today's veterinary client desires to be an active participant in decision making for the pet.(10) This mirrors the trend in human healthcare: the human patient expects to be intimately involved in formulating and following through with diagnostic and/or treatment plans.(1, 10, 17, 18) Healthcare is thus seen as an opportunity for partnership, in which the veterinarian and client come together as one team for the benefit of common ground, the patient.(19, 20)

Although the veterinarian may counsel and advise, she or he is expected to be, first and foremost, a collaborator.(1, 10, 19–22) In this role, the veterinarian is tasked with providing information and resources that are necessary for the client to make informed decisions.(21) This requires the veterinarian to consider the client's needs, preferences, and desires.(21)

Any obstacles to patient care are expected to be identified, discussed, negotiated, and remedied.(21)

Ultimately, it is the veterinarian–client partnership that decides upon a mutually agreeable diagnostic and/or therapeutic plan.(21)

In this way, the veterinarian facilitates decision making, rather than dictates it. Because the client actively participates in the decision-making process, she or he considers her or himself to be a partner in healthcare.(21) This shift away from paternalism has been termed *relationship-centered care*.(21, 23, 24)

Since clients are more involved in planning patient care, they are more likely to hold themselves accountable for the decisions that are made.(21) Because clients have a say in decision making, they exhibit greater rates of compliance and adherence to treatment recommendations.(21)

Veterinary clients that are involved in determining case outcomes are also more likely to be satisfied with the healthcare team and the services that are rendered.(21)

Increased consumer satisfaction with relationship-centered care and increased adherence are just two of the advantages that the human and veterinary health professions have witnessed as both move towards models of relationship-centered care. (21, 25–28) In addition, case outcomes and physicians' satisfaction with their chosen professions are also improved.(29–34) Litigation rates are also lower because both parties are able to articulate their concerns and carry out a mutually agreed upon plan.(21, 24–28, 35, 36)

Veterinary communication styles impact the success of companion animal practice. (1, 10, 37–40) Veterinary clients expect correspondence to convey a sense of respect for their role as decision makers.(10, 38, 41–43) Veterinary clients also expect an invitation to contribute knowledge from past experiences and to provide perspective, given their familiarity with the patient.(10, 11, 42–44)

10.2 Are Veterinary Clients Experts?

Veterinary clients may not know everything about a given disease; however, they see themselves as experts in their own right. Their areas of expertise include:

- the patient
  - what is considered normal about the patient
  - what is considered abnormal about the patient
- their financial status
  - what can they afford
  - what they cannot afford
  - what are they willing to spend
  - what they perceive to be the value of your services
- their schedule
  - which treatments are feasible
  - which treatments are not feasible
  - is there room to compromise?
- their core values and beliefs
  - for example, American pet owners have their own opinions as to whether or not it is ethical to declaw their cats
  - other pet owners may have personal or religious beliefs that prevent them from electing for euthanasia.

When it comes to knowledge about the patient, clients expect the veterinary team to defer to them:: "We know the pets better [than the veterinarian] because they live with us 24 hours per day, 7 days per week."(9)

As a result of this insider information, clients expect to be asked the following by the veterinary team.(9)

- What is best for the pet?
- What do they think is wrong with the pet?
- What concerns them most about the patient's clinical presentation?
- What has their past experience with disease "X" been?

Clients who are invited to share these areas of expertise are more likely to be receptive to new information from the veterinary team.(10, 41) In contrast, clients become dissatisfied and close off themselves to conversation when they feel that they are not being taken seriously or when their concerns have not been addressed.

Veterinary clients may be presenting the patient to us for advice. However, they are powerful contributors to the diagnosis by virtue of what they can share with us (or choose not to share) during history taking. As such, they are the gateway to information that can point us in the right direction of what ails our patient. For this reason alone, they deserve to be heard.

10.3 Setting the Stage for Relationship-Centered Care

In order for relationship-centered care to work, the veterinary team must adapt the following strategies.(20, 45–49)

- Be willing to accept the client as a partner in healthcare.
- Demonstrate respect for the client.
- Demonstrate respect for the patient.
- Recognize the role of the patient in the client's life.
- Acknowledge and accept the client's concerns as being valid.
- Be informative, yet responsive and receptive to client concerns.
- Be flexible and willing to change the game plan as necessary to provide the patient with the very best care.

Partnership breeds a two-way street of respect. If the veterinarian demonstrates respect for the client, then the client is more likely to be respectful of the veterinary team.

Relationship-centered care takes time. Time is an essential component because educating the client and building rapport are not instantaneous.(20) However, the investment of time is well worth it. Client engagement is the key to successful outcomes for veterinarians, clients, and patients alike.(24)

As professionals, it behooves us to enhance relationship-centered care. This chapter introduces the first of four supplemental communication skills that facilitate rapport-building:

1. establishing partnership
2. eliciting the client's perspective – refer to Chapter 11
3. asking for the client's permission – refer to Chapter 12
4. assessing the client's knowledge – refer to Chapter 13.

10.4 Establishing Partnership with the Client

Veterinarians are among the first to admit that their chosen discipline is, at its core, a "people profession." Although they are trained to attend to the medical and/or surgical needs of their patients, their patients cannot visit the practice on their own. Their presence within the clinic requires an active participant on the other end of the leash, someone who is observant and invested in the patient's healthcare.(50–54)

Caring for the patient ultimately requires caring for the client. After all, it is the client who determines whether or not to proceed with patient care. The way in which we interact with our clients impacts their perception of us and the practice. They judge our competence and compassion based upon our interactions, both with the patient and themselves.

It is therefore critical that we invest in getting to know the client at the very beginning of each consultation.(55) Although there was a time when this was viewed as "soft," "fluffy," or "superfluous," we recognize now that first impressions matter and play a significant role in establishing trust.(55)

A client who bonds with the veterinary team is a loyal client.(56) Loyal clients are retained by practices even when they move to a residence greater than 45 minutes away.(56) Loyal clients are less likely to switch practices due to cost of care.(56) Loyal clients are likely to see value in healthcare and adhere to recommendations, even if recommendations are pricy.(56)

Loyalty is based upon trust. Loyal clients feel supported by the veterinary team. Loyal clients trust in the team's competence and appreciate the team's compassion.

That being said:

> Communication with clients involves more than simply being kind; rather, it is about building a professional relationship such that the veterinarian's message is expressed effectively and the client feels his/her concerns are being acknowledged and addressed.(51)

Rapport-building sets the tone for what we hope will be a lifelong relationship. Accordingly, a significant amount of time should be set aside for this purpose.

A 2004 study by Shaw et al. analyzed the content of veterinary appointments. Shaw reported that a typical consultation lasted 13 minutes, of which 30% of the time, on average, was devoted to building the relationship. An additional seven percent solidified that relationship by actively engaging the client in decision making and acknowledging his or her role as a healthcare partner.(40) This contributed to the relaxed atmosphere of wellness appointments, and set the stage for social talk and laughter to mingle with the delivery of healthcare.(40)

A strong and positive working relationship is also a motivating force for clients to get onboard with recommendations, particularly those concerning preventative care.(57)

10.4.1 Phrases that Effectively Communicate Partnership

There are many ways that veterinarians can demonstrate partnership. Above all, remember the old adage, "there is no I in team." This means that we replace "I" statements with "we" statements and actually mean them.

For example, instead of saying, "I want Fluffy to get better," consider rewording your statement as such: "We both want Fluffy to get better."

Other examples of *we* statements include the following.

- "We are committed to helping Juniper lose weight."
- "We are invested in finding a solution to Harry's house-soiling."
- "We are hopeful that the biopsy results will be favorable for Newt."

Partnership statements might also make use of the phrase, *let us*, or the contraction, *let's*.

- "Let's consider what toxins Harvest may have had access to."
- "Let's decide how to reduce anxiety so that Jelly's next visit can be a good one."
- "Let's figure out the best solution to Trolley's fear of fireworks so that he is not miserable next year on July 4th."
- "Let's establish Jenny's baseline bloodwork today so that we are well-prepared for her surgery next week."
- "Let's determine which dog breed best suits your needs so that the next dog that you adopt is a good 'fit' for your lifestyle."

Sometimes, the additional word, *together*, is tacked onto the statement to further emphasize partnership.

- "Let's work together to come up with a plan that will be best for you two."
- "Let's put our heads together to figure out what most likely caused Titon's kidneys to fail."
- "Let's determine together which diagnostic test is most likely to provide the answer we are looking for."
- "Let's together create a plan that is designed to reduce Tilly's separation anxiety so that you are less likely to come home to a house that has been destroyed."

Other inclusive language includes the words *ours* and *us*.(58) Using inclusive language helps us to exceed our client's expectations for the consultation.(58)

10.4.2 Contrast Partnership Phrases with Those that Exclusively Use "I"

Partnership phrases are easy to incorporate into any conversation; however, in clinical practice, statements that exclusively use "I" are frequent substitutions that undermine the relationship. This is detrimental.

Consider how the exclusive use of "I" may sound to a new client by exploring the following clinical scenario:

> You are an associate veterinarian in a companion animal practice. You have just diagnosed a dog with a corneal ulcer, and you are outlining the treatment plan for the client.

- "Jupiter has developed an ulcer on his left eye. This is painful and infections on the surface of the eye, the cornea, can progress rapidly. I want to treat him right away."
- "I am going to prescribe antibiotic eyedrops that need to be applied every four hours."
- "I need to see Jupiter back here in three to five days."
- "I need Jupiter to wear an Elizabethan collar so that he does not further damage his eye."
- "I need to know if his eye becomes bloodshot or if his squinting becomes worse."

Note that these are all important instructions that need to be shared with the client.

However, can you see that the use of "I" makes the appointment one-sided? The use of "I" shifts the focus onto me and my plan. Instead of affording the client the opportunity to weigh in on the plan, I have short-circuited our partnership. I have replaced partnership with dictation.

- Did I allow the client to weigh in with his views?
- Did I allow the client to share what he thinks is possible in terms of treatment?
- Did I check in with him to see if he will be able to medicate?
- Did I check in to see if he is willing to go along with the treatment plan?

The ideal client might be accepting of your dictation and follow through on each and every instruction.

But would most clients? What about the average client? Or, worse, consider the client who wants to follow through, but cannot.

- Maybe he cannot medicate Jupiter without Jupiter attempting to bite him.
- Maybe Jupiter will tolerate eye drops, but the client is not in a position to administer them every four hours because he works full time.
- Maybe he can medicate Jupiter as instructed, but will be out of town during the interval when you indicated that a recheck was essential.

Because you did not ask him if your treatment plan was possible and because you did not include him in its design, you have set him up for failure.

When the client does not return for follow-up, who will you blame? We have a tendency to cast blame on the client, but is that fair? Wouldn't it be better to partner with the client to come up with a plan that you can both agree to?

10.4.3 Revisiting Partnership

Let us take a look at how that same conversation might unfold if I were to incorporate partnership statements.

> Veterinarian: Jupiter has developed an ulcer on his left eye. This is painful and infections on the surface of the eye can progress rapidly. We need to start treatment right away.
>
> [pause]
>
> Veterinarian: Treatment will require medication to be applied directly to Jupiter's eye. Let's go through the various options together so that we can decide what the best course of action is for you and Jupiter.
>
> Client: Ok.
>
> Veterinarian: Jupiter will need treatment for at least a week, possibly longer. Do you think that he will tolerate medications being applied to the surface of the affected eye?
>
> Client: Absolutely, he lets me do whatever is necessary. It's not a problem.
>
> Veterinarian: That's great! Would you prefer an eye drop that needs to be applied every four hours or an ointment that needs to be applied every 8 hours?
>
> Client: Hmmm, that's going to be tricky. I work pretty long hours. There's no way that I can come home to apply eye drops every four hours. Let's go with the ointment.
>
> Veterinarian: Sounds great. We also need to work together to keep Jupiter from pawing at his eye, which could create more damage. What are your thoughts about using an E collar at home?
>
> Client: You mean that lampshade? The cone of shame?
>
> Veterinarian: Exactly.
>
> Client: He hates it, but if it will get him better, then okay, I guess we can make it work.
>
> Veterinarian: We will do everything in our power to make sure that he gets better – and fast. To help us know that he is on track, it would help if we could visit again in three to five days for a recheck exam. Would that work for you?
>
> Client: Five days would work best for me.
>
> Veterinarian: Great, then that's what we'll do. In the meantime, please keep a close watch: if you see that eye becoming bloodshot or if the squinting gets worse, please let me know and we will adjust his medications.

Consider how this conversation flowed.

Consider the veterinarian's use of partnership statements. Partnership statements remind our client that we are in the trenches together. It's not "us" vs "them." It's an "all hands on deck" approach to the practice of medicine.

Partnership statements reinforce that our client has a say when it comes to treatment options.

Partnership statements reinforce that we are a team – and that patient care is only as effective as the team that is responsible for providing it. Our client is very much a part of that team. Partnership statements are a way for us to honor that sentiment.

Our clients value teamwork and consider being a team player to be a desirable attribute that defines "a good vet."(59)

Consider how partnership statements allowed the veterinarian to check in with the client.

Consider the veterinarian's willingness to be flexible. This flexibility made it possible for the veterinarian to adapt the treatment plan to the needs of the client in such a way that the treatment plan has the greatest chance for success.

The client is more likely to comply with the plan if he has a say in it, and the patient is more likely to improve with the plan in effect.

Note that partnership statements were not the only communication tool that was put to work here. Partnership statements often go hand in hand with another communication tool, eliciting the client's perspective. Refer to Chapter 11 for additional information on this paired communication skill.

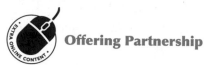 **Offering Partnership**

References

1. Shaw JR, Adams CL, Bonnett BN. What can veterinarians learn from studies of physician-patient communication about veterinarian–client–patient communication? J Am Vet Med Assoc. 2004;224(5):676–84.
2. Martin F, Taunton A. Perceived importance and integration of the human-animal bond in private veterinary practice. J Am Vet Med Assoc. 2006;228(4):522–7.
3. Timmins RP. The contribution of animals to human well-being: a veterinary family practice perspective. J Vet Med Educ. 2008;35(4):540–4.
4. Blackwell MJ. Beyond philosophical differences: the future training of veterinarians. J Vet Med Educ. 2001;28(3):148–52.
5. Brown JP, Silverman JD. The current and future market for veterinarians and veterinary medical services in the United States. J Am Vet Med Assoc. 1999;215(2):161–83.
6. Shanan A. A veterinarian's role in helping pet owners with decision making. Vet Clin North Am Small Anim Pract. 2011;41(3):635–46.
7. Timmins RP, Fine AH. The role of the veterinary family practitioner in animal-assisted therapy and animal-assisted activity programs. In: Fine AH, editor. Handbook on animal-assisted ther-

apy. San Diego, CA: Academic Press; 2006. pp. 475–86.

8. Russell RL. Preparing veterinary students with the interactive skills to effectively work with clients and staff. J Vet Med Educ. 1994;21:40–3.

9. Englar RE, Williams M, Weingand K. Applicability of the Calgary–Cambridge Guide to dog and cat owners for teaching veterinary clinical communications. J Vet Med Educ. 2016;43(2):143–69.

10. Show A, Englar RE. Evaluating dog and cat owner preferences for calgary-cambridge communication skills: results of a questionnaire. J Vet Med Educ. 2018:1–10.

11. Opperman M. The cost of a dissatisfied client. DVM management consultant's report. 1990;21:1.

12. Martin EA. Managing client communication for effective practice: what skills should veterinary graduates have acquired for success? J Vet Med Educ. 2006;33(1):45–9.

13. Radford AD, Stockley P, Taylor IR, Turner R, Gaskell CJ, Kaney S, et al. Use of simulated clients in training veterinary undergraduates in communication skills. Vet Rec. 2003;152(14):422–7.

14. Shaw JR, Lagoni L. End-of-life communication in veterinary medicine: delivering bad news and euthanasia decision making. Vet Clin North Am Small Anim Pract. 2007;37(1):95–108; abstract viii-ix.

15. Lagoni L, Butler C, Hetts S. The human–animal bond and grief. Philadelphia, PA: Saunders; 1994.

16. Adams CL, Bonnett BN, Meek AH. Predictors of owner response to companion animal death in 177 clients from 14 practices in Ontario. J Am Vet Med Assoc. 2000;217(9):1303–9.

17. Stewart M, Brown JB, Boon H, Galajda J, Meredith L, Sangster M. Evidence on patient–doctor communication. Cancer Prev Control. 1999;3(1):25–30.

18. Stewart MA. Effective physician–patient communication and health outcomes: a review. CMAJ. 1995;152(9):1423–33.

19. Shaw JR, Bonnett BN, Adams CL, Roter DL. Veterinarian–client–patient communication patterns used during clinical appointments in companion animal practice. J Am Vet Med Assoc. 2006;228(5):714–21.

20. Kuper AM, Merle R. Being nice is not enough – exploring relationship-centered veterinary care with structural equation modeling. a quantitative study on German pet owners' perception. Front Vet Sci. 2019;6:56.

21. Cornell KK, Kopcha M. Client–veterinarian communication: skills for client centered dialogue and shared decision making. Vet Clin North Am Small Anim Pract. 2007;37(1):37–47; abstract vii.

22. McArthur ML, Fitzgerald JR. Companion animal veterinarians' use of clinical communication skills. Aust Vet J. 2013;91(9):374–80.

23. Roter DL, Stewart M, Putnam SM, Lipkin M, Jr., Stiles W, Inui TS. Communication patterns of primary care physicians. JAMA. 1997;277(4):350–6.

24. Bard AM, Main DC, Haase AM, Whay HR, Roe EJ, Reyher KK. The future of veterinary communication: partnership or persuasion? A qualitative investigation of veterinary communication in the pursuit of client behaviour change. PLoS One. 2017;12(3):e0171380.

25. Hall JA, Dornan MC. Meta-analysis of satisfaction with medical care: description of research domain and analysis of overall satisfaction levels. Soc Sci Med. 1988;27(6):637–44.

26. Hall JA, Dornan MC. What patients like about their medical care and how often they are asked: a meta-analysis of the satisfaction literature. Soc Sci Med. 1988;27(9):935–9.

27. Levinson W. Physician–patient communication. A key to malpractice prevention. JAMA. 1994;272(20):1619–20.

28. Levinson W, Roter DL, Mulloly JP, Dull VT, Frankel RM. Physician–patient communication. The relationship with malpractice claims among primary care physicians and surgeons. JAMA.

1997;277(7):553–9.

29. Fraenkel L, McGraw S. What are the essential elements to enable patient participation in medical decision making? J Gen Intern Med. 2007;22(5):614–9.

30. van Dam HA, van der Horst F, van den Borne B, Ryckman R, Crebolder H. Provider–patient interaction in diabetes care: effects on patient self-care and outcomes. A systematic review. Patient Educ Couns. 2003;51(1):17–28.

31. Ward MM, Sundaramurthy S, Lotstein D, Bush TM, Neuwelt CM, Street RL, Jr. Participatory patient–physician communication and morbidity in patients with systemic lupus erythematosus. Arthritis Rheum. 2003;49(6):810–8.

32. Macfarlane J, Holmes W, Gard P, Thornhill D, Macfarlane R, Hubbard R. Reducing antibiotic use for acute bronchitis in primary care: blinded, randomized controlled trial of patient information leaflet. BMJ. 2002;324(7329):91–4.

33. Kennedy AD, Sculpher MJ, Coulter A, Dwyer N, Rees M, Abrams KR, et al. Effects of decision aids for menorrhagia on treatment choices, health outcomes, and costs: a randomized controlled trial. JAMA. 2002;288(21):2701–8.

34. Greenfield S, Kaplan S, Ware JE, Jr. Expanding patient involvement in care. Effects on patient outcomes. Ann Intern Med. 1985;102(4):520–8.

35. Shaw JR, Adams CL, Bonnett BN, Larson S, Roter DL. Veterinarian–client–patient communication during wellness appointments versus appointments related to a health problem in companion animal practice. J Am Vet Med Assoc. 2008;233(10):1576–86.

36. Roter D. The enduring and evolving nature of the patient–physician relationship. Patient Educ Couns. 2000;39(1):5–15.

37. Dysart LM, Coe JB, Adams CL. Analysis of solicitation of client concerns in companion animal practice. J Am Vet Med Assoc. 2011;238(12):1609–15.

38. Coe JB, Adams CL, Bonnett BN. A focus group study of veterinarians' and pet owners' perceptions of veterinarian-client communication in companion animal practice. J Am Vet Med Assoc. 2008;233(7):1072–80.

39. Coe JB, Adams CL, Bonnett BN. Prevalence and nature of cost discussions during clinical appointments in companion animal practice. J Am Vet Med Assoc. 2009;234(11):1418–24.

40. Shaw JR, Adams CL, Bonnett BN, Larson S, Roter DL. Use of the Roter interaction analysis system to analyse veterinarian–client–patient communication in companion animal practice. J Am Vet Med Assoc. 2004;225(2):222–9.

41. Shaw JR, Barley GE, Broadfoot K, Hill AE, Roter DL. Outcomes assessment of on-site communication skills education in a companion animal practice. J Am Vet Med Assoc. 2016;249(4):419–32.

42. Stoewen DL, Coe JB, MacMartin C, Stone EA, C ED. Qualitative study of the communication expectations of clients accessing oncology care at a tertiary referral center for dogs with life-limiting cancer. J Am Vet Med Assoc. 2014;245(7):785–95.

43. Stoewen DL, Coe JB, MacMartin C, Stone EA, Dewey CE. Qualitative study of the information expectations of clients accessing oncology care at a tertiary referral center for dogs with life-limiting cancer. J Am Vet Med Assoc. 2014;245(7):773–83.

44. Heath TJ, Mills JN. Criteria used by employers to select new graduate employees. Aust Vet J. 2000;78(5):312–6.

45. Adams CL, Kurtz SM. Skills for communicating in veterinary medicine. Oxford: Otmoor Publishing and Dewpoint Publishing; 2017.

46. Donovan JL. Patient decision making. The missing ingredient in compliance research. Int J Technol Assess Health Care. 1995;11(3):443–55.

47. Donovan JL, Blake DR. Patient non-compliance: deviance or reasoned decision-making? Soc Sci Med. 1992;34(5):507–13.
48. Abood SK. Increasing adherence in practice: making your clients partners in care. Vet Clin North Am Small Anim Pract. 2007;37(1):151–64; abstract ix-x.
49. Kanji N, Coe JB, Adams CL, Shaw JR. Effect of veterinarian–client–patient interactions on client adherence to dentistry and surgery recommendations in companion-animal practice. J Am Vet Med Assoc. 2012;240(4):427–36.
50. Adams CL, Frankel RM. It may be a dog's life but the relationship with her owners is also key to her health and well being: communication in veterinary medicine. Vet Clin North Am Small Anim Pract. 2007;37(1):1–17; abstract vii.
51. Dalley JS, Creary PR, Durzi T, McMurtry CM. An interactive teddy bear clinic tour: teaching veterinary students how to interact with young children. J Vet Med Educ.44(2):302–15.
52. Kurtz SM, Silverman JD, Draper J. Teaching and learning communication skills in medicine. Grand Rapids, MI: Radcliffe; 2004.
53. Adams CL, Kurtz S. Coaching and feedback: enhancing communication teaching and learning in veterinary practice settings. J Vet Med Educ. 2012;39(3):217–28.
54. Committee ASPS. The Association of American Veterinary Medical Colleges strategic plan, 2010–2014. J Vet Med Educ. 2009;36(2):154–7.
55. Frankel RM. Pets, vets, and frets: what relationship-centered care research has to offer veterinary medicine. J Vet Med Educ. 2006;33(1):20–7.
56. Lue TW, Pantenburg DP, Crawford PM. Impact of the owner–pet and client–veterinarian bond on the care that pets receive. J Am Vet Med Assoc. 2008;232(4):531–40.
57. Belshaw Z, Robinson NJ, Dean RS, Brennan ML. Motivators and barriers for dog and cat owners and veterinary surgeons in the United Kingdom to using preventative medicines. Prev Vet Med. 2018;154:95–101.
58. Hunter LJ, Shaw JR. How to exceed – not merely meet – client expectations. Veterinary Team Brief. 2018(March):19–22.
59. Mellanby RJ, Rhind SM, Bell C, Shaw DJ, Gifford J, Fennell D, et al. Perceptions of clients and veterinarians on what attributes constitute 'a good vet'. Vet Rec. 2011;168(23):616.

Chapter 11

Eliciting the Client's Perspective to Enhance Relationship-Centered Care

As veterinarians, we are trained to be the experts in the examination room. Clients look to us for answers concerning medicine and surgery, and we need to be able to fulfill their needs. However, there are times when we need to hear from our clients as much as they need to hear from us.

In particular, we need to be receptive to hearing client's inner dialogue. We need to know what words are rattling around in their heads: things that they may want to ask us about, but may not feel comfortable without our invitation to do so.

Eliciting the client's perspective is an important skill because it invites the client to share.(1) The client who is allowed to share is more likely to feel heard by the clinician.(1) Clients want to be heard.(2) They value two-way conversation with healthcare providers because they see it as a sign of respect.(2–13)

The client who feels heard is more likely to experience a positive outcome.(1) One of the best examples of this is research conducted by the University of Western Ontario in 1986. Researchers found that the strongest predictor of whether chronic headache symptoms would resolve within 1 year of the patient's initial visit was if the patient felt heard by the clinician.(14)

Eliciting the client's perspective often takes the form of an open-ended question.

Recall that open-ended questions and statements invite clients to share their story in greater detail.(1) In this regard, they are relationship builders. They help us to get to know our clients better. They open up doors so that we know more fully what it is that may be weighing on their minds.

Open-ended questions and statements let clients know that you value what they have to say and that you are interested in their thoughts.

For more information about open-ended questions, you may wish to revisit Chapter 8.

Let us return now to the communication skill, eliciting the client's perspective. This skill is defined as asking the client how she or he feels about a particular situation or experience. In other words, it is a way to ask where the client is coming from when she or he is tasked with decision making.

Eliciting the client's perspective can help us to understand why the client may be hesitant to pursue the proposed diagnostic or treatment plans.(15) Eliciting the client's perspective also helps us to hear our client's expectations.(16) These expectations are based upon client assumptions and desires.(16, 17)

Client expectations may relate to:(16)

- us, as doctors
- our team members
- our practice.

Client expectations may also be about today's visit.(16)

- What action plan is the client hoping to achieve?
- Which treatment outcomes does the client anticipate?
- What is the client expecting to pay for services?
- What is the anticipated timeline for recovery?

Today's veterinary clients have high expectations.(18) They are better informed than ever before.(19) They are also increasingly invested in patient outcomes because the patient is often considered to be an integral part of the family.(19–26)

If we as a profession fail to meet expectations, then we risk client dissatisfaction, client complaints, and rising claims of malpractice.(8, 21, 27–29) Clients are also more likely to be lost to follow-up, meaning that patients are unlikely to receive the care that they need.

Eliciting the client's perspective is critical if we are to meet, if not exceed, client expectations.(16) Eliciting the client's perspective ensures we are on the same page as our clients. If we understand our clients, then we are more likely to effectively partner with them to achieve the optimal outcome for our patients.(16, 30)

11.1 Phrases that Effectively Elicit the Client's Perspective

Statements that elicit the client's perspective often start with:

- tell me
- share with me
- explain to me.

Consider the following examples.

- "Tell me what concerns you most."
- "Tell me what's on your mind."
- "Tell me why you're reluctant to get Molly spayed."
- "Share with me your reservations about proceeding with Trevor's surgery."
- "Share with me what you saw when Toby was having his latest episode."

- "Share with me what's going through your mind right now."
- "Explain what you saw."
- "Explain to me why you are reluctant to proceed."
- "Explain what worries you most about my recommendation to start treatment with drug 'X'?"

11.2 Softening These Phrases

Sometimes new graduates feel awkward about eliciting the client's perspective using the phraseology that was introduced in Section 11.1 because they feel that the wording sounds forceful, like a command.

I like to remind my students that it is important to find their own cluster of words that feels most sincere so that delivery comes across as being natural.

For those students who prefer to soften these statements, consider tacking on "please" or "can."

- "Please tell me what concerns you most."
- "Can you tell me what's on your mind?"
- "Can you please tell me why you're reluctant to get Molly spayed?"
- "Please share with me your reservations about proceeding with Trevor's surgery."
- "Can you share with me what you saw when Toby was having his latest episode?"
- "Can you please share with me what's going through your mind right now?"
- "Please explain what you saw."
- "Can you explain to me why you are reluctant to proceed?"
- "Please, can you explain what worries you most about my recommendation to start treatment with drug 'X'?"

You can further soften these phrases by asking, "Would you mind …?"

This is particularly valuable when exploring topics that have a potential to be sensitive in nature. Consider, for example, the following statement:

"What scares you most about Fluffy having diabetes?"

Some new graduates are timid about asking this question in the manner that it has been phrased because they fear it is asking clients to discuss an emotion that they may be reluctant to acknowledge.

For these individuals, it may be helpful to amend the statement as follows:

"Would you mind sharing what scares you most about Fluffy having diabetes?"

This is a softer, gentler approach. It also grants the client permission to decline to answer.

Asking for the client's permission is a relationship builder that was introduced in Section 10.3 and will be covered in greater detail in Chapter 12.

11.3 What Happens When We Do Not Use This Skill

Let us take a look at how a common clinical scenario might unfold if I do not make use of the communication skill, eliciting the client's perspective.

Background

You are an associate veterinarian in clinical practice.

Your client, Mr. Smith, has recently adopted a young adolescent female cat. On physical exam, you palpate a firm, multinodular mass over the left mammary chain. You express your concerns about the possibility of a malignancy, and the need to biopsy the tissue to definitely determine the cause of the mass.

Clinical Conversation

Veterinarian: Mr. Smith, we both agree that it's important to know exactly what is causing this lump and that a biopsy under general anesthesia is the best approach.

Mr. Smith: Hmmm

Mr. Smith proceeds to avert his gaze at the mention of general anesthesia.

Veterinarian: (ignoring the client's nonverbal cues) Okay, great, so then I will get my technician to review an estimate with you. If all looks good on paper, then we can schedule that biopsy for first thing tomorrow.

How effective was this conversation? Did the veterinarian get buy-in from the client? Is the client onboard with the plan? How likely is Mr. Smith to schedule the procedure for tomorrow? How likely is he to postpone the procedure?

If the client does postpone, then we may incorrectly assume it was done on account of a limited budget when in actuality it is not the cost, but the anesthetic risk, that frightens him. If we do not successfully address the client's concerns, then he may not agree to pursue the procedure that his cat needs.

11.4 Revisiting the Same Scenario and Eliciting the Client's Perspective

Let us take a look at how that same conversation might unfold if I were to incorporate statements designed to elicit the client's perspective.

Clinical Conversation

Veterinarian: Mr. Smith, we both agree that it's important to know exactly what is causing this lump and that a biopsy under general anesthesia is the best approach.

Mr. Smith: Hmmm

Mr. Smith proceeds to avert his gaze at the mention of general anesthesia.

Veterinarian (picking up on the client's nonverbal cues): Mr. Smith, I'm sensing that you have some concerns about our plan for getting some answers about Fiji's lump. Can you share with me what's going through your mind right now?

Mr. Smith: I got my cat spayed five years ago. I loved that cat. I trusted my vet. It was a routine procedure, she said. We do it all the time. Well, guess what. My cat never woke up.

Veterinarian: I can't imagine going through something like that. No wonder you are concerned about having to face the same situation again – anesthesia.

Mr. Smith: Yes, that's it. I know we need to find out what this lump is, but I'm afraid. I don't want to lose another cat.

Veterinarian: I completely understand and yes, it is scary. I wish that anesthesia carried zero risk, but you and I both know that is not true. With any procedure, there is some risk. We do everything we can to lessen that. Would you be open to me sharing what our practice will do to monitor your cat so that we can reduce the chance that any risk will happen?

In this clinical scenario, eliciting the client's perspective gave the client the freedom to share what was weighing heavily on his mind. Eliciting his perspective also afforded you the opportunity to acknowledge and validate his concerns. You were also then able to take a step in the right direction, to hopefully reassure the client so that he feels more comfortable with proceeding with the plan.

Note that the client may still choose to decline the procedure, based upon his previous experience. However, at least now you understand why that may be so.

11.5 Eliciting the Client's Perspective Also Helps Clients Open Up about Treatment Preferences

Eliciting one's perspective also allows our clients to share their constraints concerning treatment options, in terms of what is possible versus impossible for them to achieve at home.

Let us see how this might work in clinical practice.

Background

You are an associate veterinarian.

Your client, Mr. Harris, has recently adopted a young kitten that presents to you for sneezing. On physical exam, you notice appreciable yellow-green oculonasal discharge bilaterally. The kitten is also febrile and reluctant to eat. You express your concerns about the possibility of an upper respiratory tract infection. You elect to treat with antibiotics.

Rather than ask for the client's insight, you prescribe antibiotic therapy with an oral pill that is to be given every 12 hours. Your client does not say anything, but his nonverbal cues suggest discomfort with the proposed plan.

Clinical Conversation

Mr. Harris: So what are we going to do to fix Fiji's cold?

Veterinarian: I'm going to send her home on an antibiotic, Clavamox. You'll give her one pill, twice a day, for the next two weeks. That should clear it right up.

Mr. Harris: Hmmm

Mr. Harris proceeds to avert his gaze and assumes a closed-off posture, with his arms folded across his chest.

Veterinarian: Great, then I'll have my staff draw up the medication; it should be ready in about 15 minutes.

How effective was this conversation? Did the veterinarian get buy-in from the client? Is the client onboard with the plan? How likely is Mr. Harris to administer the medication? How likely is the patient to receive the treatment that she needs to get well?

What could have gone better with this conversation to improve client compliance? I could have asked if the client has ever had to administer antibiotics to a cat before? Maybe this is his first cat. Or maybe he has never had to "pill" a cat before.

See what happens when I actually invite the client to share his experience.

Clinical Conversation

Mr. Harris: So what are we going to do to fix Fiji's cold?

Veterinarian: Fiji would benefit greatly from taking an antibiotic, Clavamox, but that requires her to receive medication at home. Have you ever had to give a cat a pill before?

Mr. Harris: Uh … No … You know, come to think of it, I don't even know how I would get her to sit still long enough for that.

Veterinarian: You're right, it is easier said than done. Would it help if I had my technician join us? She can work with you on how to get the pill into Fiji.

Mr. Harris: That would be great.

Alternatively, consider that Mr. Harris might have experience administering medication to a cat, but he is not comfortable with pilling. He would prefer liquid drops. Instead of telling him that he will give a pill because that is *your* plan, consider asking him what he would prefer.

Clinical Conversation

Veterinarian: Mr. Harris, we both agree that Fiji needs antibiotics for the next two weeks to manage her upper respiratory infection. There are two options for me to prescribe: a pill or liquid drops. Do you have a preference as to which might be easier for you to administer?

Mr. Harris: The pills never seem to work for me; to be honest, more ends up on the floor than in my cat. The liquid is much easier for me. I'd prefer that.

Note that the veterinarian gave the client an option rather than dictating the patient's healthcare plan. By inquiring about the client's preference, the veterinarian has increased the chance that the client will be compliant.

This is especially important when there are complicated medical cases that require extensive outpatient care. In these cases, the burden falls upon the owner to "get it done."

If we do not ask the client what is within reason or what is possible for him or her to achieve, then we have set the client up for failure.

It would be better to ask the client, "What would work with your schedule?" or "Is this plan possible for you to work around?"

Consider, for example, a prescription of antibiotic eye drops. You may prescribe them to be administered every 4 hours, but will that actually happen?

A client that works 12 hour shifts may only be able to administer something twice a day. Will that dosing schedule be sufficient for your plan? If not, then you need to find a way to work around the obstacle that is reasonable.

The client cannot cancel his or her shift every day for *x* number of days. That is unreasonable. So, you would have to exchange your drug of choice for one with a reasonable dosing schedule in order to make treatment possible.

Consider how this might play out.

Clinical Conversation

Veterinarian: In order to manage Fiji's eye ulcer, you are going to need to administer a medication to the affected eye often …

If I prescribe eye drops, then you will need to instill one drop into the left eye every 4 hours, so six times a day.

If I prescribe eye ointment, then you will only have to medicate three times a day.

Which would be easiest for you based upon your schedule?

Mr. Harris: I really prefer eye drops, but I'm not home often enough to make that work

---

– and I don't want her to miss doses. Let's go with the ointment. I feel confident that I can get that in three times a day.

Note that the client was given a choice; this reinforces partnership. The client was also treated as an expert in the room. The client is, in fact, an expert when it comes to what is "normal" for his or her pet; what is possible in terms of his or her own schedule; and what is possible in terms of financial investment in the patient.

We will not know what is "normal" for the pet, what is feasible in terms of client scheduling, or what is within the client's budget unless we invite them to share.

Eliciting the client's perspective is a tool that helps to achieve just that.

 Eliciting the Client's Perspective

References

1. Englar RE, Williams M, Weingand K. Applicability of the Calgary–Cambridge Guide to dog and cat owners for teaching veterinary clinical communications. J Vet Med Educ. 2016;43(2):143–69.
2. Show A, Englar RE. Evaluating dog and cat owner preferences for Calgary–Cambridge communication skills: results of a questionnaire. J Vet Med Educ. 2018:1–10.
3. Tuckett D, Boulton M, Olson C. Meetings between experts: an approach to sharing ideas in medical consultations. London: Tavistock; 1985.
4. Arborelius E, Bremberg S. What can doctors do to achieve a successful consultation? Videotaped interviews analysed by the 'consultation map' method. Fam Pract. 1992;9(1):61–6.
5. Stewart MA. Effective physician–patient communication and health outcomes: a review. CMAJ. 1995;152(9):1423–33.
6. Stewart MA. What is a successful doctor–patient interview? A study of interactions and outcomes. Soc Sci Med. 1984;19(2):167–75.
7. Shilling V, Jenkins V, Fallowfield L. Factors affecting patient and clinician satisfaction with the clinical consultation: can communication skills training for clinicians improve satisfaction? Psychooncology. 2003;12(6):599–611.
8. Bell RA, Kravitz RL, Thom D, Krupat E, Azari R. Unmet expectations for care and the patient-physician relationship. J Gen Intern Med. 2002;17(11):817–24.
9. Eisenthal S, Koopman C, Stoeckle JD. The nature of patients' requests for physicians' help. Acad Med. 1990;65(6):401–5.
10. Eisenthal S, Lazare A. Evaluation of the initial interview in a walk-in clinic. The patient's perspective on a "customer approach". J Nerv Ment Dis. 1976;162(3):169–76.
11. Little P, Everitt H, Williamson I, Warner G, Moore M, Gould C, et al. Preferences of patients for patient centred approach to consultation in primary care: observational study. BMJ. 2001;322(7284):468–72.
12. Korsch BM, Gozzi EK, Francis V. Gaps in doctor–patient communication. 1. Doctor–patient interaction and patient satisfaction. Pediatrics. 1968;42(5):855–71.

13. Kinnersley P, Stott N, Peters TJ, Harvey I. The patient-centredness of consultations and outcome in primary care. Br J Gen Pract. 1999;49(446):711–6.

14. Predictors of outcome in headache patients presenting to family physicians—a one year prospective study. Headache; 1986: Headache Study Group of The University of Western Ontario.

15. Cornell KK, Kopcha M. Client–veterinarian communication: skills for client centered dialogue and shared decision making. Vet Clin North Am Small Anim Pract. 2007;37(1):37–47; abstract vii.

16. Hunter LJ, Shaw JR. How to exceed – not merely meet – client expectations. Veterinary Team Brief. 2018(March):19–22.

17. Magalhaes-Sant'Ana M, More SJ, Morton DB, Hanlon AJ. Challenges facing the veterinary profession in Ireland: 1. Clinical veterinary services. Ir Vet J. 2017:70.

18. Coe JB, Adams CL, Bonnett BN. A focus group study of veterinarians' and pet owners' perceptions of veterinarian-client communication in companion animal practice. J Am Vet Med Assoc. 2008;233(7):1072–80.

19. Kogan LR, Schoenfeld-Tacher R, Simon A, Viera A. The internet and pet health information: perceptions and behaviors of pet owners and veterinarians. Internet J Vet Med. 2009;8(1):1–19.

20. Martin F, Taunton A. Perceived importance and integration of the human-animal bond in private veterinary practice. J Am Vet Med Assoc. 2006;228(4):522–7.

21. Shaw JR, Adams CL, Bonnett BN. What can veterinarians learn from studies of physician–patient communication about veterinarian–client–patient communication? J Am Vet Med Assoc. 2004;224(5):676–84.

22. Timmins RP. The contribution of animals to human well-being: a veterinary family practice perspective. J Vet Med Educ. 2008;35(4):540–4.

23. Blackwell MJ. Beyond philosophical differences: the future training of veterinarians. J Vet Med Educ. 2001;28(3):148–52.

24. Brown JP, Silverman JD. The current and future market for veterinarians and veterinary medical services in the United States. J Am Vet Med Assoc. 1999;215(2):161–83.

25. Shanan A. A veterinarian's role in helping pet owners with decision making. Vet Clin North Am Small Anim Pract. 2011;41(3):635–46.

26. Kedrowicz AA. Clients and veterinarians as partners in problem solving during cancer management: implications for veterinary education. J Vet Med Educ. 2015;42(4):373–81.

27. Lue TW, Pantenburg DP, Crawford PM. Impact of the owner–pet and client–veterinarian bond on the care that pets receive. J Am Vet Med Assoc. 2008;232(4):531–40.

28. Bartlett EE, Grayson M, Barker R, Levine DM, Golden A, Libber S. The effects of physician communications skills on patient satisfaction; recall, and adherence. J Chronic Dis. 1984;37(9–10):755–64.

29. Jackson JL, Chamberlin J, Kroenke K. Predictors of patient satisfaction. Soc Sci Med. 2001;52(4):609–20.

30. Stoewen DL, Coe JB, MacMartin C, Stone EA, C ED. Qualitative study of the communication expectations of clients accessing oncology care at a tertiary referral center for dogs with life-limiting cancer. J Am Vet Med Assoc. 2014;245(7):785–95.

Chapter 12

Asking Permission to Enhance Relationship-Centered Care

Historically, the practice of medicine leaned heavily on the tradition of paternalism. The Hippocratic Oath gave birth to the philosophy that "doctor knows best," thereby granting the physician the authority to act upon his instincts.(1–3) This attitude of paternalism was reinforced by the belief that the clinician possessed more knowledge and skill than the patients.(3–5) Thus, the doctor was always placed in the driver's seat.(6) It was the doctor who determined the best course of action for the patient.(6) It was the doctor who dictated case outcomes.(6–8) It was the doctor who made choices to minimize physical harm or emotional trauma.(5) The *good* doctor had a duty to protect his or her patient, however he or she saw fit.(5)

It could therefore be said that the traditional doctor took on the role of being "expert-in-charge."(9)

The "expert-in-charge" role remains a staple of emergency room medicine today, both in human and veterinary healthcare.(9) When clinical presentations are acute and/or life threatening, the physician takes charge of the situation to address the immediate threat to the patient.(9) Patients who are unstable and/or in critical condition require expedited treatment.(9) Human patients or veterinary clients may not be of sound mind to collaborate in such a way as to positively contribute to the case outcome.

Human medical scenarios that require an "expert-in-charge" approach to healthcare include presentations of diabetic ketoacidosis (DKA), myocardial infarction, head trauma, and sepsis.

Veterinary medical scenarios that require an "expert-in-charge" approach to healthcare include automobile trauma, evisceration, open fractures, urinary tract obstruction (UTO), and a panting cat in respiratory distress.

In these situations, compassion is implied by the way in which care is expedited. In the heat of the moment, the doctor cannot devote resources – particularly time – to the psychosocial aspects of care.(9) The doctor must engage the team to save a life. This is an appropriate use for the role, expert-in-charge.

As veterinarians, we often take on the role of being the "expert-in-charge" in non-emergency situations. This role is familiar to us because our clients place us in the role of expert: they pay for our consultation time and our evidence-based opinions as to how to effectively manage patient care.

However, there are times when it is both appropriate and respectful to ask permission from a client to either share our insight or to perform a procedure on the patient.(9)

Asking permission from a client means exactly what it says: asking a client if it is okay to proceed. Asking permission requires us to step outside of the more familiar "expert-in-charge" role and instead become a partner in healthcare and/or a facilitator.

Partnership was addressed in Chapter 10. Partnerships are particularly effective doctor–client–patient relationships when the patient is experiencing chronic disease, for which long-term care is indicated.(9) Consider, for example, the following list of human ailments:

- asthma
- atopy
- cancer
- chronic kidney disease (CKD)
- congestive heart failure (CHF)
- dental disease
- diabetes mellitus
- hyperadrenocorticism (Cushing's Disease)
- hyperthyroidism
- hypoadrenocorticism (Addison's Disease)
- hypothyroidism
- immune-mediated disease
- obesity
- osteoarthritis (OA).

In these clinical scenarios, partnership takes precedence over the "expert-in-charge" role because the human physician must work with the patient to effectively manage long-term healthcare. This perspective stems from the evolution of the doctor–patient relationship.(10) The physician is viewed as a collaborator or facilitator of healthcare rather than a dictator.(10) This philosophy is derived from the belief that:

> The patient is not just a group of symptoms, damaged organs and altered emotions. The patient is a human being, at the same time worried and hopeful, who is searching for relief, help and trust. The importance of an intimate relationship between patient and physician can never be overstated because in most cases an accurate diagnosis, as well as an effective treatment, relies directly on the quality of this relationship. (11)

This viewpoint humanizes medicine. It also recognizes the role that the patient plays in establishing and maintaining his or her healthcare.

The same perspective may be applied to the healthcare discipline, veterinary medicine. In order to effect change and to yield a positive case outcome, the veterinarian needs to share responsibilities for patient care with the client. The client must be given the opportunity to contribute. The veterinarian must motivate the client into action.(9) Each individual must rely upon the other to commit to treatment and to follow through.(9)

One way to motivate the client into action is to enhance connectivity. A client is more likely to comply with treatment recommendations if she or he is made to feel like part of the team. Case outcomes are more likely to improve when patients are allowed to share health-related concerns with the medical team.(12–19)

Refer to Chapter 10 for additional details on how to incorporate partnership statements into clinical conversations with clients.

Another way to introduce partnership is to ask for the client's permission. "Asking permission" statements often start with "May I?"

- "May I borrow Brandon for a moment so that we can get started on drawing the blood for those laboratory tests?"
- "May I shave the fur around the wound so that it is easier for us to keep it clean while it is healing?"
- "May I trim his toe nails when he is in the back treatment area with my technicians?"

12.1 Incorporating Permission Statements into Clinical Scenarios

Let us take a look at how this might work in clinical practice.

Background

You are an associate veterinarian in clinical practice.

Your client, Mr. Curtis, has recently adopted a beagle, Frank. This is Mr. Curtis' first visit to your clinic. He's not familiar with how your clinic operates.

You need to draw blood from Frank for a heartworm test, but you feel that it would go more smoothly if you were to take Frank away from his owner.

Let us examine this clinical scenario first, from the client's perspective, if you don't ask for permission to take Frank to the treatment area.

Clinical Conversation

Veterinarian: Okay, Mr. Curtis, everything checks out with Frank. He just needs his heartworm test and then you two will be on your way.

[Veterinarian reaches out to grab Frank's leash without explanation]

Veterinarian: We'll be back in a minute.

From the client's perspective, this is an unclear directive, particularly because this is his first experience with your clinic and he is not familiar with how the practice operates.

The client may wonder about any or all of the following:

- Where is Frank going?
- Why can't Frank stay here?
- In the meantime, what is the client supposed to do?
- Is he supposed to follow you?
- Is he supposed to wait for you in the examination room?

Asking for permission would have more respectfully transitioned the visit from the consultation to the next step: diagnostic testing.

Asking for permission would have clarified for the owner what this next step entails.

Let us revisit the same clinical scenario over again, this time asking for permission.

Clinical Conversation

Veterinarian: Okay, Mr. Curtis, everything checks out with Frank. He just needs his heartworm test and then you two will be on your way.

[pause]

Veterinarian: Would it be okay with you if I took Frank to the backroom to get his blood drawn?

Mr. Curtis: Absolutely.

Veterinarian: That's great, thank you! My technicians are all set up and ready for him. They can collect a blood sample and then bring him straight back to you to wait for the results. How does that sound?

Mr. Curtis: That works for me.

[Mr. Curtis offers up the leash]

Mr. Curtis: (to the Veterinarian) Here you go. / (to Frank) Be a good boy.

Note how much more smoothly this conversation flowed. Mr. Curtis feels respected because he was asked before the dog was taken from him. Mr. Curtis also knows what to expect: Frank will have his blood drawn and will then return to his side to wait for the results.

12.2 What if the Client Doesn't Say "Yes"?

Note that if we ask for permission, most owners will say "yes." However, if we ask for permission, we have to be prepared with a Plan B if the owner says "no."

For example, what if Mr. Curtis does not want his dog to go to the back treatment room? What could we do instead?

You will want to have a couple of options in mind so that you are prepared if and when a client says "no." Let us see how that might play out in clinical practice:

Clinical Conversation

Veterinarian: Okay, Mr. Curtis, everything checks out with Frank. He just needs his heartworm test and then you two will be on your way.

[pause]

Veterinarian: Would it be okay with you if I took Frank to the backroom to get his blood drawn?

[pause]

Mr. Curtis: You know, that kind of worries me. He's not so good around other dogs and he might get out hand if I'm not there to intervene.

Veterinarian: That's completely understandable, thank you for the heads-up. What if we were to draw the blood in here so that Frank doesn't have to leave, but you stepped out of the room for a moment. Would that work?

Mr. Curtis: Sure, I'd rather do that. I don't really want to risk him being around other dogs.

Veterinarian: Not a problem. When we finish getting Frank's sample, perhaps you and I can think about ways we might be able to improve his interactions with other dogs in the future.

Note that the veterinarian did not force the client to subscribe to his plan.

Instead, the veterinarian heard and accepted the client's reluctance to take the patient to the treatment area. Rather than pressing the issue, the veterinarian was prepared to offer a viable solution that was agreeable to both parties. In return, the client felt respected, and was willing to work with the veterinarian to achieve the end goal (diagnostic testing).

12.3 Alternative Phrasing of "May I?"

Sometimes, new graduates feel that asking, "May I?" is awkward.

Some students have told me that it feels like they are back in grade school, when they are asking the teacher, "May I use the lavatory?" If "May I?" feels unnatural, then avoid its use. Otherwise, it will come across as being stiff and stilted.

Instead, try out other appropriate phrases that are synonymous:

- "Can I?" or "Can we?"(20)
- "If I may ...?"
- "Would it be okay if ...?"
- "Are you okay if ...?"
- "Would it be alright if ...?"
- "Are you alright if ...?"

- "Would that work?"
- "What are your thoughts about …?"

These questions achieve the same communication purpose as "May I", while sounding a bit less formal and a bit more conversational.

12.4 Other Clinical Scenarios that Benefit from Asking Permission

Asking permission is beneficial in the following clinical situations.

1. When there is a fee associated with a procedure.
2. When the patient has a specific purpose (other than companion) and a procedure that you recommend may impact its ability to perform.
3. When the procedure could cause harm.
4. When sharing information via telephone.
5. When sharing patient-sensitive data with those outside of the doctor–client–patient relationship.

12.4.1 Asking Permission When There Are Fees Associated with Procedures

If there is a fee associated with a procedure, then clients have a right to know – for example, a toe nail trim that is *not* complimentary. The clinician owes it to the client to ask, "Would you like us to trim Frank's nails while he is in the treatment area? It costs $15.00, but would save you from having to trim them at home. I know how much he loves that!" The client will not appreciate *not* being asked *and* being hit with an unexpected bill.

12.4.2 Asking Permission When a Procedure Could Alter a Patient's Function

Sometimes a procedure may put a patient's function or purpose at risk.
Consider the following two populations of patients:

- show dogs and cats
- working dogs.

If the pet is a show dog or cat, it is especially important to ask for permission before shaving any fur.
There are situations in which we absolutely have to shave fur off in order to provide

gold standard care – for example, when placing intravenous catheters. However, if you shave a show dog or cat's limb without asking for permission first, your client will not look favorably upon your actions.

Better for you to prepare the client, "If we place an IV catheter, then we are going to have to shave Felicia's front leg. I know she has a prized coat, but it is really the only way to rehydrate her. Are you okay with that?"

Alternatively, consider working dogs, such as those among the Beagle Brigade. The Beagle Brigade is a team of dogs and their human handlers who are employed by the US Department of Agriculture to inspect luggage in airports. These dogs are heavily relied upon as gatekeepers at checkpoints for US Customs and Border Protection to prevent the introduction of prohibited agricultural products (and their associated diseases) into the country. Thanks to their keen sense of smell, canine team members contribute to 75,000 seizures of prohibited products annually.(21)

For these patients, sense of smell is essential for their continued employment. Any procedure that threatens to disrupt their ability to carry out their job description should be avoided at all costs. The burden falls upon the veterinarian to alert the client of reasonable alternatives whenever possible so as to safeguard these dogs' sense of smell. For example, the veterinarian might suggest that Beagle Brigade team members be vaccinated against *Bordetella bronchiseptica* using an injectable or oral formulation as opposed to the intranasal one.

If the client has presented the patient for the intranasal vaccination, then asking permission to share alternative options will facilitate a discussion about what is considered best practice for the patient.

The veterinarian might approach this conversation any number of ways, including the following.

- "May I share with you a new formulation that may be more appropriate for your dog, given that his work relies upon preserving his excellent sense of smell?"
- "If it's okay with you, can we discuss a new type of *Bordetella* vaccination that will protect your dog just as well as the intranasal one, but without affecting his sense of smell?"

12.4.3 Asking Permission Before Performing Procedures that Could Cause Physical Harm

If the procedure that you are going to perform has the potential to cause harm to your patient, then you should ask for permission to proceed.

For instance, something as benign as a toe nail trim could result in a bloody foot or even transient lameness, as from trimming nails too short. If you do not ask the client for permission – and then the patient returns from the treatment area with a bloodied foot, this is a problem. If you do not ask the client for permission – and then the patient has an altered gait, this is a problem. Better for you to ask the client for permission first, "Would it be okay if we trimmed her nails today?"

True, the patient could still be injured in the process, but you have at least given the client the opportunity to say, "No" before you got started on something that the client may not have wanted in the first place.

12.4.4 Asking Permission to Share Information via Telephone

In an ideal world, we would always be able to share information about the patient with the client face to face. However, in reality, the practice of veterinary medicine often requires us to reach out to clients outside of the examination room. This may be due to time constraints in clinical consultations. Appointments average 13 minutes in clinical practice.(22) It is impossible to address every client concern within this time frame. Follow-up consultations and/or telephone conversations are essential in order for patient care to be thorough and in order for veterinary recommendations to be comprehensive.

We may also need to reach out to clients by telephone to discuss:

- anatomic pathology diagnostic test results
  - gross necropsy findings
  - histopathology
- clinical pathology diagnostic test results
  - bloodwork
  - fecal analysis
  - urinalysis
- imaging diagnostic test results
  - radiographs
  - ultrasound
  - computed tomography (CT)
  - magnetic resonance imaging (MRI)
  - contrast-enhanced imaging
- patient's recovery from a medical or surgical procedure
- patient's response to treatment
- referrals.

When I first graduated from Cornell University College of Veterinary Medicine in 2008, my expectation was that clients would be waiting by the telephone to hear from me. I expected that clients would be available and eager to chat. I expected that clients would stop whatever it was they were doing to take my call, and that they would listen intently.

I awoke to a harsh reality.

Clients did not always pick up the telephone. More often than not, I would be forced to leave a voicemail. On other occasions, clients would take my call, but they would be abbreviated in speech, short with me, or overtly distracted. Much of what I said was not heard. Much of what I said had to be repeated the next day, or to another member of the family.

This frustrated me until I realized that it was not the client's fault. It was mine. I had never taken the time to ask the client if she or he was available to speak.

I would have done better to have asked the client for permission to share information. For example, after introducing myself on the telephone, I could have said:

- "Is now an okay time to chat about Fievel?"
- "I just got a report from the pathologist. Is now a good time to discuss the results of Jesse's biopsy?"
- "I have some updates to share about Genevieve. Do you have time to discuss these?"
- "If it's okay with you, I'd like to go over Forest's bloodwork results."
- "If it's alright with you, can we talk about next steps for Simba?"

These statements demonstrate that you, the clinician, respect the client and value his or her time. They also acknowledge that you recognize the client may or may not be free to chat in the moment. They give the client the opportunity to decline speaking now and postpone a necessary conversation to a date and time when it will be more convenient.

Postponing the conversation does not mean that the client does not care. Postponing the conversation is the client's way of expressing that she or he cares what you have to say and wants to wait until a time when she or he can truly listen.

Maybe the client is unable to talk right now because:

- She's at work.
- He's handling something urgent at the office.
- She's off to a meeting and only has a "few seconds."
- He's in the middle of an urgent conversation on the other line.
- She's on her way out the door.
- He's in the car driving from point A to point B.
- She's boarding an airplane.
- He's picking up the kids from school.

The possibilities are endless.

It doesn't matter why the client cannot talk.

What matters is that we give the client the freedom to express that now is really not a good time – and that we do not take this personally. Instead, we remain flexible and willing to work with the client to come up with a better day or time. By doing so, we set the stage for a conversation in which the client will be actively present, rather than focused on something or someone else.

If now is not a good time to chat for the client, then be prepared to inquire when it would be convenient.

Alternatively, you may suggest other days and times.

- "Would it be more convenient if I telephoned tomorrow over the lunch hour?"
- "I can telephone on Monday morning between 10 and 11 am. Would that work?"
- "I could make myself available to telephone tomorrow night, between 5–6 pm. Would that be easier for you?"

Do not be reluctant to express your needs. If you do not, then you may resent the client for something that really is not the client's fault.

If the client offers up an alternate date and/or time that does not work for you, it is okay to say "No." Just be polite about it. For example:

- "I wish I could make that work, unfortunately I will be seeing another appointment at that time. Could I telephone immediately after I finish up with that client? That would be approximately 4 pm."
- "Unfortunately, I'm tied up with work at that hour. What about an hour after that? Would that work better for you?"

It may take a couple of tries to find a mutually agreed upon time. That is okay. It is well worth the investment now to plan ahead for later.

12.4.5 Asking Permission to Share Patient-Sensitive Data with Those Outside of the Veterinary Team

Sometimes we may wish to share patient-sensitive data with others outside of the veterinary team. Maybe we want to consult informally with a colleague about the root of a patient's problem. Maybe we want to make use of a patient as a case study for a conference or a write-up in a professional journal or popular press magazine. Maybe we are an instructor at a veterinary college and wish to share a patient's case history, bloodwork results, and/or diagnostic images within the classroom setting.

In any of these cases, we are first and foremost bound to the rules that our administration has established concerning the sharing of patient-specific data. However, beyond the established criteria for what constitutes acceptable sharing of information, it is appropriate and considered common courtesy to ask the client for permission to share.

Asking permission may take the form of one of the following statements:

- "Like you, I, too, am concerned about Sadie being put under anesthesia, given her age and advanced heart disease. If it's okay with you, I would like to reach out to a colleague who is a veterinary anesthesiologist. She is well equipped to make recommendations that will improve the safety of Sadie's procedure. Would that be alright with you?"
- "Peeta's case serves as a great reminder why history taking is such an important part of the appointment. Had you not shared with me what Peeta had access to, in the garage, we may never have realized he had ingested rat poison until it was too late.

Would you mind if I referenced Peeta's case in the classroom so that students can learn to ask the right questions and to listen to the clients?"

- "Finnick definitely looks like he read the textbook: his bloodwork perfectly demonstrates how urinary tract obstructions impact electrolytes. May I share this with my students so that they can make clinical connections between what they are learning in the classroom and real-life cases? I think that his bloodwork would really help them to better understand the consequences that disease has on the body."

- "As we've discussed, this is the first case of slipped capital femoral epiphysis (SCFE) in a cat that I have ever seen. In fact, very few case reports have been reported in the medical literature. I think that Joey's case could help many of my colleagues treat other cats with the same condition if they read about it. Would it be okay with you if I wrote up Joey's case for the *Journal of the American Veterinary Medical Association* (JAVMA)?"

- "I am so happy for you that little Penelope found you as her Forever Home! Our hospital director is looking to showcase happy endings, such as this one, on our practice's monthly newsletter. Would it be alright if I passed along your information so that she can reach out?"

Asking for permission in these clinical situations demonstrates respect for your client.

Asking for permission demonstrates that you are deferring to your client. You are acknowledging to the client that she or he is the gatekeeper for patient-specific data. You are admitting aloud that, despite your wishes to share information, at the end of the day it is up to the client to decide if sharing is acceptable.

Clients appreciate the opportunity to authorize or refuse information sharing. Clients appreciate the sense of respect that asking for permission conveys.

12.5 The Clinical Importance of Asking for Permission among Dog and Cat Owners

A focus group pilot study was conducted by my research team in 2016 to evaluate the clinical importance of communication skills within companion-animal practice.(23) This study evaluated dog owners and cat owners separately to better understand their communication preferences and needs. All dog owners in the study rated the skill of asking for permission as "very to extremely important." (23) Dog owners expressed the importance of asking for permission in the following circumstances: (23)

- prior to performing the physical examination
- prior to vaccinating the patient
- prior to attempting venipuncture.

When asked why this skill was so important, dog owners expressed that they felt responsible for preparing their dog for what is going to happen next. One owner said it best:

"Dogs pick up on a lot. If I know what's going to happen, I can give him a little pep talk." (23)

I conducted a follow-up study in 2018 using survey questionnaires to reach a broader audience.(24) Asking permission was again considered to be of primary importance to dog owners.(24) In this study, cat owners were also in agreement that they valued this communication skill.(24) Asking permission was viewed as a demonstration of respect for the client by the veterinary team.(24)

Respect is an integral part of relationship building.(25) Today's veterinary client expects to be respected. Respect denotes their value to the veterinary team, and enhances relationship-centered care.(24–26)

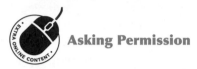 **Asking Permission**

References

1. McCullough LB. Was bioethics founded on historical and conceptual mistakes about medical paternalism? Bioethics. 2011;25(2):66–74.
2. Weiss GB. Paternalism modernized. J Med Ethics. 1985;11(4):184–7.
3. Tan NHSS. Deconstructing paternalism: what serves the patient best? Singapore Med J. 2002;43(3):148–51.
4. Nuland SB. Autonomy run amuck: review of patient heal thyself: how the 'new medicine' puts the patient in charge, by Robert M. Veatch. The New Republic. 2009;240(11):48–51.
5. Buchanan A. Medical paternalism. Philos Public Aff. 1978;7(4):370–90.
6. Bradley G, Sparks B, Nesdale D. Doctor communication style and patient outcomes: gender and age as moderators. J Appl Soc Psychol. 2001;31(8):1749–73.
7. Burgoon M, Birk TS, Hall JR. Compliance and satisfaction with physician–patient communication – an expectancy-theory interpretation of gender differences. Hum Commun Res. 1991;18(2):177–208.
8. Savage R, Armstrong D. Effect of a general-practitioners consulting style on patients' satisfaction – a controlled-study. Brit Med J. 1990;301(6758):968–70.
9. Lussier MT, Richard C. Because one shoe doesn't fit all – a repertoire of doctor–patient relationships. Can Fam Physician. 2008;54(8):1089–92.
10. Kaba R, Sooriakumaran P. The evolution of the doctor–patient relationship. Int J Surg. 2007;5(1):57–65.
11. Hellin T. The physician–patient relationship: recent developments and changes. Haemophilia. 2002;8(3):450–4.
12. Simpson M, Buckman R, Stewart M, Maguire P, Lipkin M, Novack D, et al. Doctor–patient communication – the Toronto Consensus Statement. Brit Med J. 1991;303(6814):1385–7.
13. Kaplan SH, Greenfield S, Ware JE, Jr. Assessing the effects of physician–patient interactions on the outcomes of chronic disease. Med Care. 1989;27(3 Suppl):S110–27.
14. Predictors of outcome in headache patients presenting to family physicians—a one year prospective study. Headache; 1986: Headache Study Group of The University of Western Ontario.
15. Orth JE, Stiles WB, Scherwitz L, Hennrikus D, Vallbona C. Patient exposition and provider

explanation in routine interviews and hypertensive patients' blood pressure control. Health Psychol. 1987;6(1):29–42.

16. Ha JF, Longnecker N. Doctor–patient communication: a review. Ochsner J. 2010;10(1):38–43.

17. Arora NK. Interacting with cancer patients: the significance of physicians' communication behavior. Soc Sci Med. 2003;57(5):791–806.

18. Lee SJ, Back AL, Block SD, Stewart SK. Enhancing physician–patient communication. Hematology Am Soc Hematol Educ Program. 2002:464–83.

19. Kindler CH, Szirt L, Sommer D, Hausler R, Langewitz W. A quantitative analysis of anaesthetist–patient communication during the pre-operative visit. Anaesthesia. 2005;60(1):53–9.

20. Hunter LJ, Shaw JR. How to exceed – not merely meet – client expectations. Veterinary Team Brief. 2018(March):19–22.

21. Querna B. U.S. Beagle Brigade is first defense against alien species. National Geographic Society [Internet]. 2001. Available from: https://archive.is/20130421101019/http://news. nationalgeographic.co.uk/news/2001/06/0607_beaglebrigade.html.

22. Shaw JR, Adams CL, Bonnett BN, Larson S, Roter DL. Use of the Roter interaction analysis system to analyse veterinarian–client–patient communication in companion animal practice. J Am Vet Med Assoc. 2004;225(2):222–9.

23. Englar RE, Williams M, Weingand K. Applicability of the Calgary–Cambridge Guide to dog and cat owners for teaching veterinary clinical communications. J Vet Med Educ. 2016;43(2):143–69.

24. Show A, Englar RE. Evaluating dog and cat owner preferences for Calgary–Cambridge communication skills: results of a questionnaire. J Vet Med Educ. 2018:1–10.

25. McArthur ML, Fitzgerald JR. Companion animal veterinarians' use of clinical communication skills. Aust Vet J. 2013;91(9):374–80.

26. Shaw JR, Adams CL, Bonnett BN. What can veterinarians learn from studies of physician–patient communication about veterinarian–client–patient communication? J Am Vet Med Assoc. 2004;224(5):676–84.

Chapter 13

Enhancing Relationship-Centered Care by Assessing the Client's Knowledge

During a veterinary consultation, we spend a great deal of time in the consultation room explaining the following to our clients:

- clinical findings
- the patient's diagnosis
- the patient's prognosis
- proposed treatment plans
- expected patient outcome.

The amount of information that each client needs in order to make confident, informed decisions about patient care varies depending upon what each client already knows about a certain disease or disease process.

Some clients need to know much more information before they feel comfortable with making decisions. Others are much farther along in their understanding and need only a few key facts to prompt a decision.(1)

Clients expect us to tailor our delivery of healthcare to their wants and needs.(2) This was conveyed best in a focus group study by my research team in 2016 that evaluated communication preferences of companion animal-owning clients. Respondents acknowledged that healthcare needs vary client to client, and emphasized the importance of receiving individualized care from veterinary team members.

- "We're not just another person. Treat me as my own person."(2)
- "Treat each person as an individual and cater to their needs."(2)
- "Get to what our needs are."(2)

How do we know which client is seated before us in the consultation room?

We can make use of communication to assess the client's knowledge. Assessing the client's knowledge allows us to gauge the depth of our client's understanding about any number of topics.(3) These include:

- clinical signs
- diagnoses
- diagnostic plans
- diseases
- medications
- surgical approaches
- treatment plans.

Assessing the client's knowledge gives the client the opportunity to share what they know about a given topic.(3)

Veterinary clients may be knowledgeable about a condition or disease from past experiences.(1) Perhaps the veterinary condition also occurs in people, and our client actually has the diagnosis. A good example would be diabetes mellitus. Or perhaps the client does not him/herself have the disease, but has previously owned a pet with the same condition.

Firsthand knowledge provides a foundation or starting point for us to launch into more descriptive discussions about a particular condition, diagnostic modality, treatment recommendation, or alternative approach to care.

If the client is correct, then we can validate his or her understanding and build onto pre-existing knowledge to round out the clinical picture. If the client is incorrect about his or her knowledge base, then we can use the consultation as a gentle learning opportunity in a safe, supportive environment to clarify misinformation. If the client is unsure, then we know that we need to make use of consultation time to fill in the gaps where knowledge is unclear.

Statements that assess the client's knowledge often begin as follows.

- "Are you familiar with ...?"
- "What do you know about ...?"
- "Did you know that ...?"
- "Are you aware that ...?"
- "What is your understanding of ...?"
- "How much do you know about ...?"
- "Have you ever heard of ...?"
- "Do you know ...?"

Here are some examples from clinical practice that make use of this phraseology.

- "Are you familiar with lymphoma?"
- "What do you know about lymphoma in cats?"
- "Did you know that dogs can become diabetic?"
- "Are you aware that diabetic cats may go into remission?"
- "What is your understanding of insulin therapy to manage diabetes?"
- "How much do you know about diabetes in dogs?"

- "Have you ever heard of hypoglycemia?"
- "Do you know how to recognize the signs of hypoglycemia in a cat?"
- "Do you know how to administer insulin to a dog?"

In clinical scenarios that involve medical management of a chronic disease, such as hypertension, it is particularly important to assess the patient's knowledge.(4) Effective management of hypertension in human healthcare requires extensive patient education and buy-in to multiple avenues of treatment.(4) These include:(4)

- polypharmacy
- lifestyle modifications
  - exercise
  - stress reduction
  - weight loss
- modifications to diet
  - limiting salt intake.

Effective management of diabetes mellitus in human healthcare also requires an extensive understanding of the disease process as well as various avenues for intervention:(4)

- dietary modification
- potential use of oral hypoglycemic agents, such as glipizide
- injectable insulin therapy
- at-home blood glucose monitoring
- potential sequelae.

Adequate knowledge about medications is essential in order for patients to take medications, as instructed.(5–7) Yet studies from the human literature suggest that patients do not always understand why they are instructed to take a particular medication.(5) Patients do not always understand the correct action to take if they miss one or more doses of medication.(5) Furthermore, patients are often unaware of medication side effects.(5, 8)

Knowledge of drug regimens varies immensely among our population of patients, yet we often make assumptions about what patients do and do not need to hear from us.(5)

Patients that actively seek out information will ask for clarification or will research areas of uncertainty to gain clarity.(5) However, others will act upon misunderstandings or misinterpretations of healthcare recommendations.(5) This could have deleterious effects on patient health and wellbeing.

Knowledge is therefore key to adherence to treatment, particularly when it comes to prescription medications.(9, 10)

Successful case outcomes in veterinary medicine equally depend upon effective communication between the veterinarian and the client.(11) Given that veterinary consultations are typically on the order of 10–15 minutes, it is challenging to cover all aspects of care in a single office visit.(11)

Consider a 2019 study by Albuquerque et al. that evaluated owners' perceptions and priorities about the medical management and monitoring of their diabetic cats. Ninety-one percent of respondents acknowledged that insulin treatment was discussed at the time of initial diagnosis; and 73% recalled discussing the frequency of rechecks.(11)

However, many topics were poorly addressed.(11)

- Only 46% of veterinarians discussed clinical signs that might suggest difficulty with regulating diabetes.
- Only 41% of veterinarians discussed the possibility of diabetic remission.
- Only 40% of veterinarians discussed the possibility of home blood glucose monitoring.

Moreover, many clients felt deficient in knowledge or in technical skills that were deemed necessary for successful case outcomes.(11)

- Only 45% of clients felt comfortable recognizing or treating hypoglycemia.
- One-quarter of clients had not been shown how to draw up insulin.
- 27% of clients had not been shown how to administer insulin.
- Only 49% of clients were supervised by the veterinary team when administering their first injection to their cat.

It is impossible to educate a client about every aspect of a medical condition and every angle of care at a single consultation, particularly those of abbreviated lengths.(11)

However, if clients are asked to share pre-existing knowledge with the veterinary team, then we as professionals are better equipped to gauge how much education is necessary. We also will be better able to serve the needs of our patients.

We will be able to recognize those clients who are least knowledgeable and therefore most likely to struggle with patient care. These clients can be flagged in the system so that they are more carefully followed and monitored.

Additional opportunities for education and hands-on learning can be provided so as to set these clients up for success, taking care to welcome their involvement rather than portray it as a burden on the veterinary team.

These new learners can become our best clients, if we are willing to demonstrate patience and commitment to care.

13.1 What Happens When We Do Not Assess the Client's Knowledge?

How does assessing the client's knowledge work in a clinical setting?

For the purpose of providing contrast, let us first consider a clinical scenario in which the clinician fails to assess the client's knowledge. Doing so will allow you to see first-hand how this omission adversely impacts the flow of the conversation.

Background

You are an associate veterinarian in clinical practice. You have just diagnosed a cat with diabetes mellitus.

Clinical Conversation

Veterinarian: Cupid has diabetes. Most cats require insulin injections in order to manage their diabetes. There are a few products that are available on the market for cats, but personally, I've had the most success with using human insulin, glargine. Glargine is typically administered subcutaneously twice per day. We will see how she responds to insulin injections and may have to adjust her dose several times before we find the right dose for her.

Client: I know. I've owned five diabetic cats in my lifetime.

Note how the veterinarian failed to assess the client's knowledge. In this case, the client was pleasant enough about pointing out his knowledge to the veterinarian. But not all clients will be so cordial.

In truth, this client probably knows more than I do about the day-to-day logistics of managing a diabetic cat than I do, because I have never personally owned one.

It would have been better for me to have asked the client what he knew about the disease and treatment options, to assess his knowledge base and where to begin a conversation that was appropriate for his level of education.

13.2 Revisiting the Same Scenario to Assess our Client's Knowledge

Let us revisit the same clinical scenario over again, this time taking time to assess our client's knowledge.

Clinical Conversation

Veterinarian: Cupid has diabetes. Are you familiar with diabetes in cats?

Client: I think you could say that I've owned my fair share. Cupid will be my sixth diabetic cat.

Veterinarian: Oh wow! Then you definitely know what you're getting into! Can you share with me a bit about what management of your diabetic cats has involved?

Client: They all did well on insulin. That human insulin, glargine, seemed to work best

---

for us. Once we got them regulated on the right dose, it was easy to manage.

Veterinarian: That's great! Then you're ahead of the game. I definitely think that glargine would be an appropriate choice for Cupid. Let's talk about what dose would work best to start.

Note how efficiently we were able to recognize that this client has some baseline knowledge about diabetes in cats, including product names and medication regimes.

Note that we still will need to review doses, injection sites, risks of treatment, and signs of an insulin overdose with the client, but at least now we have a starting point.

We also took the time to recognize and honor his experience with the condition. This demonstrates our baseline level of respect. We are, in a sense, recognizing that he is, in his own right, a content area expert.

13.3 Other Reasons to Assess our Client's Knowledge

In clinical practice, we often assess the client's knowledge about a disease or a disease-related process. However, it is equally important to assess the client's understanding of a particular procedure or medical regime.

* Have you ever administered injections to dogs before?
* Have you ever given your dog a shot?
* Have you ever given sub-q fluids before?
* Have you ever had to pill your cat?
* Have you ever needed to give your dog eye drops?
* Have you administered transdermal medication?
* Have you applied topical ear medication before?
* Have you ever taken your dog's rectal temperature?

You can also assess the client's knowledge about certain medications.

* How familiar are you with the drug, metronidazole?
* Are you aware of this drug's potential side effects?
* Have you ever given your dog cephalexin?
* Did your dog ever experience any ill effects related to cephalexin therapy?
* I am going to prescribe prednisone to your dog to reduce the intensity of his itch while his skin condition is resolving. Are you familiar with the dosing schedule of this drug?
* Are you aware what will happen if you discontinue this drug abruptly?

13.4 Assessing Knowledge Is Respectful

Assessing the client's knowledge is an important communication tool that helps you to explore what your client knows about a disease, disease process, diagnostic or treatment plan, medication, therapy, or prognosis.

When you invite your client to share their knowledge with you, you are accepting them as contributors to the conversation and to patient care.

This demonstrates respect. The client feels welcome to share his or her knowledge base. The client may also feel less reluctant to share that he or she does not know something.

If the client is asked, "Are you familiar with …?", the client may be more likely to answer honestly because the question is conversational.

Assessing the client's knowledge is intended to have a relaxed feel. The purpose is not to interrogate your client. The purpose is to showcase what your client knows so that you know where to begin and you can build on from there.

 Assessing the Client's Knowledge

References

1. Show A, Englar RE. Evaluating dog and cat owner preferences for Calgary–Cambridge communication skills: results of a questionnaire. J Vet Med Educ. 2018:1–10.

2. Englar RE, Williams M, Weingand K. Applicability of the Calgary–Cambridge Guide to dog and cat owners for teaching veterinary clinical communications. J Vet Med Educ. 2016;43(2):143–69.

3. Hunter L, Shaw JR. What's in your communication toolbox? Exceptional Veterinary Team. 2012(November/December):12–7.

4. Williams MV, Baker DW, Parker RM, Nurss JR. Relationship of functional health literacy to patients' knowledge of their chronic disease. A study of patients with hypertension and diabetes. Arch Intern Med. 1998;158(2):166–72.

5. Ascione FJ, Kirscht JP, Shimp LA. An assessment of different components of patient medication knowledge. Med Care. 1986;24(11):1018–28.

6. Becker MH. Understanding patient compliance: the contributions of attitudes and other psychosocial factors. In: Cohen SJ, editor. New directions in patient compliance. Lexington, MD: Lexington Books; 1979. pp. 1–31.

7. Leventhal H, Meyer D, Gutmann M. The role of theory in the study of compliance to high blood pressure regimens. In: Haynes RB, Mattson ME, Engebretson TO, editors. Patient compliance to prescribed antihypertensive medication regimens: a report to the national heart, lung, and blood institute. Washington, DC: United States Department of Health and Human Services; 1980. pp. 1–15.

8. Kay EA, Bailie GR, Bernstein A. Patient knowledge of cardio-respiratory drugs. J Clin Pharm Ther. 1988;13(4):263–8.

9.   Okuyan B, Sancar M, Izzettin FV. Assessment of medication knowledge and adherence among patients under oral chronic medication treatment in community pharmacy settings. Pharmacoepidemiol Drug Saf. 2013;22(2):209–14.

10. Akici A, Kalaca S, Ugurlu MU, Toklu HZ, Iskender E, Oktay S. Patient knowledge about drugs prescribed at primary healthcare facilities. Pharmacoepidemiol Drug Saf. 2004;13(12):871–6.

11. Albuquerque CS, Bauman BL, Rzeznitzeck J, Caney SM, Gunn-Moore DA. Priorities on treatment and monitoring of diabetic cats from the owners' points of view. J Feline Med Surg. 2019:1098612X19858154.

Chapter 14

Mapping Out the Clinical Consultation

Signposting

Have you ever found yourself in a strange city far from home? Have you ever journeyed to an exotic location and had to navigate to an unfamiliar destination? Maybe you had to navigate through the airport of another country, or through the customs and border control of a foreign land. Maybe you had to navigate through the metro or direct a taxi cab to pick you up in an unfamiliar part of town, without benefit of a GPS system. Or maybe construction walled off your usual way home and now you have to find an alternate route.

If you are blessed with a sense of adventure or "street smarts," then you will be undeterred by navigation. In fact, navigation may excite you. You may even look forward to new sights along the way, as well as the sense of accomplishment that comes from knowing you could find your way. Maybe you have a knack for reading roadmaps or compasses, and directions like "point yourself 30 degrees North of West" make sense to you. Maybe you're blessed with technology. You keep your smartphone tied to your waist and are a daily subscriber of Google Maps.

But what if you don't have any of these resources? Or worse, what if you're like me, and you can't find your way out of a cardboard box? If so, then you know that dreadful feeling of being unable to find your way. Think about how being lost makes you feel. Think about the growing knot in the pit of your stomach. Think about how little you can think about other than the growing questions inside of you:

- How will I find my way?
- How will I find help?
- How will I get home?

How does this feeling of being lost relate to the practice of veterinary medicine?

Our clients may also get lost in the course of a consultation. Consultations are rarely simple. Most of the time, they are complex because medicine is complicated. So, too, are our patients. Patients rarely present to us with a single primary complaint. They may have two or three. I have encountered some with a couple dozen.

Patients often present to us with complex histories. Patients may present to us with a multitude of related or unrelated clinical signs. Clients may have more than one concern. We may or may not be able to address every concern at every visit. All of these factors lead to potentially choppy waters. Appointments are brief, and they often end in a blur.

At the end of a consultation, clients may be left reeling from information overload. They may left pondering unanswered questions.

- Which topics did we cover today?
- Which topics can we cover tomorrow?
- Which topics did we table for next time?
- What information do we now know, from diagnostic testing?
- Which information are we still waiting on?
- Do we know the diagnosis?
- What is the diagnosis?
- What is the prognosis?
- Why did we elect not to treat with drug "X"?
- Which treatment did we decide upon?
- Why did we decide to treat?
- What will happen if we do not medicate?
- When do we need to schedule a recheck examination?
- What will follow-up involve?
- Will the condition be chronic or is the condition expected to resolve?
- What do I need to do to appropriately manage the issue?
- What can I do to speed its resolution?

These questions may be difficult to answer, and clients may not be able to access all the answers on their own.

The problem is that all of these questions roll around in their minds and cloud their judgement. They may seem overwhelming. They may jumble our clients' perspective of the situation.

Clients may have a difficult time remembering what was said because it all seems to blur together.(1) Clients may become frustrated. They may be at a loss to differentiate what they know versus what they do not. When clients become confused, they stress out. Stressed clients are more likely to become emotional. They are more likely to react with strong emotions, as opposed to acting rationally.

What can we do to alleviate some of this stress and uncertainty? We can create a roadmap. Recognize that although we, as veterinarians, may understand the course of the consultation, our clients may be unfamiliar with the terrain – that is, they may not understand one or more of the following.

- How are the clinical signs related to the diagnosis?
- What do the diagnostics test for?
- What does the diagnosis mean for the patient?

- How does the diagnosis impact the client?
- What is the prognosis?
- Which treatment options exist?
- What does the gold standard treatment involve?
- What are the potential side effects of therapy?
- What is the anticipated cost of therapy?
- What does follow-up involve?

These are easy questions that we, as doctors, can answer in our sleep. But clients may not be as familiar with medical conditions and how to manage disease.

In order for clients to understand the process, they often need assistance with navigating the consultation. This is particularly important when clinical cases get tough or when emotions run high. Mapping out the consultation is a communication skill that provides the sense of direction that is otherwise all too often lacking from the examination room.

14.1 Defining the Consultation Map

Mapping out the consultation is sometimes referred to as signposting.(2–6) What signposting means is that we verbally provide structure to the consultation.(2, 3, 6) We acknowledge openly where the conversation is headed and what we are choosing to discuss now versus that which we will discuss later.

Mapping out the consultation is therefore a way of orienting the client. Just like a compass tells you which direction you are facing, a consultation map may tell the client the order in which consultation events will happen.(2, 3, 5–7)

Mapping statements that outline the order of a consultation often begin with:

- "First …"
- "Second …"
- "Third …"
- "Fourth …"
- "Fifth …"

Usually, statements are limited to the first three bullet points, so as not to overwhelm the client.

- "First I'll take a patient history from you so that I am on the same page in terms of what you're noticing at home that is unusual."
- "Second, I'll examine your dog to see what, if anything, strikes me as out of the ordinary."
- "Third, we'll chat about any abnormal findings."

Alternatively, mapping statements that outline the order of a consultation may begin with transitional words or phrases:

- "At the beginning …"
- "Next …"
- "Then …"
- "Finally …"

Consider how this might be phrased in clinical practice.

- "At the beginning of our appointment, I will ask you specific questions to gather a patient history."
- "Next, I will examine your dog."
- "Then, we will talk about any important findings from the physical exam."
- "Finally, we'll decide whether or not laboratory tests or imaging studies are appropriate to get to the bottom of what is going on with your dog."

Other appropriate transitional words or phrases that structure the consultation in terms of the order of events include:

- before
- after
- afterward
- at the end.

Let us take a look at how signposting the order of a consultation may work in a clinical vignette.

Background

You are an associate veterinarian in clinical practice.

You have already greeted and introduced yourself to the client, who is a first-time pet-owner.

Clinical Conversation

Mr. Smith: Thank you so much for seeing us today, Doc. I've never had to go to a vet before. This is my first time.

Veterinarian: That's wonderful! Welcome to our clinic family – it's always a pleasure to visit with new friends. Might it be helpful for me to review how a typical appointment works here so that you know what to expect?

Mr. Smith: That would be great.

Veterinarian: Perfect. First, I'll ask some questions about you and Fluffy so that I get a general picture of how things are at home. Then I'll examine Fluffy. You'll have a chance to ask any questions that you may have. Finally, we'll come up with a plan of what kind of care Fluffy needs – and what that looks like over time. How does that sound to you?

14.2 Using Signposting to Outline Differentials

Mapping statements may also be used to outline the clinician's thought process when discussing differential diagnoses.

For example, the veterinarian may outline his or her concerns about neoplasia aloud, using signposting: "There are three main types of oral cancer that I am worried about in Fifi: melanoma, squamous cell carcinoma, and fibrosarcoma."

The veterinarian might then go on to describe each one in a bit more detail. Let us take a look at how this might work in practice.

Background

You are an associate veterinarian in clinical practice.

You are presented with a dog that has a 3-day history of ptyalism (hypersalivation). The dog has blood-tinged saliva and seems reluctant to eat.

Oral examination reveals an irregular, friable tumor that is located at the right caudol-ateral pharynx. The dog is tolerant enough to allow you to show the client what the lesion looks like, when his mouth is opened.

Clinical Conversation

Mr. Smith: That looks really bad, Doc. What could it mean for him?

Veterinarian: I agree with you that it is very concerning. To be honest, I am concerned about the possibility of it being cancerous.

Mr. Smith: I was afraid you might say that. What kind of cancer could it be?

Veterinarian: In dogs, there are three main types of oral cancer.

The first type is melanoma.

The second type is squamous cell carcinoma.

The third is fibrosarcoma.

14.3 Using Signposting to Discuss Treatment Plans

Mapping statements may also be used to outline the clinician's thought process when discussing treatment plans.

Consider, for example, a senior cat that is newly diagnosed with chronic kidney disease. The cat is clinically ill and requires hospitalization. Mapping helps the client to understand the order and the priority of treatments that you are recommending for the patient.

As the clinician of this case, you may prepare the client for hospitalization and all that follows by taking them through the steps.

- "Our first priority is to resolve your cat's dehydration, which at this point is life-threatening. We do this by administering IV fluids."
- "A second priority is to correct imbalances in electrolytes that are contributing to your cat feeling punky and depressed."
- "A third priority is to transition from injectable to oral medications to be certain that your cat can tolerate at-home medications."
- "Finally, when we are confident that your cat can be managed safely at home, we will discharge your cat to your care."

Mapping helps this client to understand that this is not going to be an instant fix. It is going to take time and care to get the patient back to health. Even then, when all is said and done, the emphasis is on getting the patient back to his or her "new normal" as opposed to finding a clinical cure.

Mapping helps the client to recognize that treatment will have to be continued when the cat transitions from inpatient to outpatient care.

14.4 Using Signposting to Rein in a Chatty Client

Mapping statements can also help to re-focus a client who is verbose and/or has a tendency to stray from the topic at hand.

For example, consider the client of a cat who presents acutely ill, inappetent, lethargic, and dehydrated. The cat is subsequently diagnosed with DKA.

This cat requires expedited care to survive this metabolic insult. You have stressed the urgency of the situation with the client. However, the client is not quite comprehending that time is of the essence.

While you are in the process of discussing the severity of the cat's condition, the client nonchalantly makes mention of the fact that, oh by the way, the cat is marking inappropriately around the house.

This is important to the client. It is weighing on the client's mind. Clearly, this topic is a part of the client's agenda that the client would like to discuss in depth.

You agree that this is something you will need to discuss about the patient. However, you know that this is not urgent, whereas treatment of the cat for DKA is.

Signposting is one way for you to acknowledge the concern so the client will know that she or he is heard, but to indicate respectfully that you will address the concern at a later point in time. In other words, in the moment, you are making an executive decision to table it.

Let us see how that might work in clinical practice, using this case of the cat with DKA.

Clinical Conversation

Mr. Smith: I didn't mention this before, but Bobby has been peeing on and off around the house.

Veterinarian: It could be related to his unmanaged diabetes – all that sugar spilling into

---

his urine has caused him to have a urinary tract infection, which we will need to treat.

Mr. Smith: No, I don't think that's it. A neighbor just moved in down the street. He has an outdoor cat that likes to roam. Bobby pees every time that this cat shows up on our porch. We really need to fix that because I can't keep cleaning up the rugs. It's a big problem.

Veterinarian: Yes, I imagine it would be – how very frustrating!

[pause]

Veterinarian: We can and will most definitely talk about Bobby's urinary habits … But first, we really need to focus on pulling him through this condition. DKA is very serious and can be life threatening. Let's concentrate our energy on getting him stable now – and then let's revisit this topic. Would that be okay with you?

Note how signposting was used to redirect the client's attention back to the primary problem.

Signposting is not about ignoring the client's concerns. In this clinical scenario, you are not telling the client that his or her concerns do not matter. You are simply saying that this concern does not take precedence. This concern can and will be addressed once the cat is stable.

In this regard, mapping is an effective, time-efficient tool to help keep a consultation on track.

If the consultation goes off course, mapping is a gentle way of streamlining the conversation so that you can prioritize talking points now and come back to other "lesser" concerns at a later point in time.

It lets the client know: "I hear you … and we're going to chat about it … We just can't chat about it now."

14.5 Using Signposting to Preface Actions, Such as Reviewing the Medical Record

In order for the veterinarian–client–patient relationship to be productive and long lasting, the client must feel bonded to the practice and to the practitioner. This bond is strengthened when the client perceives a sense of investment, that is, that the practice and the doctor are both invested in case outcomes.

The perception that the doctor cares stems from what the doctor shares aloud, through verbal communication, and from what the doctor does not say, but implies, through nonverbal cues and gestures.

Recall from Chapter 7 that we, as clinicians, often overestimate the significance of verbal communication and overlook the role that nonverbal cues play in our clients' assessment of our practice.

As much as 80 to 90% of clinical communication is nonverbal.(8–12) Nonverbal communication influences how the spoken word is received.(13–15) When nonverbal communication contradicts what is said aloud, clients have a tendency to believe the former.(7, 8, 15–17)

Nonverbal communication can convey interest in a clinical conversation, as when the veterinarian makes eye contact with and faces the client, leans slightly forward, and maintains an open posture.(11, 12, 18–23)

Conversely, nonverbal cues can also communicate disengagement, as when the veterinarian breaks eye contact.(11, 18)

There are many barriers in the consultation room that can disrupt clinical conversations, from the perspective of the client. Although the medical record is an essential database for a patient's health history, it can also become obtrusive when it interrupts the flow of dialogue.

Historically, the medical record was written on paper. Over time, a patient's chart could become quite bulky and might require the clinician to flip through page after page to find the appropriate data to reference.

This fumbling for information is a distraction in the examination room. It breaks eye contact between the veterinarian and client, and takes precious time away from an already abbreviated consultation slot.

As more and more clinics transition to using EMRs, the paper barrier has been replaced by the computer. The computer was introduced to the examination room to enhance efficiency as both a means of data-entry and a repository for the EMR. However, it may also detract from clinical communication.(24–27)

A 2006 study by Margalit et al. found that computer use during medical consultations could consume a significant fraction of the office visit. Of consultation time, 35 to 42% was spent with the doctor facing the computer screen, and one-quarter of all visits involved extensive typing by clinicians.(28)

If the clinician appears to have more face-time with the computer than the client, particularly during instances when the client is verbalizing his or her concerns, then the client may feel that the clinician is not listening. This may lead to a sense of dissatisfaction with the visit.

The client may also begin to abbreviate his or her answers if she or he feels that they are falling upon deaf ears. This ultimately undermines history taking. The veterinarian does not learn everything that she or he needs to know about the patient. Because 80% of cases can be diagnosed based upon history alone, diagnostic errors are likely to occur when patient histories are incomplete or inaccurate.(29–33)

Signposting can be an effective communication tool that acknowledges the medical record and explains to the client the doctor's reason for examining it in the midst of a consultation.(34–37) Signposting is a way of communicating that "I am not distracted" and "I am still listening."

A doctor who takes copious notes during an office visit should signpost this to the client as a means of explanation: "I'm going to take a lot of notes during our visit to help us get to the bottom of your ailment, but I assure you, I'm listening."

A notetaker may also blend signposting with an "asking for permission" statement: "If it's okay with you, I am going to take notes as you share the sequence of events with me so that I make sure to get it right." Refer to Chapter 12 for additional information on the communication skill, Asking for Permission (Section 12.4).

A doctor who wants to reference the medical record should signpost this need to the client. Signposting may take one or more of the following forms.

- "First, I'm going to ask you a series of questions about your cat. I am going to type your answers as you share them with me."
- "I apologize for having to turn my back to you while I type up the information that you just shared with me."
- "I am going to turn away from you just now to type up a visit summary, but once I am done, I am happy to take any questions that you may have."
- "I'm going to need a minute to review the information that your referring doctor just faxed over."
- "If you give me a moment, I can pull up your latest bloodwork just now so that we can reference it when deciding upon a plan to manage your schnauzer's high cholesterol."
- "Please forgive me for a moment while I review the results of your cat's at-home blood sugar curve."
- "Please hold that thought while I find the pathology report on the computer."
- "Hang on for a moment, if you will, while I access the surgical report."
- "Before I forget, I need to print out some information that I typed up before your visit that I want you to take home with you today."
- "Please allow me to input your request for Pfiefer's prescription into the system so that by the time our appointment is complete, the medication will be ready for pick-up at our pharmacy."

When technology works, it has the power to expedite tasks and increase efficiency within the practice.

When technology fails, it has a domino effect on the system and its employees. Be upfront about technological glitches with clients, and signpost your intentions so that they feel you have everything under control.

- "The computer is really slow today, so rather than make you wait for it to catch up, I am going to handwrite my notes today. I will later input them into the system for safekeeping."
- "The server is down, so I am unable to send an electronic prescription to the pharmacy of your choice. After we finish our consultation, I will handwrite a script for you that you can then deliver to the pharmacy at your convenience. Will that work?"

14.6 Using Mapping Statements as Caution Signs, So-Called "Warning Shots"

Up to this point, we have likened signposts to road signs that identify location (that is, at what point are we in the clinical consultation?) or distance (that is, which steps do we take, and in what order?).(4) However, signposting may also be used to indicate that the client ought to proceed with caution.(7) In other words, there are hazards up ahead.(4) When signposts identify hazards, they are called "warning shots."

A warning shot is a preparatory statement: it prepares the listener for the news that you are about to deliver.(38) It is essential for bad news delivery. Bad news delivery includes the relaying of news that is unsettling or unexpected.

Consider, for example, the following clinical scenarios.

Unexpected Diagnosis

- A client presents a geriatric patient for evaluation of a cough, hoping that the dog has an upper respiratory infection; in reality, the dog is in congestive heart failure (CHF).
- A client presents a feline patient for evaluation of open-mouth breathing, hoping that the cat has medically manageable asthma; in reality, the cat has pleural effusion.
- A client presents a dog for evaluation of lameness, hoping that the patient sustained a sprain after rigorous activity in the park; in reality, the dog has osteosarcoma of the pelvic limb.

Unexpected death

- An elderly patient that is boarding at the hospital passes away in its kennel overnight.
- A young patient experiences cardiopulmonary arrest (CPA) during recovery from routine ovariohysterectomy (OVH); CPR is not effective.

Medical error

- A patient is inadvertently given a dose of cefovecin sodium (Convenia®) instead of maropitant citrate (Cerenia®).
- A patient is inadvertently given an overdose of insulin: she was due to receive a dose of 1.0 units (1.0 u); however, an inexperienced team member misread the chart and administered 10.
- Maropitant citrate (Cerenia®) is accidentally administered intravenously; it was supposed to be administered subcutaneously.
- The patient's right ear was supposed to be cleaned with sterile saline; instead, an inexperienced team member substituted isopropyl alcohol for saline.
- The patient was scheduled to undergo tendonectomy; instead, the surgeon performed an onychectomy.
- The patient was scheduled to undergo dewclaw removal; the surgeon accidentally performed an orchiectomy, which was not authorized, at the same time.

A warning shot lets the listener know that this is serious. It tells the listener, "this is really important" and "I need you to pay attention." An effective warning shot should be direct. Its wording should be clear rather than vague so as not to create more confusion during a time that may already be tense.

An effective warning shot is also brief, so as not to prolong the sharing of news, which could lead to a build-up of anxiety within the client.(39)

Examples of effective warning shots include the following.

- "I've got some bad news …"(38)
- "I've got some very difficult news to share with you."(40)
- "I have some difficult news to share with you about …"(39)
- "I need to talk to you about something serious."
- "About Jesse's biopsy … it isn't good news …"
- "Listen, about Jesse's biopsy … it isn't the news that we had been hoping for …"
- "I'm afraid that I don't have very good news to share about the biopsy results."
- "I know that what I'm about to share with you will be very hard to take in."
- "I know this isn't what you expected."
- "I know this may be difficult to hear …"
- "This is hard for me to tell you, but …."
- "This isn't easy for me to say …"
- "I need you to hear what I'm about to say …"
- "What I'm about to say may come as a shock …"

The warning shot sets the stage for bad news delivery.

Note that it does not remove emotion from the equation. Deliverers of bad news are likely to be stressed and anxious about what to say and how they anticipate the client will respond.(40)

Clients are also likely to be emotional. Situations that involve bad news delivery are often highly charged. Emotions may run the gamut from shock and numbness to anger and rage.

The warning shot does not eliminate feeling from the clinical picture. What it does achieve is helping both parties to focus on a conversation that must take place.(40)

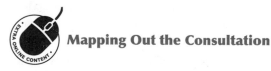 **Mapping Out the Consultation**

References

1. Kaufman G. Patient assessment: effective consultation and history taking. Nurs Stand. 2008;23(4):50–6, quiz 8, 60.
2. Englar RE, Williams M, Weingand K. Applicability of the Calgary–Cambridge guide to

dog and cat owners for teaching veterinary clinical communications. J Vet Med Educ. 2016;43(2):143–69.

3. Silverman J, Kurtz S, Draper J. Skills for communicating with patients. Oxford: Radcliffe Medical Press; 2008.

4. Best C. Building strong client partnerships through communication. AAEP Business Education [Internet]. 2013. Available from: https://professionalfarriers.com/docs/Building_Strong_Client_Partnerships_Through_Communication.pdf.

5. Radford A, Stockley P, Silverman J, Taylor I, Turner R, Gray C. Development, teaching, and evaluation of a consultation structure model for use in veterinary education. J Vet Med Educ. 2006;33(1):38–44.

6. Hunter L, Shaw JR. What's in your communication toolbox? Exceptional Veterinary Team. 2012(November/December):12–7.

7. Adams CL, Kurtz SM. Skills for communicating in veterinary medicine. Oxford: Otmoor Publishing and Dewpoint Publishing; 2017.

8. Shaw JR. Four core communication skills of highly effective practitioners. Vet Clin North Am Small Anim Pract. 2006;36(2):385–96, vii.

9. Kurtz SM, Silverman JD, Draper J. Teaching and learning communication skills in medicine. Grand Rapids, MI: Radcliffe; 2004.

10. Carson CA. Nonverbal communication in veterinary practice. Vet Clin North Am Small Anim Pract. 2007;37(1):49–63; abstract viii.

11. Caris-Verhallen WM, Kerkstra A, Bensing JM. Non-verbal behaviour in nurse-elderly patient communication. J Adv Nurs. 1999;29(4):808–18.

12. Gross D. Communication and the elderly. Phys Occup Ther Geriatr. 1990;9(1):49–64.

13. Cocksedge S, George B, Renwick S, Chew-Graham CA. Touch in primary care consultations: qualitative investigation of doctors' and patients' perceptions. Br J Gen Pract. 2013;63(609):e283–90.

14. Hall JA, Harrigan JA, Rosenthal R. Nonverbal behavior in clinician patient interaction. Appl Prev Psychol. 1995;4(1):21–37.

15. Roter DL, Frankel RM, Hall JA, Sluyter D. The expression of emotion through nonverbal behavior in medical visits: mechanisms and outcomes. J Gen Intern Med. 2005;21(Suppl 1):S28–34.

16. Koch R. The teacher and nonverbal communication. Theory Pract. 1971;10(4):231–42.

17. McCroskey JC, Larson CE, Knapp ML. An Introduction to interpersonal communication. Englewood Cliffs, NJ: Prentice Hall; 1971.

18. Heintzman M, Leathers DG, Parrott RL, Cairns I. Nonverbal rapport-building behaviors' effect on perceptions of a supervisor. MCQ. 1993;7(2):181–208.

19. Burgoon K. Nonverbal signals. In Knapp ML, Daly JA, editors. The SAGE handbook of interpersonal communication. Thousand Oaks, CA: SAGE Publications; 1994. pp. 229–71.

20. Collier G. Emotional expressions. Hillsdale, NJ: Erlbaum; 1985.

21. von Cranach M. The role of orienting behaviour in human interaction. In: Esser AH, editor. Behaviour and environment. New York: Plenum Press; 1971. pp. 217–37.

22. Rosenfeld HM. Conversational control functions of nonverbal behaviour. In: Siegman AW, Feldstein S, editors. Nonverbal behaviour and communication. New York: Wiley; 1978. pp. 291–328.

23. Reece MM, Whitman RN. Expressive movements, warmth, and verbal reinforcement. J Abnorm Soc Psychol. 1962;64:234–6.

24. Noordman J, Verhaak P, van Beljouw I, van Dulmen S. Consulting room computers and their effect on general practitioner–patient communication. Fam Pract. 2010;27(6):644–51.

25. Ridsdale L, Hudd S. Computers in the consultation – the patients view. BJGP. 1994;44(385):367–9.

26. Als AB. The desk-top computer as a magic box: patterns of behaviour connected with the desk-top computer; GPs' and patients' perceptions. Fam Pract. 1997;14(1):17–23.

27. Lelievre S, Schultz K. Does computer use in patient-physician encounters influence patient satisfaction? Can Fam Physician. 2010;56(1):e6–12.

28. Margalit RS, Roter D, Dunevant MA, Larson S, Reis S. Electronic medical record use and physician–patient communication: an observational study of Israeli primary care encounters. Patient Educ Couns. 2006;61(1):134–41.

29. Bordage G. Why did I miss the diagnosis? Some cognitive explanations and educational implications. Acad Med. 1999;74(10 Suppl):S138–43.

30. Faustinella F, Jacobs RJ. The decline of clinical skills: a challenge for medical schools. Int J Med Educ. 2018;9:195–7.

31. Wiener S, Nathanson M. Physical examination. Frequently observed errors. JAMA. 1976;236(7):852–5.

32. Frankel RM. Pets, vets, and frets: what relationship-centered care research has to offer veterinary medicine. J Vet Med Educ. 2006;33(1):20–7.

33. Lipkin MJ, Frankel RM, Beckman HB, Charon R, Fein O. Performing the interview. In: Lipkin MJ, Putnam SM, Lazare A, editors. The medical interview. New York: Springer-Verlag; 1995. pp. 65–82.

34. Silverman J, Kinnersley P. Doctors' non-verbal behaviour in consultations: look at the patient before you look at the computer. Br J Gen Pract. 2010;60(571):76–8.

35. Duke P, Frankel RM, Reis S. How to integrate the electronic health record and patient-centered communication into the medical visit: a skills-based approach. Teach Learn Med. 2013;25(4):358–65.

36. Swinglehurst D, Roberts C, Li S, Weber O, Singy P. Beyond the 'dyad': a qualitative re-evaluation of the changing clinical consultation. BMJ Open. 2014;4(9):e006017.

37. Alkureishi MA, Lee WW, Lyons M, Press VG, Imam S, Nkansah-Amankra A, et al. Impact of electronic medical record use on the patient–doctor relationship and communication: a systematic review. J Gen Intern Med. 2016;31(5):548–60.

38. Ptacek JT, Leonard K, McKee TL. "I've got some bad news …": veterinarians' recollections of communicating bad news to clients. J Appl Soc Psychol. 2004;34(2):366–90.

39. Garrett LD. CVC Highlight: How to break bad news to veterinary clients. DVM 360 [Internet]. 2013. Available from: http://veterinarymedicine.dvm360.com/cvc-highlight-how-break-bad-news-veterinary-clients?id=&sk=&date=&pageID=2.

40. Bateman SW. Communication in the veterinary emergency setting. Vet Clin N Am-Small. 2007;37(1):109–21.

Chapter 15

Communication Skills that Facilitate Client Comprehension

Summarizing and Checking in with the Client

Think back to the last lecture you attended. If you're a veterinary student, maybe you just sat through a 60 or 90-minute dictation on the principles of anatomy or physiology. If you're a veterinarian, maybe you last sat in the audience at a conference for continuing education (CE).

Consider the presentation itself.

- Was the content appropriate for its audience?
- Was the content relatable?
- Was the content understandable?
- Was the content engaging?

Were any content areas unclear or difficult to follow? If so, how did that make you feel? Could you keep up with the rest of the presentation, or did you find yourself distracted by what you did not comprehend?

After the presentation, did the content stick? How much material did you recall:

- within the first 5 minutes that followed the presentation
- within the first hour
- 1 day later
- 1 week later
- 1 month later
- 1 year later?

If you are like most people, recall is poor when learning is passive, and rapidly diminishes over a short period of time.(1, 2) A passive audience member who sits through a 1 hour lecture is likely to recall only three facts immediately following the presentation.(2)

How does this relate to the practice of veterinary medicine?

Veterinarians are responsible for delivering a large amount of information to the client in a relatively short amount of time. If we are not careful, this delivery of material can feel like a lecture: a one-way transfer of information in which we recite material faster than our clients can absorb.

Clients are just like us, whether we are veterinary students, faculty, or practicing veterinarians. Their attention spans are finite. They cannot be expected to sit as a captive audience and remember every word that we say. There is simply too much material and too little time.

Consider, for instance, the wellness examination for a new kitten or puppy. The content areas that need to be addressed exceed the time allotted for most consultations, and include, but are not limited to:

- acquisition of the pet
- purpose of the pet
  - companion
  - show dog or cat
  - hunter
  - athlete
  - working dog
  - therapy dog
- household
  - who interacts with the pet?
    - other people
    - conspecifics
    - other species
  - who is responsible for daily pet care?
- environmental safety
- environmental enrichment
- anticipated lifestyle of pet
  - exclusively outdoor
  - exclusively indoor
  - indoor/outdoor
- travel history
- dietary history
- weight management
- behavioral history
- elimination habits
- reproductive planning
- breed predispositions to disease
- preventative medicine
  - ectoparasites
  - endoparasites

- vaccinations
- dental care

Try as we might to cover all of these topics, we cannot.

At most, we often merely touch upon a subject, without having the time or the ability to delve deep in discussion. Often, due to time constraints, we are forced to rely upon patient histories to determine how urgent it is to address a particular topic today or whether it can be tabled until the next visit.

Even if time were infinite, our clients still could not be expected to have perfect recall. At most, they will absorb bits and pieces of our conversation. Some of those bits will make perfect sense and they will hold onto these nuggets of information for the long term. Other pieces of conversation may be taken out of context or misinterpreted. Others details may create confusion.

The information that we share may seem obvious to us, but remember, we have been bathed in medical knowledge for years before we find ourselves on the other side of the examination room table, as clinicians.

To many of our clients, the information that we share is new. It may be the first time that they are hearing about recommendation "X" or drug "Y." Or maybe they have heard about it in the past, but today is the first time that it is truly sinking in.

Clients take time to hear us. They take time to process information and to absorb. This requires us to be patient. We cannot expect them to know everything and hold onto our every word. What we can hope for is that the most important aspects of our dialogue are retained.

We can facilitate client comprehension and recall by making use of the following communication techniques:

- summarizing
- checking in.

15.1 Summarizing

From the standpoint of clinical communication, summarizing is defined as providing a brief review of key points.(3) Summarizing is a way to review what was discussed with the hopes that by recapping take-away messages, they stick.(4, 5) Summaries often lead to a check-in statement.(5) This type of statement will be discussed in Section 15.4.

There are two types of summaries that appear in clinical consultations:(3, 6, 7)

- internal summaries
- end-of-consultation summaries.

15.2 Internal Summaries, Defined

Internal summaries are used to wrap-up a specific part of the consultation or transition between two segments of the office visit.(3, 6) For example, they may be used to review:

- case history that the client provided
- our list of concerns for a given patient
- our differential diagnoses
- the diagnostic plan
- the order of diagnostic tests that will be performed
- our medical and/or surgical findings
- the diagnosis
- preventative care recommendations, including the proposed vaccination schedule
- treatment plans for inpatients or outpatients
- recommendations for follow-up.

15.2.1 Using Internal Summaries to Review Case History

As a clinician, I use summarizing most often to review case history and treatment plans, as well as to summarize new patient visits.

Let us take a look at how this might play out in clinical practice, beginning with the use of summarizing to review case history.

Background

You are an associate veterinarian in clinical practice.

Your client, Mr. Jones, has presented his Jack Russell Terrier, Stu, to you on a Saturday morning for evaluation of gastrointestinal upset.

Clinical Conversation

Veterinarian: I understand that Stu has been vomiting. Can you tell me more about that?

Mr. Jones: Stu had a great day with me at the park on Tuesday. I had the day off work, so we both went for a 3-mile hike. It was like old times. I'd forgotten how much we both enjoyed getting out of the house. By the time we'd finished our hike, it was awfully hot. So, we both went for a swim in the lake. Stu must've been really thirsty because he gulped down a gallon or two of water from the lake. Then we got some ice cream down at the corner store.

Veterinarian: The dog version of ice cream?

Mr. Jones: No way! That stuff tastes like cardboard. I mean the good stuff, the real stuff

---

– Ben and Jerry's. He likes chocolate chip cookie dough, just like me. Anyhow, he ate about half a pint. That night, we both slept like babies.

Veterinarian: I bet!

Mr. Jones: The next day Stu seemed a bit put out, but I just chalked it up to him being tired. He didn't really want his breakfast, he just kind of pushed it around in his bowl. That night, he ate one or two bites, but then it all came up about a half-hour later. It was just a mess of food and liquid. He threw up twice more overnight – I know because both times were on my bed and woke me up. He's vomited at least 5 times since then and his appetite is still iffy.

Veterinarian: Wow, it sounds as if you and Stu have been through quite a lot! Let me see if I got this right…

[pause]

Veterinarian: To summarize, Stu went for a long hike and a swim at the lake on Tuesday. He drank lake water and ate cookie dough ice cream. His appetite hasn't been the same since. He vomited three times Tuesday into Wednesday, and five more times between then and now. Am I understanding that correctly?

Mr. Jones: Yes, that's right … About the vomiting … But Stu has also been having diarrhea …

Let us reflect upon this clinical vignette. In this case, summarizing the patient history helped me to know that I understood correctly about Stu's vomiting, including the timeline.

Summarizing allowed me to check in with the client to see if I heard right. Summarizing also allowed the client to recognize that there were gaps in my understanding of the case because I had only been informed about Stu's vomiting. Summarizing therefore prompted the client to remember to share that Stu was also exhibiting diarrhea. Summarizing was a means of jogging the client's memory. Now the client is ready and able to share important details about this second clinical sign.

15.2.2 Using Internal Summaries to Review Key Physical Exam Findings

Internal summaries serve as important recaps of patient history. They can be used throughout the consultation. For example, they may be used at the conclusion of the physical examination to review key findings. Coming back to Stu's case, the veterinarian may have chosen to make use of an internal summary to relay his physical exam findings:

Stu is depressed on exam today. He acts like he's tired or in a fog. He's also quite dehydrated because his skin tents and his eyes are sunken in. I can tell he doesn't feel well because when I push on his belly, he tenses up. Did you see how he lowered his front end to the floor and raised his butt end in the air? That tells me that the part of his abdomen that is nearest to his rib cage is uncomfortable. He's also licking his lips when I push in on his abdomen, which tells me that he's still quite a bit nauseous."

15.2.3 Using Internal Summaries to Review the Diagnosis

Internal summaries are an important means of reviewing the patient's diagnosis, particularly in complicated cases.

For example, a feline patient that presents on emergency for evaluation of acute UTO may have an extensive problem list when he is triaged:

- lateral recumbency
- obtundation
- distended, turgid, painful urinary bladder
- grossly visible urethral plug at penile tip
- discolored, cyanotic penis
- dehydration
- significant bradycardia (heart rate <100 bpm)
- hypothermia
- clin path abnormalities
  - azotemia
  - hyperphosphatemia
  - hyperkalemia
- EKG abnormalities
  - lengthened PR intervals
  - flatted P waves
  - tall and tented T waves
  - widened QRS complexes.

For seasoned clinicians, this amount of detail makes perfect sense and in fact reinforces our understanding of anatomy, physiology, and pathophysiology.

However, for the client, this amount of detail may be overwhelming. After reviewing the problem list and preliminary diagnostics with the client, it may be beneficial to provide an internal summary to recap the most important details:

"Your cat is in critical care because a plug of mucous and crystals obstructed his urethra and prevented him from being able to urinate. When the urethra became blocked, his body could no longer remove toxins from the bloodstream or maintain normal levels of electrolytes. As a result, he is very ill. The high levels of toxins are causing him to appear very depressed, and the high levels of potassium are having a serious impact on his heart. We need to intervene right away to remove the obstruction from his urinary tract so that we can reverse the problem areas on his bloodwork."

An internal summary is an effective way to put the patient's condition in perspective. It emphasizes the areas that are most important for the client to understand so that the client is able to make an informed decision about proceeding with medical care.

15.2.4 Using Internal Summaries to Review Treatment Recommendations

Internal summaries also play an important role in reviewing what the client agreed to in terms of medical treatment. Consider how this might take shape in the consultation, if we were to draw our attention back to Stu's case.

Clinical Conversation

Veterinarian: We've covered a lot of ground today and I agree that Stu's indigestion is most likely due to overeating rich foods that he often doesn't get to sample. Because he hasn't vomited since you stopped feeding him, we agreed that a conservative approach to his care is safe at this time.

[pause]

Veterinarian: To summarize, we are going to send Stu home with you today. We will start to reintroduce food to his diet tonight, beginning with small amounts of boiled chicken and rice, offered every three or four hours. As long as Stu keeps it down, he will not need to come back to see us. But if Stu vomits more than once after eating, then we will need to proceed with bloodwork and X-rays. How does that sound to you?

Mr. Jones: Sounds good to me.

In this clinical scenario, an internal summary was used to wrap up the conversation about Stu's treatment plan, and remind the client of three key aspects of at-home care.

1. Bland diet will be introduced tonight, with small meals offered more frequently.
2. If Stu keeps the food down, then no further diagnostics are indicated.
3. If Stu vomits more than once, then he must return for a more complete work-up.

The internal summary set the stage for expectations for care. The client now knows what to do at home to care for Stu and what signs to look for that might indicate Stu is declining, rather than improving. As a result, the client knows when it is appropriate for Stu to return to the clinic for additional tests.

The client is also more likely to recall this information because it has been emphasized. The clinician can further assist with recall by providing these instructions in writing.

15.3 End-of-Consultation Summaries

Although internal summaries are helpful in wrapping up a specific part of the consultation, we also need to incorporate end summaries into clinical conversations.

Think of the content of a clinical conversation as a gift, and the end-of-consultation summary as a bow. The end-of-consultation summary ties the clinical conversation together into one pretty little package.

Why are end-of-consultation summaries necessary? In clinical practice, during the course of a single office visit, there is much discussion that takes place. Just as audience recall from a lecture dwindles over the course of the presentation, so, too, does the client's ability to pay attention to each and every detail that we may wish to share with him or her.

End-of-consultation summaries provide one last opportunity to ensure that both parties – veterinarian and client – are on the same page and that there is closure.(3) End-of-consultation summaries allow us to check for accuracy, one last time, and therefore increase the odds of adherence.(3, 8)

Client adherence in companion animal practice is especially concerning.(9) According to a 2003 study that was conducted by the American Animal Hospital Association (AAHA), adherence to preventative care recommendations is much lower than healthcare providers anticipated.(10) This includes recommendations by the veterinary team for core vaccinations, dental prophylaxis, heartworm testing, and heartworm prevention.(10)

Clients claim that they would be more likely to act on recommendations if the veterinary team took the time to check in with them.(9, 10)

End-of-consultation summaries provide the opportunity for veterinarians to do just that.

15.3.1 Using End-of-Consultation Summaries to Conclude Wellness Visits

Recall from the beginning of this chapter that new patient visits, such as wellness examinations for kittens and puppies, can result in information overload. There are so many content areas to cover, particularly when the client is unfamiliar with the needs and expectations of this new arrival. This can be overwhelming for new pet parents.

Sending clients home with information kits, so-called kitten and puppy "packs," can help to reinforce key concepts before the next visit. However, the use of an end-of-consultation summary is an effective tool to highlight key topics of interest that you do not want the client to forget.

Let us see how this might work in clinical practice.

Background

You are an associate veterinarian.

Your client, Mr. Brown, has presented his new kitten, Penelope, to you for a new patient wellness examination. You have taken a case history and have completed your examination. You have spent the past 30 minutes consulting with Mr. Brown about the new addition to his family and what the next several months will look like in terms of veterinary care. You are getting ready to conclude the preventative care aspects of the conversation.

Clinical Conversation

Veterinarian: Thank you so much for the opportunity to meet Penelope! She's a great new addition to our clinic family!

[pause]

Veterinarian: We talked a lot today about what Penelope needs to maintain her health and prevent disease.

[pause]

Veterinarian: We agree that she needs her first feline distemper shot today, and that she will return every 3–4 weeks for two additional boosters. You will provide us with a sample of her stool as soon as possible, so that we can screen her for gastrointestinal parasites, and we will get her started on a monthly topical flea and tick preventative today.

[pause]

Veterinarian: You're also going to work with her on nail-trimming at home and we'll see how that is going for you at her next visit. After she is fully vaccinated, we will plan to have her spayed. Does that sound like a good plan?

Mr. Brown: Yes, I'll get that next visit scheduled before I leave the office today. I'd also like to buy a pair of nail trimmers while I'm here so that I can get started on that right away.

Veterinarian: That's great. I'll let the technician know so that she can get you started on the right foot.

Mr. Brown: Perfect.

Using an end-of-consultation summary facilitated Penelope's visit. The veterinarian took the time to review key aspects of veterinary care. Important areas of emphasis for Penelope's preventative health regimen included:

* updating vaccinations
* initiating endoparasite and ectoparasite control
* learning how to trim claws
* discussing spaying after her boosters have been completed.

The client is more likely to remember these key points because they were repeated, rather than said just once in passing.

The veterinarian can further reinforce these agenda items by sending the client home with complimentary pamphlets or brochures that support the treatment plan.

15.3.2 Using End-of-Consultation Summaries to Conclude Problem Appointments

An end-of-consultation summary is also an effective strategy for wrapping up problem appointments. Problem visits may include:

- mystery illness – that is, one for which the diagnosis remains unclear
- new diagnosis
- recurrent illness
- chronic disease
- acute-on-chronic presentations.

Problem visits have a tendency to be complex because they are very rarely associated with a single presenting complaint. More often than not, clients present additional concerns in a patient with multiple problems. Consider, for instance, the hyperthyroid cat with chronic kidney disease (CKD). Both conditions require long-term medical management, and treatment of each is a balancing act. What works most efficiently to manage one condition may sabotage treatment for the other. In order to provide the highest level of care, clinicians must work closely with clients to customize treatment recommendations to the patient, and adjust the plan as needed. This often requires an extensive list of instructions, including the following.

- Which medications to give, by which route of administration, at which dose and at what dosing frequency.
- When, if ever, to reduce the dose of medication.
- When to discontinue medications, for instance, if side effect "X" occurs.
- When to contact the veterinary clinic by telephone with concerns.
- When to present the patient for recheck examination.
- When to present the patient on emergency.

This list of instructions would be challenging for anyone to recall, particularly for those who are not in the medical field or who have never had to manage disease "X" or disease "Y," let alone both diseases concurrently.

The stakes are high. If instructions are miscommunicated or misinterpreted, then the patient's health – and potentially the patient's life – are in jeopardy.

End-of-consultation summaries help to crystallize key take-away messages so as to reduce the chance that messages are lost in translation.

Let us see how this might work in clinical practice, keeping in mind the case of the cat with concurrent hyperthyroidism and CKD.

Background

You are an associate veterinarian in clinical practice.

Your client, Ms. Myers, is a longtime client. Together, you've shared a professional working relationship for the past 12 years.

Ms. Myers is one of your best clients in terms of compliance. She follows through with every recommendation you make, and is always on schedule in terms of preventative care for her three geriatric cats.

Three months ago, Ms. Myers presented her oldest cat, Tasha, a 15-year-old Burmese, for evaluation of weight loss.

Despite Tasha's reportedly increased appetite, she had lost 2.5 pounds since her visit last year.

On physical examination, there was a palpable thyroid "slip." A complete work-up confirmed your index of suspicion: Tasha had developed hyperthyroidism.

At that time, Tasha's renal function – urine specific gravity (USG), blood urea nitrogen (BUN), and creatinine – appeared to be adequate.

You had discussed treatment options with Ms. Myers, including the potential for hyperthyroidism to mask renal disease.

After careful consideration, Ms. Myers elected to start Tasha on methimazole therapy.

You had prepared Ms. Myers that as cats were medically managed for hyperthyroidism, it was not uncommon to see elevations in renal parameters. You told her that you would need to keep a close watch on those values.

Tasha presents to you today with a history of intermittent, but progressive vomiting. Ms. Myers also reports an increase in the size and number of urine clumps that Tasha is producing in the litterbox.

Diagnostic tests confirm that Tasha has CKD. According to the International Renal Interest Society (IRIS) guidelines, her condition is best characterized as stage 3, borderline proteinuric, and severely hypertensive.

After a lengthy conversation about new medications for Tasha as well as how CKD is likely to impact Tasha's quality of life, the visit draws to an end.

Because you recognize that this is a significant amount of information to process and retain, you decide that an end-of-consultation summary would be helpful.

Clinical Conversation

Veterinarian: I know we've covered a lot of new material today. To recap, Tasha's increased vomiting and changes in urination habits prompted you to bring her in

---

today. The good news is that her hyperthyroidism appears to be stable on methimazole: she is tolerating the medication well and she has actually gained back half a pound. Unfortunately, as we had discussed at the time of her initial diagnosis, her hyperthyroidism was masking kidney disease. Now that her thyroid is better controlled, her kidneys are no longer able to hide the fact that they are struggling to perform their job. Because of this, Tasha is urinating larger amounts of urine more often, which has caused her to become dehydrated. Her kidneys are also not adequately filtering out toxins, so they are building up in the bloodstream, which is causing her to feel unwell. We decided that Tasha would benefit from fluid therapy.

[pause]

Veterinarian: In addition to her methimazole, you are going to give her SubQ fluids every day, and these three medications:

Tumil-K® to increase her potassium level

Amlodipine besylate to reduce her blood pressure

Aluminum hydroxide to reduce her phosphorus level.

[pause]

Veterinarian: I'm going to provide you with all of the medication instructions in writing, and then we will need to recheck Tasha within the next 1–2 weeks – sooner if her frequency of vomiting increases, rather than decreases.

The end-of-consultation summary serves as the final wrap-up for the case.

When cases are complicated by one or more disease processes, an end-of-consultation summary is essential to recap take-away messages. The end-of-consultation summary that was provided here, by way of example, covered the following content areas concerning Tasha's care:

- her chief (presenting) complaint
- her diagnosis
- an explanation of how her diagnosis relates to her clinical signs
- an outline of modifications to her treatment plan
- an overview of drugs and their mechanisms of action.

Note that this is still a lot of information for the client to absorb. In many cases, it may still be too much.

An end-of-consultation summary is essential, but it needs to be tailored to the client. When we visit with longstanding clients, we have some sense as to how much information is too much and what they can handle. When we visit with new clients, we are not so sure.

As new graduates, we learn the art of communication much like we learn the practice of medicine, through trial and error. We give what information we feel is necessary, and then we see how well it is received.

How can we more effectively bring a consultation to an appropriate point of closure? Is there a way to trim down an end-of-consultation summary in complex cases?

Absolutely.

We can make use of an additional skill called "chunk and check."

15.4 "Chunk and Check"

"Chunk and check" is a communication tool that reminds us that consultations are more effective when we break down what we have to say into segments.(4, 5, 7, 8, 11, 12) Each segment or "chunk" represents two or three sentences of material that we want to convey.(13) We deliver that chunk.(13) Then we "check in" with our client.(13)

Why do we check in with our client? (7, 12, 14)

- We are checking that the client is on the same page. In other words, we are checking for mutual understanding.
- We are checking for accuracy: did we hear the client correctly?
- We are demonstrating our willingness to be responsive to the client's needs
- We are ensuring that the conversation is a dialogue rather than a monologue: the client has the opportunity to participate in the conversation, and share his or her needs with the veterinary team.

We do not move on to the next chunk until we have checked in with our client. This prevents us from losing our client. This prevents us from getting to the end of the consultation, only to have the client say, "I didn't catch any of that, can you start over?"

Chunk and check may seem like time-killers, but they are actually time-savers.(15) Chunk and check help you to identify sources of misunderstanding early. You can correct misconceptions before it is too late.

15.4.1 Checking in May Take the Form of a Pause

The simplest form of checking in may be a pause in conversation. Let us see what that might look like in practice:

Background

You are an associate veterinarian. You have just diagnosed a cat with hyperthyroidism. You are discussing options for medical management with your client.

Clinical Conversation

Veterinarian: If we do not treat Tulip's hyperthyroidism, then she will continue to eat ravenously, yet lose weight. Her body cannot sustain itself in the long run.

[pause]

[Client nods to demonstrate understanding]

Veterinarian: We can treat Tulip's condition in one of two ways: We can either use radioactive iodine to destroy the cells in her thyroid that are overactive, or we can administer a lifelong medication that prevents the thyroid from overworking.

[pause]

[Client nods to demonstrate understanding]

Pausing is an effective way to allow for a "breath" in the conversation. It allows the client to follow your train of thought and catch up. It gives the client time to digest what you have shared.

15.4.2 Checking in May Require Words

Sometimes, during a clinical consultation, you may want to do more than just pause in order to make sure that you have been clear. In these situations, your version of a check in might be a phrase or statement.

Check in statements include the following.

- "Does that make sense?"
- "How does that sound to you?"
- "Does that sound reasonable?"
- "Are you with me?"
- "Is that clear?"

Let us revisit the same clinical scenario as was introduced in Section 15.4.1 to demonstrate the effective use of check in statements.

Clinical Conversation

Veterinarian: If we do not treat Tulip's hyperthyroidism, then she will continue to eat ravenously, yet lose weight. Her body cannot sustain itself in the long run. Does that make sense?

Client: Yes.

Veterinarian: Great, so if we choose to treat Tulip's condition, we can select one of two ways: we can either use radioactive iodine to destroy the cells in her thyroid that are overactive, or we can administer a lifelong medication that prevents the thyroid from overworking. How does either option sound to you?

Client: I am a bit concerned about side effects that the iodine treatment might cause for Tulip.

Veterinarian: That makes sense. The good news is that the risks to Tulip are low. Cats

---

with radioiodine therapy do not have any increased incidence of cancer as a result of their treatment.

[pause]

[Client nods to demonstrate understanding]

Veterinarian: The greater risk would be managing your exposure to Tulip when she is still considered radioactive. We would need to limit your exposure to her initially by having her board within a special facility. How does that sound?

15.4.3 Be Cautious about Overusing Check-ins

Note that check-in statements can be overused. If we check in after *every* statement, then we may come across as being stiff, unfeeling, and robotic. It may also seem to the client that we do not feel they understand *anything*, particularly if we continue to ask, every two or three sentences, "Does that make sense?"

The trick is to use check-in statements *sparingly*.

Sprinkle them into the conversation at key points when it is most important for you to check your client's understanding – for example, after discussing a diagnosis or prognosis – or after reviewing treatment options.

When you are not using check-in statements, read your client's body language. Recall from Chapter 7 that your client's nonverbal cues are a good indicator of how receptive they are to the conversation and whether or not they are following you.

 Sectioning the Conversation into Bite-Sized Chunks

References

1. Steinert Y, Snell LS. Interactive lecturing: strategies for increasing participation in large group presentations. Medical Teacher. 1999;21(1):37–42.
2. Robertson LJ. Twelve tips for using a computerized interactive audience response system. Medical Teacher. 2000;22(3):237–9.
3. Adams CL, Kurtz SM. Skills for communicating in veterinary medicine. Oxford: Otmoor Publishing and Dewpoint Publishing; 2017.
4. Englar RE, Williams M, Weingand K. Applicability of the Calgary–Cambridge Guide to dog and cat owners for teaching veterinary clinical communications. J Vet Med Educ. 2016;43(2):143–69.
5. Radford A, Stockley P, Silverman J, Taylor I, Turner R, Gray C. Development, teaching, and evaluation of a consultation structure model for use in veterinary education. J Vet Med Educ. 2006;33(1):38–44.

6. Best C. Building strong client partnerships through communication. AAEP Business Education [Internet]. 2013. Available from: https://professionalfarriers.com/docs/Building_Strong_Client_Partnerships_Through_Communication.pdf.

7. Silverman J, Kurtz S, Draper J. Skills for communicating with patients. Oxford: Radcliffe Medical Press; 2008.

8. Hunter L, Shaw JR. What's in your communication toolbox? Exceptional Veterinary Team. 2012(November/December):12–7.

9. Englar RE, Show-Ridgway A. Post-appointment follow-up: what veterinary clients say they want. DVM 360 [Internet]. 2018. Available from: http://veterinarynews.dvm360.com/post-appointment-follow-what-veterinary-clients-say-they-want.

10. The path to high quality care: practical tips for improving compliance. Lakewood, CO: American Animal Hospital Association (AAHA); 2003.

11. Moffett J. The modern, evidence-based approach to veterinary communication skills. Veterinary Practice [Internet]. 2010. Available from: https://veterinary-practice.com/article/the-modern-evidence-based-approach-to-veterinary-communication-skills.

12. Gray C, Moffett J. Handbook of veterinary communication skills. Chichester: Wiley-Blackwell; 2010. xviii, 198 p. p.

13. Bonvicini KA, Cornell KK. Are clients truly informed? Communication tools and risk reduction. Compendium. 2008(November):572–6.

14. Shaw JR, Hunter LJ. Communicating pet health information to veterinary clients. Clinician's Brief. 2017(May):37–40.

15. Ettinger S. A cancer diagnosis is not a death sentence. Today's Veterinary Practice. 2017(January/February):103–7.

Chapter 16

Communication Skills that Facilitate Compliance

Contracting for Next Steps

Think back to the last time that you were required to complete a group project.

If you are a veterinary student, maybe you were assigned a region of the canine body to dissect and present to the class. If you are a faculty member, maybe you were assigned to a task force to review the admissions process or create a proposal for curricular revisions.

How did you feel about the process of teamwork?

- Did you enjoy your team?
- Was your team productive?
- Was your team well-managed?
- Did everyone on the team understand their role?
- Did everyone on the team accomplist their assigned tasks?

Teamwork can be challenging. Each of us brings to the table differences in terms of:

- personality
- attitude
- past experiences
  - obstacles
  - failures
  - successes
  - lessons learned
- leadership style
  - directing
  - coaching
  - supporting
  - delegating
- performance strengths
- performance weaknesses

- response to stress
- response to feedback.

Teamwork can be made more challenging when team members' roles are not defined.

Have you ever left a team meeting unclear about who was in charge of which task? What is the impact of that uncertainty on you? How does the uncertainty impact the rest of your team? How does uncertainty impact productivity? For those who prefer structure, uncertainty can breed discontent and even discomfort. More importantly, if tasks are not well-defined, then how likely is it that they will be accomplished? The same situation can crop up in the examination room.

The trend towards relationship-centered care in the practice of veterinary medicine has effectively created a partnership between your practice and your client.(1) In effect, you have forged a team that includes:

- the patient
- the client
- the client's support system
- your support staff
- your colleagues
- your practice manager
- your hospital director.

You are no longer a team of one. You are no longer considered to be the sole expert in the consultation room. You are no longer the dictator of care, but rather, a partner in care.

Patient/client autonomy is now central to the practice of medicine in modern day human and veterinary healthcare.(2) Physicians and veterinarians are essential providers of information; however, they no longer hold the authority to exert complete control over patient fates and clinical outcomes.(2) Instead, their purpose on the team is to provide options and information that will facilitate decision making by the patient/client.(2)

In addition, physicians are responsible for eliciting the patient's perspective and being open to hearing the patient's thoughts, feelings, ideas, and values.(3–6) This requires the physician to:(3)

- give the floor to the patient/client, so that the patient/client can lead off the consultation with an uninterrupted opening statement
- acknowledge and validate the patient's/client's experience
- be supportive and non-judgmental
- provide information that is easy to understand
- provide resources that are easily accessible by the patient/client
- provide strategies that will facilitate, rather than hinder, patient care.

Ultimately, teamwork and collaboration drive outcomes.(2)

In order for patient outcomes to be successful, veterinary clients must be:

- informed
- allowed to actively participate in healthcare decisions
- given the opportunity to question healthcare recommendations
- given the opportunity to seek clarification before making a decision.

Veterinary clients that are active participants are more likely to express "buy-in" and commit to action plans.

However, in order for follow-through to occur, each team member must fully understand who is responsible for which action. This communication skill is termed "contracting for next steps." It is an essential part of teamwork, without which treatment recommendations are likely to fail.

16.1 Defining "Contracting for Next Steps"

Patient care is a two-way street. Veterinarians are responsible for advising clients about proper care. However, it is ultimately up to both clients and veterinarians to provide the care that has been recommended.

Patient care can therefore be thought of as a contract between caregivers.(7–13) The client authorizes the veterinary team to initiate patient care.(7, 9) The veterinary team thus takes responsibility for those services that have been outlined and agreed to, either verbally or in writing.(9) These services may include:

- data gathering, through history taking
- patient handling and restraint
- whole-body physical examination
- organ- or systems-specific examination
    - fundoscopy
    - neurologic examination
    - ophthalmoscopy
    - orthopedic examination
    - otoscopy
    - prostatic examination
    - rectal examination
    - vaginal examination
- venipuncture
- blood pressure assessment
- diagnostic imaging
- administration of drugs
    - injectable
        - intramuscular (IM)

- – intravenous (IV)
- – subcutaneous (SQ)
    - ▪ intranasal
    - ▪ oral
    - ▪ transdermal
- • catheterization
    - ▪ IV
    - ▪ urinary
- • hospitalization
- • anesthesia
- • analgesia
- • surgical interventions
- • complementary medicine.

In exchange for the services that have been rendered, the client agrees to compensate the veterinary team.(9) Financial compensation is facilitated by the provision of an estimate before care has been delivered so that clients agree to costs upfront.

In addition to paying for veterinary services, the client may also agree to take on patient care responsibilities.(7, 9) This is particularly true of clinical scenarios in which pet owners agree to conservative management on an outpatient basis.

Patient care responsibilities, for the client, may include:

- • observing the patient in its home environment
- • charting changes in appetite or voiding (urination/defecation)
- • reporting vomiting or diarrhea
- • administering oral medications
- • restricting patient activity
- • keeping patient bandages dry.

Patient care responsibilities should also be outlined in terms of what the client should do if things do not go according to plan.(7, 14)

- • By when should the client see an improvement in the patient?
- • At what point should the client become concerned about the patient's lack of improvement?
- • Who should they contact? And when?
    - ▪ during office hours?
    - ▪ after hours?
- • Under which circumstances?

Patient care responsibilities, for the client, are not always easy. They may be time or labor intensive:

- administering multiple medications, several times a day
- preparing a home-cooked diet
- bathing or otherwise grooming a patient one or more times a week
- cleaning ears on a regular basis
- expressing anal glands
- administering injectable medications, particularly those that take more than just a few seconds to give, such as SQ fluids
- administering a prescription product through a feeding tube
- performing at-home blood glucose (BG) monitoring
- manually expressing the patient's urinary bladder
- slinging a towel underneath a recumbent patient to support him as he rises.

Each client has a different threshold in terms of what they consider to be reasonable versus care.

Regardless of which actions the veterinarian and client agree to, their agreement is a form of a contract.

16.2 Examples of Contracting for Next Steps in Clinical Practice

16.2.1 The Veterinarian Outlines the Care Plan

At its simplest, contracting for next steps is about who pays who for which services. But contracting for next steps is not always about money. It is often about dividing up patient care responsibilities so that everyone has the same patient care expectations.

Contracting for the next steps may require the veterinary team to research a given disease process for novel treatment modalities. Contracting for the next steps may require the client to provide additional information, such as vaccination records or the ingredient label for the brand of dog food that is being fed.

Contracting for the next steps is *always* about who is doing what, in the best interest of the patient. Let us take a look at how this communication skill may be used by the veterinarian to outline his or her responsibilities to a given patient.

> **Background**
>
> You are an associate veterinarian in clinical practice.
>
> Your client, Mr. Rogers, has presented his Boston terrier, Gemstone, to you for paint-ball ingestion. This is an unusual toxicosis that has caused the patient to succumb to extreme hypernatremia. This imbalance of sodium has resulted in seizure activity. The patient has been stabilized in the moment; however, you are concerned about progres-

sion of clinical signs. You and the client agree to admit the patient to the hospital for continued observation and management of abnormal neurological activity.

Clinical Conversation

Veterinarian: Gemstone is in good hands. We will continue to administer IV fluids and monitor her sodium level every two hours so that it is dropping at a rate that is safe enough for her body to handle. I will also reach out to our local Poison Control Center to see if there are any additional suggestions for supportive care.

In the example above, the veterinarian has outlined the role she will play in Gemstone's care. The veterinarian has acknowledged that Gemstone's inpatient care will consist largely of IV fluid therapy and blood-draws to track the patient's sodium levels.

The veterinarian has made it clear that the rate at which sodium drops is critical to the patient's recovery, and that sodium levels cannot drop too quickly. To prevent this, sodium levels will be assessed every 2 hours.

In addition, the veterinarian will make contact with toxicologists to determine if any other treatments are indicated.

16.2.2 The Veterinarian Asks for the Client's Help

The conversation in Section 16.2.1 is a prime example of the veterinarian using the communication skill, "contracting for next steps," to tell the client what she or he plans to do to care for the patient. However, "contracting for next steps" may also involve asking the client to agree to a patient care plan. Consider, for instance, a clinical scenario in which a West Highland White Terrier presents to you for presumptive food allergies.

Background

You and the client agree to a 12-week elimination diet, meaning that the patient will be fed a novel protein and carbohydrate source – and nothing else – to assess the skin's response.

In order to create this novel diet, the veterinarian needs to know precisely what the patient has been fed during the course of its lifetime.

This is where "contracting for next steps" comes in handy.

Clinical Conversation

Veterinarian: We are in agreement that the best next step for Finnegan is to start him on an elimination diet that exposes him to a carbohydrate and protein that his body has never before experienced.

[pause]

Veterinarian: For this to have the best success rate, we need to work together to come up with a diet that is truly new to him.

[pause]

Veterinarian: I am going to need you to provide me with a list of all foods that he has eaten in the past, including treats and brand name items, so that we truly pick something that he has never had before. Would you be able to email the clinic this list by next Monday?

Client: Definitely, that is doable.

Veterinarian: Great! Thank you. Once I get the list from you, I will come up with a plan that we can discuss by telephone. Once we agree to the plan, this diet is *all* that Finnegan will eat for the next 12 weeks. No treats. No table scraps. Just this diet. It's going to be tough, but it's worth it.

Note that in this clinical scenario, contracting for next steps involved the veterinarian outlining his or her expectations for the client's role in patient care. In order for the veterinarian to formulate a new diet, the veterinarian needs a list of items that Finnegan has consumed.

The veterinarian is making a contract with the client: if the client can provide the list by a certain date, then the veterinarian can fulfill his end of the bargain.

The order of events is also made very clear.

- In order for the diet to be formulated, the client must provide the veterinarian with a list of ingredients.
- Once the list of ingredients has been created, then the veterinarian can tailor the diet to suit the patient's needs.
- Once the veterinarian formulates the diet, then the veterinarian will telephone with instructions for how to proceed.

16.3 Contracting for Next Steps Tells the Client What to Expect

Contracting for next steps may sound *formal,* but it is really just about setting expectations. It is about telling the client what you need to do your job effectively. For instance, the following statements involve contracting for next steps so that the client has a clear expectation as to what she or he needs to do.

- "Please provide us with your cat's stool sample at your earliest convenience so that we can screen him for worms."

- "Please email us a copy of your dog's vaccination records so that we know which vaccines require updating."
- "Please call us with a status update in two or three days so that we know if your pet is on track."
- "Please schedule a recheck appointment in 7–10 days so that we can re-examine his eye."
- "Please bring him in on emergency if he vomits more than three times in the next hour."

16.4 Contracting for Next Steps Reinforces Our Role in Patient Care

Contracting for next steps also reinforces what we have agreed to do on behalf of our patient as part of the patient's healthcare team. The following statements demonstrate proper use of this communication tool as it relates to our patient care responsibilities.

- "I will provide you with an estimate for his dental cleaning so that you can be prepared two months from now when he really needs it."
- "I will give you a call as soon as the bloodwork is back from the lab. I expect the results to be back by the weekend."
- "I will contact you with the biopsy results as soon as the lab provides me with the finalized report."
- "I will contact the university to see if there are any therapeutic trials that we could enroll your dog in."
- "I will provide you with a script that you can take to your local pharmacy to have the medication filled there."

16.5 Modifying How Contracting for Next Steps Is Phrased

Contracting for the next steps can be softened by placing a "please" in front of the request, as demonstrated in the sample phases – or by following up on the statement with a check-in.
    For example, let us re-examine the statement:

"I will provide you with a script that you can take to your local pharmacy to have the medication filled there."

A proper check-in statement might be:

- "Is that okay?"
- "Is that alright?"
- "How does that sound?

- "Will that work?"
- "Does that work for you?"

This gives the client the opportunity to express content or discontent with the plan.

For more information on check-in statements, please refer to Chapter 15.

16.6 Be Prepared for the Client to Say "No" to the Initial Plan

Let us consider what might happen if you ask the client, "Does that work for you?" For instance, maybe you are currently involved in a case that involves a feline corneal ulcer. The ulcer is deep, and you have expressed concerns that conservative (topical) therapy may be insufficient. If the ulcer deepens much further, then the globe risks perforation, with loss of vision. In order to keep a close watch on the eye, you have recommended that the cat be rechecked in 2–3 days.

You ask the question, "Does that work for you?" The client responds, "No, that's not going to work." You are taken back by the candid nature of the client's response. You were not expecting that.

In truth, you need to expect that sometimes clients will not agree. Just because you have a clear idea in your mind of what constitutes standard of care does not necessarily mean that your client shares the same vision.

Or maybe your client does want to follow through, but other life circumstances are getting in the way of compliance. Maybe the client has business meetings that must be attended to and cannot simply cancel them. Maybe the client took off from work today, and does not have any additional "sick leave" to use to return again to your practice in 2–3 days. The possibilities could be endless.

Rather than judge the client, we need to be receptive to their needs. That does not mean we have to agree to a day and time that will not work for us. For example, just because it may be most convenient for a client to visit us on a Sunday afternoon does not mean that we must rise to the occasion and meet them then.

However, it does require us to be flexible. If the client cannot meet us in 2–3 days, for whatever reason, then when would it be convenient for the client? Can you and the client work out a compromise? Can the client find a way to make a visit 4–5 days from now possible?

As veterinarians, we need to think outside of the box and be creative. Maybe the client can ask a family member to bring the cat in to see you.

Or maybe the client can schedule a drop-off appointment and deliver the cat to the clinic on his way into the office. Maybe you can then discuss the cat's condition and care when he or she picks the cat up on his or her way home from work.

The bottom line is that the burden falls upon the veterinary team to modify patient care plans in a way that is mutually agreeable.(12) In such circumstances, the tone of the veterinary team is very important. If you ask the client, "Does that work for you?" and the client says, "No," then you have to be okay with finding an alternative solution.

If you offer an alternative solution, but do so in a tone that conveys annoyance, then the client will pick up on your disgruntled state. The client may then question the sincerity of future attempts, on your part, to elicit his or her perspective. A frustrated tone is corrosive to relationship-centered care and works against rapport, rather than in favor of it.

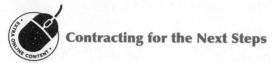

Contracting for the Next Steps

References

1. Frankel RM. Pets, vets, and frets: what relationship-centered care research has to offer veterinary medicine. J Vet Med Educ. 2006;33(1):20–7.
2. Chin JJ. Doctor–patient relationship: from medical paternalism to enhanced autonomy. Singapore Med J. 2002;43(3):152–5.
3. Makoul G. Essential elements of communication in medical encounters: the Kalamazoo consensus statement. Acad Med. 2001;76(4):390–3.
4. Novack DH, Suchman AL, Clark W, Epstein RM, Najberg E, Kaplan C. Calibrating the physician. Personal awareness and effective patient care. Working Group on Promoting Physician Personal Awareness, American Academy on Physician and Patient. JAMA. 1997;278(6):502–9.
5. Makoul G, Curry RH, Novack DH. The future of medical school courses in professional skills and perspectives. Acad Med. 1998;73(1):48–51.
6. Makoul G, Schofield T. Communication teaching and assessment in medical education: an international consensus statement. Netherlands Institute of Primary Health Care. Patient Educ Couns. 1999;37(2):191–5.
7. Adams CL, Kurtz SM. Skills for communicating in veterinary medicine. Oxford: Otmoor Publishing and Dewpoint Publishing; 2017.
8. Stewart M, B.J. B, Donner A, McWhinney IR, Oates J, Watson W. The impact of patient-centered care on patient outcomes in family practice. London, ON: Thames Valley Family Practice Unit; 1997.
9. Englar RE, Williams M, Weingand K. Applicability of the Calgary–Cambridge Guide to dog and cat owners for teaching veterinary clinical communications. J Vet Med Educ. 2016;43(2):143–69.
10. Silverman J, Kurtz S, Draper J. Skills for communicating with patients. Oxford: Radcliffe Medical Press; 2008.
11. Gray C, Moffett J. Handbook of veterinary communication skills. Chichester: Wiley-Blackwell; 2010.
12. Radford A, Stockley P, Silverman J, Taylor I, Turner R, Gray C. Development, teaching, and evaluation of a consultation structure model for use in veterinary education. J Vet Med Educ. 2006;33(1):38–44.
13. Hunter L, Shaw JR. What's in your communication toolbox? Exceptional Veterinary Team. 2012(November/December):12–7.
14. Neighbour R. The inner consultation: how to develop an effective and intuitive consulting style. Lancaster: MTP Press; 1987.

Chapter 17

Agenda-Setting and the Final "Check-In"

Like most new graduates, when I walked across that stage at Cornell University in 2008, with three shiny new letters after my name (DVM), I faced a laundry list of "firsts and fears," as we referred to them, in those days.

The "firsts" were all those things that I had yet to experience as a doctor. The "fears" were the frets that went along with the realization that I was now responsible for managing them all.

Most of the firsts and fears centered on procedural medicine:

- performing an adrenocorticotropic hormone (ACTH) stim test
- performing a cesarean section
- performing a cryptorchid orchiectomy
- performing a splenectomy
- performing an owner-present euthanasia solo in the examination room
- surgically correcting a gastric dilatation-volvulus (GDV)
- tapping a joint
- unblocking a tomcat
- using Ivomec® (1% ivermectin) off-label as a parasiticide for dogs with demodectic mange, and having to calculate the appropriate dose so as not to induce neurotoxicity.

Few firsts and fears were based on communication concerns.

Yet there was a single question that I had been trained to avoid asking because I did in fact fear the client's answer. That question took several forms, depending upon which faculty member you asked, but at its core, it was an invitation to the client to prolong the appointment.

- "Do you have any other questions for me at this time?"
- "Is there anything else that you need?"
- "Is there anything that I did not answer?"
- "Is there anything else that you want to add before I admit Oscar to the hospital?"

In our teaching hospital, many of the interns, residents, and chiefs of service avoided asking this question, or any variation of it.

When students asked why this question was not openly aired at the end of each consultation, these same clinicians cringed. If you asked them to explain their visceral reaction, they responded that this line of questioning led to "oh, by the way ..." appointments.

Their fear was that, if given the opportunity, the client would not stop talking. These clinicians were the same ones who feared asking open-ended questions, for similar reasons. In the past, they had been burned by asking the simple appointment wrap-up question, "Is there anything else that I can do for you today?"

All they could recall was that one client who said, "Yes," and proceeded to share an extensive list of concerns that could not possibly be covered within the timeframe of a single consultation.

"Is there anything else that I can do for you today?" seemed harmless, on the surface. However, all that question achieved – in their minds – was angst and frustration, as well as the growing realization that they were going to fall behind schedule for the rest of the day, all because that one client would not shut up.

At the time, their fear of the "runaway train" became my fear, and so I avoided the question altogether when I could. When I could not, I asked it quickly, followed by a minimal pause so that the client hardly had the time to answer. I am not proud of it, but that is the way it was in the earliest days of my career.

I saw it as self-preservation. I practiced what I had been taught, and because many of my leaders modeled this belief that checking in with the client at the end of the appointment was dangerous, I followed suit. I effectively shut clients down and shut clients out, without recognizing that I was wrong.

What I didn't know then was that this question had a name – the final check-in – and that it was actually a communication skill hidden in disguise. It was not until I began attending conferences for continuing education that I began to realize my mistake. The final check-in was in fact a valuable way to wrap up any appointment.(1–5) The final check-in was not only said to be polite. It was intended as one last opportunity to demonstrate partnership. It was a way of expressing the following to the client.

- "I am checking in because I am here to serve you and your pet."
- "I am checking in because I care."
- "I am checking in because I want to be sure that your concerns were addressed."
- "Hopefully, your concerns were covered today, but just in case they were not, I want you to tell me, so that I can remedy it."

The doctor who actively solicits the client's concerns at the beginning of the appointment has little to fear.(4, 6) Concerns are less likely to arise late in the consultation if the client has been allowed to disclose them upfront.(4, 6, 7)

By contrast, the doctor who interrupts the client's opening statement and/or redirects the client's disclosure of concerns is likely to experience backlash when she or he asks, "Is there anything else you need?"

Interruptions are frequent occurrences in the consultation room.(6) Human medical doctors often take over the conversation after the patient has only spoken for 12–23 seconds.(8–10) Doctors may also unintentionally direct the flow of conversation away from opportunity areas for clients to share additional concerns with the medical team. (8–10) They may hear a single concern and delve straight into addressing it, when in fact the patient often has more than one concern to share.(11–15)

Interruptions are not unique to human healthcare.(6) A 2011 study by Dysart et al. analyzed how well client concerns are solicited in companion animal practice, and concluded that veterinarians interrupted clients in 55% of appointments.(6) Interruptions occurred after a median of 11 seconds and a mean of 15.3 seconds.(6) When client concerns were not flushed out at the beginning of an appointment, on account of interruptions, it was four times more likely that a new concern would arise at the end of the consultation.(6)

It makes sense that if a client does not have the opportunity early on in the appointment to share what is on his or her mind, she or he will hold onto that concern through the appointment. That same client is likely to air the concern at the appointment's end, when the opportunity arises.

When this occurs, it is usually not so much our client's fault as it is our own. The fault falls upon the doctor, who failed to structure the appointment carefully.

17.1 The Value of Agenda-Setting

Agenda-setting is the process by which the healthcare team establishes the patient's/client's presenting complaint(s).(8, 9, 16) Sometimes, it is referred to as the "survey of problems."(17) Its purpose is to gain understanding as to why the patient/client is seeking medical care.(9, 16–20)

Each patient/client is unique, and most enter into the consultation with more than one concern. If the physician is to be complete, then she or he must invite the patient/client to share all concerns, while ignoring the temptation to limit discussion to just one.(9, 16–20)

Agenda-setting often begins with an open-ended solicitation.(6, 9) Examples include the following.

* "What can I do for you today?"
* "What can I help you with?"
* "How can I help you?"(9)
* "What brings you in today?"(6, 9)
* "What seems to be the trouble?"
* "What's going on?"
* "Anything else?"(9)

Note that agenda-setting is often phrased in a way that elicits the patient's/client's perspective. Refer to Chapter 11 to review this communication skill.

By eliciting the patient's/client's perspective, the patient/client is more likely to share what is on his or her mind.(6, 21)

By using open-ended phrasing, the patient/client is invited to tell his or her story. It may be tempting to interrupt the story, and indeed, many clinicians do.(8–10) A 1999 study by Marvel et al. confirmed that only one-in-four human patients are allowed to complete their opening statement.(9) Yet, patient's opening statements are not typically verbose.(9) If allowed to complete their thoughts, patients on average only speak for 6 seconds more than those who are interrupted.(9)

Follow-up questions play an important role in agenda-setting.(9) For instance, consider the open-ended solicitation, "How can I help you today?" If this is a veterinary scenario, the client may respond as follows: "Tabitha seems to have hurt her leg. She hasn't walked right on it since last Thursday."

It behooves the clinician to follow-up on this response with a focused open-ended question, for example, "Tell me more about the leg issue."(9) This invites the client to provide additional details. A receptive client may respond to the clinician's encouragement by sharing the following:

> It's her right back leg. It seems to be getting worse. I had some Rimadyl® (carprofen) leftover from her spay surgery six months ago, so I gave her a dose or two. It seemed to help for a few hours after giving it, but her lameness always comes back. It seems particularly painful when she gets up after a nap.

It may be tempting to shut down all other avenues of communication to focus solely on Tabitha's lameness. However, the client may have more to share. It is important that you make another inquiry to flush out any additional concerns that the client may have, whether or not they are related to the pelvic limb.

Consider the open-ended solicitation, "Is there anything else that you would like to discuss today?"

The client might add:

> I know this doesn't have anything to do with her leg, doc, but I also felt a lump at her right shoulder. We were watching TV together last night and when I was petting her, I felt something there that has never been there before. She didn't seem to care that I was touching it, but it seems big to me. It seems like I should have noticed it before now. Can you take a look?

Simply by inviting open-ended answers, we have established that Tabitha has two presenting complaints:

1. right pelvic limb lameness
2. right shoulder lump.

This clinical scenario serves as an effective reminder that our patients do not present in a bubble. In other words, Tabitha is not presenting to us with just an isolated limb to evaluate. Tabitha presents as an entire being.

Although time constraints require us to prioritize chief complaints and for that reason today's consultation may emphasize the limb, we must keep any and all additional problems on our radar. It is up to us to address each as they arise, even if this requires staging the appointment. The most important aspect of agenda-setting is that each problem is identified and acknowledged.

Agenda-setting is a valuable tool. It conveys respect for the client as a valuable resource and member of the healthcare team. It grants the client the floor to share what is weighing on his or her mind.

We are not mind readers. We only know what is weighing on our clients if we ask them. Consider, for example, a 2019 study by Albuquerque et al. that evaluated client concerns about the medical management of diabetic cats at initial diagnosis, in which it was found that: (22)

- 77% of clients were concerned about finding boarding facilities and/or pet sitters that could manage a diabetic patient during vacations and holidays
- 69% of clients expressed concern about cost of care
- 41% of clients worried about how managing diabetes might impact their lives
- 40% of clients feared that management would corrode the human–animal bond.

Sharing concerns between members of the veterinary team is valuable. By sharing, the client is more likely to focus on what we have to say. Thus, the efficiency of the consultation improves.(9) The veterinarian is also able to consider a complete clinical picture. This allows the veterinarian to prioritize those problems that require immediate attention.(9)

Gaining a complete clinical picture also allows the veterinarian to consider potential barriers to treatment. For example, if clients are afraid that they will be unable to find competent care for their pets during vacations or holidays, then they may be reluctant to pursue medical management. This drives home the importance of us working with our clients to address their concerns. Maybe we need to offer medical boarding as a viable solution for managing patient care when the client is out of town. Or maybe we need to make a list of diabetic-friendly boarding facilities and vetted pet sitters. Only then may our client be ready to commit to management.

A second benefit of agenda-setting is that the clinician no longer has to make assumptions about what the client wants or needs, because she or he has invited the client to share.(9) This allows the clinician to make the best use of time. The clinician hears every concern, want, or need, in the words of the client, and makes certain to acknowledge each. When each concern is acknowledged and a plan for how to address each is discussed during the visit, fewer new concerns are voiced by the client at the end of the consultation.(9)

Agenda-setting is a time saver. When done well, it makes the final check-in a non-event.

17.2 The Final Check-In as a Relationship Builder

Just as first impressions count, so, too, do final ones. The way we conclude a visit creates a lasting impression in the eyes of our clients.

Many of us do not know how to end an appointment because it was never taught to us. Even though veterinary curricula have evolved over time to incorporate key aspects of clinical communication into the classroom, not all programs are able to address this content area in depth.

Furthermore, because many practicing veterinarians graduated long before communication skills were considered to be a core competency, some still struggle with ending an appointment well.

It is advisable for us as a profession to rework how we conclude an appointment so that we strengthen our clinical practice of relationship-centered care. It is important for our clients to feel heard and valued as team members. The final check-in leaves a lasting impression that our clients' agendas matter to us and that what they have to say counts.

17.3 Pairing the Final Check-In with Appropriate Nonverbal Cues

If you commit to the final check-in, then you must commit yourself to hearing (and accepting) the client's answer. There is little in clinical communication that is worse than asking a final check-in, only to override it with nonverbal cues that suggest your disinterest or disengagement from the conversation.

Recall from Chapter 7 that nonverbal cues carry more weight than the spoken word in clinical conversations.(23–27) Nonverbal communication influences how verbal exchanges are received.(28–30) When nonverbal communication contradicts what is said aloud, clients put trust in the former.(4, 23, 30–32)

During the final check-in, three nonverbal cues in particular are distracting and may take away from the message that you are attempting to convey: "I care." These cues include:

- physically turning away from the client, to face the door
- placing your hand on the doorknob
- looking at your watch or phone.

These actions may be unintentional or unconscious. However, they do not go unnoticed by the client.

When these actions occur at the same time that the clinician is presenting the final check-in, "Is there anything else that you need?" the client gets the impression that the doctor is disingenuous. The client assumes that the doctor does not really want to hear what she or he has to say. The client assumes that the doctor is disinterested and ready to move on. In other words, the consultation is over.

This client may be easily deterred from providing a candid answer. The client may have wanted to say, "Yes, I do need …":

- "… more information"
- "… more time"
- "… an estimate"
- "… help with a nail trim"
- "… advice about …?"

However, if clients do not feel welcome to share, most will remain silent. They may answer "No," but not really mean it.

They are likely to leave the office dissatisfied. They may feel cheated. They may feel that they did not get out of the visit what they had hoped. They did not receive what they had paid for.

The bottom line is not to attempt a final check-in unless you are receptive to hearing the answer and are able to display that receptivity in body language. If you ask a final check-in, then it is critical for you to invite an honest answer.

This means that you should be facing the client when you are speaking. You should demonstrate engagement in the conversation by connecting to the client through appropriate eye contact. You should focus on the client, and you should pause after your check-in statement.

Let us see how this might play out in clinical practice.

Clinical Conversation

Veterinarian: Is there anything else that I can do for you today?

[pause]

Client: Actually, *yes*. It would really help if you could trim Tuffy's nails when you take him to the back for his blood to be drawn. I've tried to do them myself and it's an epic fail, every time.

Veterinarian: Not a problem. It will be our pleasure. A nail trim costs $15. Would that be okay?

Client: Certainly. $15 is worth not having to struggle.

Veterinarian: Excellent, then consider it done.

Let us examine another instance in which the final check-in is used appropriately and elicits a client's concern. Not only is the concern heard, it is addressed by the veterinarian in a way that suits the client's needs and meets expectations.

Clinical Conversation

Veterinarian: Do you have any other questions before we perform Jenny's surgery?

Client: She'll be okay, won't she, doc? I don't know what I would do if we lost her.

> She's all I've got.
>
> Veterinarian: I know how important she is to you, and I will do everything in my power to keep her safe. Surgery's a big deal and yes, it can be very scary. What can we do to make this easier on you?
>
> Client: Could you have someone call me as soon as she's awake? I really need to know that she pulled through.
>
> Veterinarian: Absolutely. I will call you as soon as she is in recovery. How does that sound?
>
> Client: That would be a big help. Thank you.

In this clinical scenario, the final check-in opened up the door to one last exchange between the client and the veterinarian. The client was able to express his concern about the pet's ability to survive the procedure. The veterinarian was able to hear that what this individual really wanted was reassurance.

This final check-in gave the client the opportunity to share his needs. This final check-in gave the veterinarian the chance to agree to a simple, but powerful request: the promise of a telephone call once the patient had recovered from surgery.

Therefore, consider final check-ins to be relationship builders for the practice. Allow final check-ins to be opportunities to cement the veterinary–client bond. Use them to make the client feel respected and heard. It does not take long to check in and honor most clients' requests.

17.4 What If the Client Does Not Stop Talking?

Many veterinarians are reluctant to ask the final check-in statement. They worry that it invites dialogue at a time when the appointment needs to wrap up. I would argue that:

> Late presentation of problems may reflect a failure of the physician to facilitate disclosure earlier as patients report waiting for the "right" moment or opportunity to present their "real" problems.(33)

In truth, we can prevent most appointments from spiraling down the "Oh, by the way ..." path if we are conscientious with agenda-setting at the beginning of the appointment.

Agenda-setting may seem labor intensive. Many clinicians worry that it will eat up too much of the appointment time. In reality, the fear that a client will never stop talking has been blown out of proportion. One human medical study reported that when opening statements were uninterrupted, the most that a patient talked for was 1 minute and 40 seconds.(34, 35)

That being said, we cannot prevent the runaway train in all situations. Medicine is imperfect. So, too, are our clients. The truth is that, yes, it is possible that a client will see the final check-in as an open door to invite more conversation that has no direction.

The reality is, this kind of client will find a way to make that happen, whether or not we ask the final check-in. The loquacious client will talk about whatever, whenever, for however long. Thankfully, this type of client is in the minority.

Do not let isolated encounters with verbose clients make you reluctant to complete the final check-in. Do not give that one client that kind of power. Do not allow that one client to shut down your opportunity to conduct the final check-in.

The final check-in is essential. It is the last impression that we leave with the client. It is their last memory of us as in our role within a customer service industry. We are here to serve. The final check-in demonstrates that we are not only present, we are *still* listening.

But what about the loquacious client? What is your best approach to managing your time in the consultation room with them? Signposting is the best tool to manage those clients who talk a lot and take a great many tangents. Refer to Chapter 14 for more information on how to incorporate signposts into your consultation to improve the flow of conversation and redirect it respectfully when necessary.

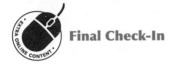 **Final Check-In**

References:

1. Englar RE, Williams M, Weingand K. Applicability of the Calgary–Cambridge Guide to dog and cat owners for teaching veterinary clinical communications. J Vet Med Educ. 2016;43(2):143–69.
2. Silverman J, Kurtz S, Draper J. Skills for communicating with patients. Oxford: Radcliffe Medical Press; 2008.
3. Radford A, Stockley P, Silverman J, Taylor I, Turner R, Gray C. Development, teaching, and evaluation of a consultation structure model for use in veterinary education. J Vet Med Educ. 2006;33(1):38–44.
4. Adams CL, Kurtz SM. Skills for communicating in veterinary medicine. Oxford: Otmoor Publishing and Dewpoint Publishing; 2017.
5. Hunter L, Shaw JR. What's in your communication toolbox? Exceptional Veterinary Team. 2012(November/December):12–7.
6. Dysart LM, Coe JB, Adams CL. Analysis of solicitation of client concerns in companion animal practice. J Am Vet Med Assoc. 2011;238(12):1609–15.
7. Baker LH, O'Connell D, Platt FW. "What else?" Setting the agenda for the clinical interview. Ann Intern Med. 2005;143(10):766–70.
8. Beckman HB, Frankel RM. The effect of physician behavior on the collection of data. Ann Intern Med. 1984;101(5):692–6.
9. Marvel MK, Epstein RM, Flowers K, Beckman HB. Soliciting the patient's agenda: have we improved? JAMA. 1999;281(3):283–7.
10. Rhoades DR, McFarland KF, Finch WH, Johnson AO. Speaking and interruptions during primary care office visits. Fam Med. 2001;33(7):528–32.

11. Robinson JD, Tate A, Heritage J. Agenda-setting revisited: when and how do primary-care physicians solicit patients' additional concerns? Patient Educ Couns. 2016;99(5):718–23.

12. Braddock CH, 3rd, Edwards KA, Hasenberg NM, Laidley TL, Levinson W. Informed decision making in outpatient practice: time to get back to basics. JAMA. 1999;282(24):2313–20.

13. Heritage J, Robinson JD, Elliott MN, Beckett M, Wilkes M. Reducing patients' unmet concerns in primary care: the difference one word can make. J Gen Intern Med. 2007;22(10):1429–33.

14. Middleton JF, McKinley RK, Gillies CL. Effect of patient completed agenda forms and doctors' education about the agenda on the outcome of consultations: randomized controlled trial. BMJ. 2006;332(7552):1238–42.

15. Rost K, Frankel R. The introduction of the older patient's problems in the medical visit. J Aging Health. 1993;5(3):387–401.

16. Smith RC. The patient's story: integrated patient–doctor interviewing. Boston, MA: Little Brown & Co. Inc.; 1996.

17. Lipkin M. The medical interview. In: Feldman MD, Christensen JF, editors. Behavioral medicine in primary care: a practical guide. Stamford, CT: Appleton & Lange; 1997. p. 1–7.

18. Coulehan JL, Block MR. The medical interview: mastering skills for clinical practice. Philadelphia, PA: FA Davis Co Publishers; 1997.

19. Levinson DL. A Guide to the clinical interview. Philadelphia, PA: WB Saunders Co; 1987.

20. Frankel RM, Beckman HB. Evaluating the patient's primary problem(s). In: Stewart M, Roter D, editors. Communicating with medical patients. Newbury Park, CA: SAGE Publications; 1989. pp. 86–98.

21. Abood SK. Effectively communicating with your clients. Top Companion Anim Med. 2008;23(3):143–7.

22. Albuquerque CS, Bauman BL, Rzeznitzeck J, Caney SM, Gunn-Moore DA. Priorities on treatment and monitoring of diabetic cats from the owners' points of view. J Feline Med Surg. 2019:1098612X19858154.

23. Shaw JR. Four core communication skills of highly effective practitioners. Vet Clin North Am Small Anim Pract. 2006;36(2):385–96, vii.

24. Kurtz SM, Silverman JD, Draper J. Teaching and learning communication skills in medicine. Grand Rapids, MI: Radcliffe; 2004.

25. Carson CA. Nonverbal communication in veterinary practice. Vet Clin North Am Small Anim Pract. 2007;37(1):49–63; abstract viii.

26. Caris-Verhallen WM, Kerkstra A, Bensing JM. Non-verbal behaviour in nurse-elderly patient communication. J Adv Nurs. 1999;29(4):808–18.

27. Gross D. Communication and the elderly. Physical and Occupational Therapy in Geriatrics. 1990;9(1):49–64.

28. Cocksedge S, George B, Renwick S, Chew-Graham CA. Touch in primary care consultations: qualitative investigation of doctors' and patients' perceptions. Br J Gen Pract. 2013;63(609):e283–90.

29. Hall JA, Harrigan JA, Rosenthal R. Nonverbal behavior in clinician patient interaction. Appl Prev Psychol. 1995;4(1):21–37.

30. Roter DL, Frankel RM, Hall JA, Sluyter D. The expression of emotion through nonverbal behavior in medical visits: mechanisms and outcomes. J Gen Intern Med. 2005;21(Suppl 1):S28–34.

31. Koch R. The teacher and nonverbal communication. Theory Pract. 1971;10(4):231–42.

32. McCroskey JC, Larson CE, Knapp ML. An introduction to interpersonal communication. Englewood Cliffs, NJ: Prentice Hall; 1971.

33. White J, Levinson W, Roter D. Oh, by the way ... – the closing moments of the medical visit. J Gen Intern Med. 1994;9(1):24–8.
34. Langewitz W, Denz M, Keller A, Kiss A, Ruttimann S, Wossmer B. Spontaneous talking time at start of consultation in outpatient clinic: cohort study. BMJ. 2002;325(7366):682–3.
35. Blau JN. Time to let the patient speak. Brit Med J. 1989;298(6665):39-.

Chapter 18

Defining Two New Skills that Companion-Animal Clients Value

Compassionate Transparency and Unconditional Positive Regard

Evidence-based research has proven that the delivery of healthcare and patient out-comes is dependent upon effective communication.(1) Accordingly, communication is now viewed as a teachable skill. To facilitate the development of this skill, clinical communication has been integrated into the curricula of most veterinary programs, and both the classroom and teaching hospital are now considered to be valuable training grounds.

It is no longer a question of whether communication should be taught to healthcare providers, including veterinarians. The leading question has become *how* to teach it best.

There is quite a bit of variability in terms of how medical programs approach this content area.(2–8)

Methodologies that are currently in use include: (2–11)

- didactic presentations as a platform for lecturing about communication
- online educational modules
- interactive workshops
- leadership retreats
- mock interviews
- team-building exercises
- small-group discussions
- live role play between students
- simulated appointments with standardized patients/clients
- videotape review of interactions with real patients
- objective structured clinical examinations (OSCEs)
- on-the-clinic-floor learning with real-life patients.

Assessment of students' communication skills is critical. We need to know if what we are teaching them is effective and promotes their successful transition, as new graduates, from the classroom into clinical practice.

Many of the communication skills that are taught by veterinary educators in the present day are adapted from human healthcare models. Perhaps the most influential of these is the Calgary–Cambridge model, which Radford et al. adapted in 2002 for use in veterinary medicine.(12–14)

As communications training continues to evolve and we begin to understand more about the psychology of our consumers, the veterinary profession owes it to clients to consider their needs.

- Do all Calgary–Cambridge skills matter to the veterinary client?
- Do some skills matter more than others?
- Does the perceived value of a given skill vary depending upon:
  - the species of animal owned?
  - the purpose of the animal?
  - the age of the client?
  - the gender of the client?
  - the clinical circumstances or scenario?

Few studies exist in the veterinary literature concerning the preferences of the consumer.

Two prominent studies in veterinary medicine were published by Coe et al. in 2007 and 2008.(15, 16) These were among the first of their kind to emphasize client perceptions and preferences concerning patient care.

Coe's 2007 focus group study was conducted to compare veterinarians' and pet owners' expectations concerning the cost of care.(15) The following conclusions about the client's perspective were made.(15)

- Clients expect veterinarians to prioritize patient care over cost. When cost is an obstacle, veterinary clients expect partnership with veterinarians to find a viable solution.
- Clients expect veterinarians to initiate conversations about cost of care, and to be upfront about even the most basic of costs so that clients are able to plan ahead and budget.
- Clients expect veterinarians to explain how cost relates to the patient's health and prognosis. In other words, what is the value associated with procedure "X"? What is the cost-to-benefit ratio?
- Clients expect veterinarians to consider vaccine and heartworm recommendations in light of what they themselves choose to do for their own pets.

One pet owner expressed that:

283

I wish that veterinarians would … say "do as I do, not as I say", because I feel that veterinarians are taught to do certain things, but then, [when you] ask the veterinarian, "what do you do?" they don't do that!(15)

In sum, veterinary clients expected transparency concerning cost of care.(15)
In 2008, Coe et al. conducted a second focus group study to compare veterinarians' and pet owners' expectations concerning clinical communication.(16) The following themes about veterinarian-client communication emerged.(16)

- Clients expect veterinarians to be proficient at history taking so that the right questions are asked to expedite patient care.
- Clients expect veterinarians to be a source of information that is easily understood.
- Clients expect veterinarians to provide information in different forms, such as:
  - handouts
  - pamphlets
  - information packets
  - written discharge instructions.
- Clients expect veterinarians to be upfront about diagnosis, treatment, and cost.
- Clients expect to be given options for management of patient care.
- Clients expect veterinarians to respect their final decisions about patient care.
- Clients expect veterinarians to partner with them to facilitate patient care.

According to Coe's focus group participants, breakdowns in communication resulted from the following.(16)

- Client perceptions that they were given misinformation.
- Client perceptions that there was miscommunication about cost.
- Client perceptions that they were being unfairly judged by the veterinary team.
- Veterinary perceptions that there was insufficient time in the consultation room.

Coe's research serves as an important reminder to the profession that care needs to be customized. While certain communication skills exhibit universality, others may be more or less important to different sectors of the population. We will never know what those skills are – or if certain skills are missing from our communication toolbox – unless we ask the consumer directly.

As a veterinary educator who was trained in the Calgary–Cambridge model, I am familiar with teaching the skills that have already been addressed throughout the preceding chapters:

- Greeting the Client (Chapter 4)
- Reflective Listening (Chapter 5)
- Empathy (Chapter 6)
- Nonverbal Cues (Chapter 7)

- Open-Ended Questions (Chapter 8)
- Reducing Medical Jargon (Chapter 9)
- Enhancing Relationship-Centered Care through Partnership (Chapter 10)
- Eliciting the Client's Perspective (Chapter 11)
- Asking Permission (Chapter 12)
- Assessing the Client's Knowledge (Chapter 13)
- Mapping Out the Consultation (Chapter 14)
- Internal and End-of-Consultation Summaries (Chapter 15)
- Checking In (Chapter 15)
- Contracting for Next Steps (Chapter 16)
- Agenda-Setting (Chapter 17)
- The Final Check-In (Chapter 17).

I wanted to determine if this skillset was considered complete in the eyes of companion-animal clients. To answer this clinical question, I conducted a pilot study involving focus groups composed of dog and cat owners.(12) Six dog owners and seven cat owners participated.(12)

Participants were asked to develop a "top ten" list of "must have" communication skills that they expected the veterinary team to possess.(12) Participants were then introduced to the Calgary–Cambridge curriculum, as outlined above, and asked to rank the skills in order of importance.(12)

When participants compared their expectations against those skills that I taught at Midwestern University (MWU), they agreed that all skills were applicable to dog and cat owners.(12)

However, participants unanimously agreed that the MWU communication skillset was not comprehensive.(12) Participants identified two areas in which the skillset could be expanded: (12)

1. compassionate transparency
2. unconditional positive regard.

18.1 What Is Transparency in Healthcare?

The concept of transparency in human healthcare emerged nearly two decades ago, when the Institute of Medicine released a controversial report, *To Err is Human*, in 1999. This report estimated that 44,000–98,000 people die annually in the United States from medical errors that could have been prevented.(17) These errors include:(17)

- delays in diagnosis or treatment
- procedural error
- equipment failure

- pharmaceutical mistakes
  - miscalculations in dosing
  - accidental administration of the wrong medication.

This publication hoped to shed light on the fact that medicine is imperfect, but can be improved when dialogue is initiated about error-reduction strategies.

In 2001, the Institute of Medicine published a follow-up report, *Crossing the Quality Chasm: A New Health System for the 21st Century*. This report outlined strategies for making healthcare more reliable and responsive to patient needs.(18) One overriding principle was fostering transparency in healthcare performance. Positive patient outcomes depended upon transparency with regards to:(18)

- patient coverage
- malpractice insurance
- standard operating procedures (SOPs)
- medical errors
- communication between clinicians
- communication between other members of the healthcare team
- communication between the healthcare team and hospital administration
- diagnostic testing and capabilities
- treatment options.

The emphasis on patient safety was intended to inspire clinical conversations so that patients would be better informed. When information about services is provided openly rather than withheld, patients and their families are afforded choices about the care that they will receive. They are also better equipped to handle decision making when things go wrong. If patients and their families feel included in decision making, then they are more likely to impart trust in the medical team. Trust promotes patient satisfaction and compliance with healthcare recommendations.(19)

In addition to promoting patient safety, transparency drives accountability. Accountability drives the setting of standards to make sure that clinicians, practices, hospitals, and referral centers are delivering safe, high-quality care. When mistakes occur, SOPs may need to be recalibrated to drive improvements in patient safety and to reduce risk of recurrence.(19)

18.2 Barriers to Transparency in Healthcare

Although embracing a culture of safety sounds good on paper, healthcare providers must overcome a steep hill of fear to bring it about.

Transparency implies disclosure. Disclosing information to patients means that providers must relinquish control over the knowledge that they have. Providers are no longer the "sage on the stage" or the sole expert in the room. Instead, they are one piece of the healthcare team. They must partner with the patient to come to a joint decision.(19)

Transparency also implies open communication, even when the topic makes the provider uncomfortable. For example, transparency requires open discussions about medical errors. This creates an ethical dilemma for the provider. The provider may feel morally obliged to share, yet fear retribution.(19)

18.3 Transparency in Veterinary Medicine through Words

Medical mistakes are not unique to human healthcare. Although incidence reports in the literature are infrequent, one study in the UK confirmed that veterinary errors are relatively common: 78% of graduates admitted to making at least one mistake that adversely impacted patient care.(20, 21) When such errors occur, veterinarians are encouraged to disclose what happened and why, the impact on the patient, and how the error will be prevented in the future.(21)

However, medical mistakes are not the only circumstance in which transparency may be required.

When dog and cat owners are asked to express their communication needs, they specifically mention the importance of transparency when veterinarians are discussing a patient's illness.(12) In particular, dog owners do not want facts sugar coated or withheld from them.(12) Even bad news delivery, such as a cancer diagnosis, was desired so that the client could be prepared for the decisions that s/he would have to make. One participant captured this perspective best:

> Don't beat around the bush. I already know it's cancer. I know what that means. So get to the point of what needs to be done. We know what needs to be done. We just need to hear you say it.(12)

Directness was particularly valued:

> Get right to it. Don't soften things up. I want to know exactly what's happening with the dog and what the worst outcome could be.(12)

Dog owners feel offended when information about prognosis or diagnosis is withheld.(12)

Dog owners misinterpret the veterinarians' intentions to shield them from harm. Clients worry that the veterinary team does not feel that they are capable of handling the facts. Dog owners also feel that their ability to make informed decisions about their pet's care is hindered because they lack the details that would have facilitated decision making. (12)

Directness is also prized by cat owners.(12) Cat owners want the veterinary team to be honest about what it does not know:

> I want them to say, "No, I really don't know." The test for [diagnosing this condition] is $300, the medicine is $100, let's just give the medicine and see what happens. And if it doesn't work, we'll move on to something else. Be open to saying, "I don't know, but this is the best course to try."(12)

18.4 Transparency in Veterinary Medicine through Actions

Sometimes, transparency is less about words and more about actions. For example, transparency can be physically present within a practice through the use of open floor plans to reduce barriers between the front and back staff, and also between veterinary clients and the rest of the veterinary team.

Other means of transparency in a practice setting include performing procedures such as acupuncture, nail trims, or venipuncture in front of the client, and incorporating spaces within the layout of the treatment area for clients to visit hospitalized pets.

Consider glass partitions rather than walls. Consider a hospital design that emphasizes approachability.(22)

18.5 Veterinary Clinical Scenarios that Involve Transparency

Veterinarians may try to soften blows, particularly when clients are emotionally distraught, in an effort to decrease the amount of pain that is felt.

Based upon my research, most clients prefer that veterinarians be open and upfront with them concerning:

* the diagnosis
* the prognosis
* the patient's quality of life
* whether or not the patient is perceived to be suffering.

Clients do not want veterinarians to be callous, cold, and unfeeling. At the same time, they don't want them to skirt around the truth either.

"Be kind, but be honest," one client shared with me. "Tell me the news straight up. If it could be cancer, then don't be afraid to use the 'C' word – cancer. I need to hear the truth. I may not *want* to hear it, but I need to hear it in order to process and ultimately accept it."(12)

Being transparent is important to clients so that they can anticipate what obstacles they may face along the way. Clients want to be prepared. Clients want time to know how they might react.

Compassionate transparency is a skill. Some veterinary disciplines may require it more than others. Consider, for instance, veterinary emergency and critical care medicine, or veterinary oncology.

Bad news delivery is never fun. However, bad news delivery is facilitated when you are ready, able, and willing to discuss the elephant in the room. Illness and death are scary, so much so that we may want to hide from them.

Compassionate transparency is about facing them head on. It is about acknowledging the figurative elephants so that our client can come up with the best plan in a bad situation.

Examples of compassionate transparency often begin with a "warning shot." Refer to Section 14.6 for more information about warning shot usage. As preparatory statements, warning shots help the client to pause and absorb that a blow is about to hit home.

In addition to preparatory statements, clinicians may encourage nonverbal cues that are more conducive to listening. For example, the clinician might ask the client, "Would you like to sit down?" Alternatively, the veterinarian may model the behavior and take a seat.

18.6 Example of a Situation that Would Have Benefited from Transparency

To better understand the skill, compassionate transparency, let us consider a clinical vignette, in which the clinician and client could have benefited from its use.

Background

You are an associate veterinarian in clinical practice. Your client presented his 8-year-old Rottweiler to evaluate acute onset of weight-bearing lameness on his right pelvic limb. On physical exam, there is appreciable swelling over the right stifle joint. Radiographs confirm the presence of an aggressive bony lesion. The top differential diagnosis is bone cancer, osteosarcoma.

Clinical Conversation

Veterinarian: I took a look at Duke's X-rays. The good news is that there does not appear to be a fracture. The bad news is that there's a lot of damage to the knee joint. I don't want to label it without more tests, but we need to investigate it further.

Client: What are you saying? Could it be cancer?

Veterinarian: Right now it's too early to tell. It could be … But let's not get ahead of ourselves. Forget about cancer for now. Don't worry. Let's think about all the other things that it could be that are a lot more treatable.

In the moment, it might seem that the veterinarian is doing right by her client. She is buffering the client's concern until more information is known about the definitive diagnosis.

However, it is the client's right to know the extent of what is possible, particularly when the client is asking directly for that type of information. Hiding the presumptive diagnosis from him or her may feel good in the moment, as if we are protecting him or her. However, when he or she finds out that cancer was the likely outcome all along, the veterinarian's plan may backfire. The client may feel misled or misguided. The client may feel hurt. The client may feel angry that he or she did not have time to prepare for the inevitable.

Let us explore now how the use of compassionate transparency might have benefited the same clinical scenario.

Clinical Conversation

Veterinarian: I took a look at Duke's X-rays. There is no fracture to explain his limp, but what I saw on the films concerned me greatly. There's no easy way to tell you this, but I am very worried that Duke may have bone cancer.

[pause]

Client: Cancer?

[pause]

Veterinarian: Yes … There is a specific type of bone cancer called osteosarcoma. It tends to prefer this location. It causes a great deal of destruction – and grows very quickly. If Duke has osteosarcoma, there is a chance that it has spread to other tissues. We need to expand our search. It is possible that it could have spread to the lungs. With your permission, I would like to take a few X-rays of his chest.

Client: And if it has spread?

Veterinarian: If it has spread, then there are limits to what we can do in terms of curing him. We would shift our focus onto doing what we can to keep him comfortable.

Note that this conversation is not easy to have, but the veterinarian is doing her part to be upfront. The client now has the opportunity to absorb the possibility of this diagnosis.

At the same time, the clinician was honest, without being cold or callous. The clinician was compassionate, without disguising the truth.

This is what we mean when we say that a situation calls for the use of compassionate transparency. Compassionate transparency means that we have no choice but to address the elephant in the room.

And so we face it. But we face it together.

18.7 Unconditional Positive Regard in Healthcare

Unconditional positive regard is a concept that was coined by Carl Rogers, a mental health expert.(23) Although it is referenced most often in the fields of psychiatry, social work, counseling, and psychology, unconditional positive regard can be ascribed to all human health professionals.

The practice of unconditional positive regard suggests that the clinician approaches each patient as an individual.(12) Patients are to be respected, rather than judged, and to be accepted for who they are rather than to be held to standards that are impossibly high to meet.(12)

Even patients that are "difficult" should not be labeled as such. Rather than focusing on good versus bad qualities, the clinician should focus on shared common ground:

what do both patient and provider wish to achieve and how can they work together to that end?(24)

Unconditional positive regard is challenging to demonstrate in clinical practice because judgment is a part of human nature. It is relatively easy for us to label people, including clients, or to judge them for their thoughts or actions.

It is especially difficult to demonstrate unconditional positive regard if the clinician is in disagreement with the patient. In such circumstances, it is important to remember that:

> Individual practitioners do not have to morally agree with an individual's behavior, nor should we avoid counseling for fear of intruding on individual values, but we must never view the individual as unworthy of conscientious care.(25)

18.8 Unconditional Positive Regard in Veterinary Medicine

Judgments about people and circumstances are not unique to human healthcare. The veterinary team often judges clients for their beliefs and actions.

Veterinary clients fear being judged. This fear may handicap them from participating in frank dialogue about patient care. They may worry about full disclosure, particularly if they feel that their actions will be disrespected, either to their face or behind closed doors.

Companion-animal owners want to be respected, rather than judged.(12) In particular, cat owners want us to understand that they have good intentions, even if in some cases their actions are inappropriate.(12)

One focus group participant in my 2015 study explained it best:

> Have you ever done something stupid with your cat and you've got to go tell the vet you did something stupid? [Good vets] don't look at you like you're crazy. They understand that we make mistakes.(12)

Another participant gave an example of dietary indiscretion to demonstrate the use of unconditional positive regard:

> [When] the cat [eats] a cardboard box and [swallows] it, [good vets] don't say, "why on earth did you let him eat the cardboard box?"(12)

Respect for the client as an individual appeared again and again in my focus group discussions.(12)

- "We're not just another person. Treat me as my own person."
- "Treat each person as an individual and cater to their needs."
- "Get to what our needs are."

Dog owners also want to be respected as individuals. However, they expect that respect to extend to the patient. One participant expressed this outright:

Respect my dog. Get on the floor with him if he's more comfortable.(12)

It matters to clients how they perceive themselves as being treated. It also matters to clients how they perceive their pets are being treated. Both perceptions impact their view of the veterinary profession and determine their level of satisfaction with the services provided.

Remember that respect is a two-way street. If veterinary clients feel respected, then they are more likely to respect the veterinary team. If veterinary clients feel disrespected, then they are more likely to disrespect us. One participant explained this simply: "When [the veterinarian] cuts me off, I'm not willing to listen to what he has to say."(12) Note that in order for our demonstration of unconditional positive regard to be effective, it has to be genuine.

Genuine use of unconditional positive regard has the potential to strengthen the veterinarian–client–patient relationship.(26) It also provides the client with a sense of autonomy.(26)

18.9 Veterinary Clinical Scenarios that Involve Unconditional Positive Regard

In companion-animal practice, unconditional positive regard may come in handy in the following circumstances.

* A client did not pursue veterinary care as soon as they ought to have.
* A client administered the wrong medication or the wrong dose of a medication, by accident.
* A client forgot to administer the right medication according to the instructions that you provided – and so the presenting complaint has not resolved.
* A client failed to return to your office for a recheck appointment, diagnostic testing, or for medication refills – and now the patient's condition has worsened.
* A client administered a medication without being instructed to, hoping that it would help
* A patient accidentally ingests an item at home that the client did not know was toxic.
* A patient is intentionally fed something at home that the client did not know was toxic.

Consider, for example, the client who mistakenly gives the cat Tylenol® (acetaminophen or paracetamol) because the cat was in pain and you did not offer emergency care overnight. Consider the client whose cat ingested lilies, and who didn't seek medical care right away because she did not know that lilies were nephrotoxic. Consider the client who accidentally ran over his dog, or the client who did not realize that his dog ingested antifreeze until it was too late.

All of these clients might be feeling different things when they present their pet to you. Guilt is a common denominator. They may also be angry at themselves. They may blame themselves for what happened, whether or not they were responsible.

Unconditional positive regard is not about letting them off the hook and rewarding bad behavior. It is about recognizing that they did what they could in the moment. It may not have helped. It may have even hurt the situation. But you understand *why* they did what they did. Or why they *did not*.

Unconditional positive regard also demonstrates that you are willing to move beyond these factors to deliver the care that the patient needs.

Unconditional positive regard statements may take the following forms.

- "You were only trying to help."
- "You did the best you could."
- "You did what anyone would have done in your shoes."
- "You did what you thought was best."
- "Of course, you didn't mean to …"
- "How would you have known …"
- "I could have done the same thing …"
- "I have done the same thing …"
- "It happens – let me work with you to make this better."

Let us take a look at how unconditional positive regard may appear in clinical practice.

Background

You are an associate veterinarian. Your client presents his 5-year-old cat for acute onset of vomiting.

When taking a history, you realize that the cat was given two 500 mg tablets of acetaminophen on Sunday afternoon because the cat came in from outside limping on his left pelvic limb. The clinic was closed, and the client didn't know what else to do. When he is in pain, he takes Tylenol®. He thought it would help his cat, too.

On physical exam, the patient is dehydrated and icteric. You are concerned about liver failure. The patient is also exceptionally tender at the cranial abdomen on superficial and deep palpation. You are concerned about stomach ulcers. You express this to the client. Let's take a look at how the client responds.

Clinical Conversation

Client: I'm so stupid, I should have waited before giving him anything. This is all my fault.

Veterinarian: It is true that Tylenol® didn't help the situation – but how could you have known?

Client: I should have asked you first.

Veterinarian: Hindsight is always 20/20. Before I went to vet school, I might have done

---

the exact same thing. The important thing is that you are here now.

[Pause]

Veterinarian: Let's work together to get to the bottom of his limping – and get his liver back up to health.

[Pause]

Veterinarian: It is going to be an uphill battle – but we're in this together. I know that you were only trying to help.

Client: Yes, I just didn't want him to hurt any more.

Veterinarian: Of course you didn't. I completely understand.

Some veterinarians worry that unconditional positive regard rewards bad behavior.

What I would say to my colleagues is that this is not about casting blame or letting anyone off the hook. It is about what we can do collectively as a team to get the patient back to health.

It is true that the client in the clinical vignette (above) needs to be engaged in a discussion, after the cat recovers, about what is and is not acceptable as pain relief. But in the moment, is it going to help to actively blame the client for an action that was well intentioned?

If we are to effectively manage the patient, then what we need most of all is for the client to be onboard. We need the client to feel understood and supported. We need the client to feel welcome as a member of the healthcare team, rather than penalized and put in "time out."

In order for us to actively accept our client, we need to put aside our differences and connect over how we will together move forward with patient care.

Unconditional positive regard is not easy. It may not always feel genuine. It may sometimes even feel forced. When it is, ask yourself: "If I were in the client's shoes, would I have done the same thing? Could I have ever imagined myself doing the same thing?"

If the answer is "Yes," then that alone is sufficient common ground for shared understanding.

Again, it does not mean that the client was *right*. It just means that you accept what they did or why they did it. Their heart was in the right place. At the end of the day, that has to count for something.

 Compassionate Transparency and Unconditional Positive Regard

References

1. Burt J, Abel G, Elmore N, Campbell J, Roland M, Benson J, et al. Assessing communication quality of consultations in primary care: initial reliability of the Global Consultation

Rating Scale, based on the Calgary–Cambridge Guide to the medical interview. BMJ Open. 2014;4(3):e004339.

2. Englar RE. A novel approach to simulation-based education for veterinary medical communication training over eight consecutive pre-clinical quarters. J Vet Med Educ.44(3):502–22.

3. Kurtz SM, Silverman JD, Draper J. Teaching and learning communication skills in medicine. Grand Rapids, MI: Radcliffe; 2004.

4. Shaw JR, Adams CL, Bonnett BN. What can veterinarians learn from studies of physician–patient communication about veterinarian–client–patient communication? J Am Vet Med Assoc. 2004;224(5):676–84.

5. Radford AD, Stockley P, Taylor IR, Turner R, Gaskell CJ, Kaney S, et al. Use of simulated clients in training veterinary undergraduates in communication skills. Vet Rec. 2003;152(14):422–7.

6. Chun R, Schaefer S, Lotta CC, Banning JA, Skochelak SE. Didactic and experiential training to teach communication skills: the University of Wisconsin-Madison School of Veterinary Medicine collaborative experience. J Vet Med Educ. 2009;36(2):196–201.

7. Rickles NM, Tieu P, Myers L, Galal S, Chung V. The impact of a standardized patient program on student learning of communication skills. Am J Pharm Educ. 2009;73(1):4.

8. Barrows HS. An overview of the uses of standardized patients for teaching and evaluating clinical skills. AAMC. Acad Med. 1993;68(6):443–51; discussion 51–3.

9. Englar RE. Using a standardized client encounter to practice death notification after the unexpected death of a feline patient following routine ovariohysterectomy. J Vet Med Educ. 2019:1–17.

10. Veterinary communication. Institute for Healthcare Communication (IHC); 2019 [Available from: https://healthcarecomm.org/veterinary-communication/.

11. Egnew TR, Mauksch LB, Greer T, Farber SJ. Integrating communication training into a required family medicine clerkship. Acad Med. 2004;79(8):737–43.

12. Englar RE, Williams M, Weingand K. Applicability of the Calgary–Cambridge Guide to dog and cat owners for teaching veterinary clinical communications. J Vet Med Educ. 2016;43(2):143–69.

13. Adams CL, Ladner LD. Implementing a simulated client program: bridging the gap between theory and practice. J Vet Med Educ. 2004;31(2):138–45.

14. Radford A, Stockley P, Silverman J, Taylor I, Turner R, Gray C. Development, teaching, and evaluation of a consultation structure model for use in veterinary education. J Vet Med Educ. 2006;33(1):38–44.

15. Coe JB, Adams CL, Bonnett BN. A focus group study of veterinarians' and pet owners' perceptions of the monetary aspects of veterinary care. J Am Vet Med Assoc. 2007;231(10):1510–8.

16. Coe JB, Adams CL, Bonnett BN. A focus group study of veterinarians' and pet owners' perceptions of veterinarian-client communication in companion animal practice. J Am Vet Med Assoc. 2008;233(7):1072–80.

17. Kohn LT, Corrigan JM, Donaldson MS, editors. Washington, DC: Institute of Medicine (US) Committee on Quality of Health Care in America; 2000.

18. Makoul G. Essential elements of communication in medical encounters: the Kalamazoo consensus statement. Acad Med. 2001;76(4):390–3.

19. Wachter R, Kaplan GS, Gandhi T, Leape L. You can't understand something you hide: transparency as a path to improve patient safety. Health Affairs Blog [Internet]. 2015. Available from: http://healthaffairs.org/blog/2015/06/22/you-cant-understand-something-you-hide-transparency-as-a-path-to-improve-patient-safety/.

20. Mellanby RJ, Herrtage ME. Survey of mistakes made by recent veterinary graduates. Vet Rec. 2004;155(24):761–5.

21. Bonvicini KA, O'Connell D, Cornell KK. Disclosing medical errors: restoring client trust. Compend Contin Educ Vet. 2009;31(3):E5.

22. Lewis HE. Building a transparent veterinary practice – with glass, open spaces, and values. DVM360 [Internet]. 2014. Available from: http://veterinaryhospitaldesign.dvm360.com/building-transparent-veterinary-practice-with-glass-open-spaces-and-values.

23. Amadi C. Clinician, society and suicide mountain: reading Rogerian doctrine of unconditional positive regard (UPR). Psychological Thought. 2013;6(1):75–89.

24. Gibson S. On judgment and judgmentalism: how counselling can make people better. J Med Ethics. 2005;31(10):575–7.

25. Larkin GL, Iserson K, Kassutto Z, Freas G, Delaney K, Krimm J, et al. Virtue in emergency medicine. Acad Emerg Med. 2009;16(1):51–5.

26. Patterson TG, Joseph S. Development of a self-report measure of unconditional positive self-regard. Psychol Psychother. 2006;79(Pt 4):557–70.

Part III

Applying Communication Skills to Everyday Conversations in Clinical Practice

Chapter 19

Using Communication Skills to Initiate the Consultation

Clinical consultations are the bread and butter of companion-animal practice. They establish professional relationships between the client and the veterinary team, both of whom come together for the sake of delivering medically sound, high-quality healthcare to the patient.

No two clients are alike, just as no two practitioners are alike, and each consultation is unique. Clinical conversations may overlap in terms of content. However, the people and the patients change. This means that each appointment represents an opportunity to forge new relationships or strengthen pre-existing ones. Additionally, clients' needs change. So, too, do those of our patients.

There is no cookie-cutter approach to the art of conversation as it pertains to the practice of medicine.

There are, however, strategies that facilitate conversational flow and improve connectivity between veterinary team members. The overriding strategy for this section of the text, Part III, takes the shape of the Calgary–Cambridge model.

Recall from Chapter 3 that the Calgary–Cambridge Referenced Observation Guides were outlined by Kurtz and Silverman in 1996 as a skills-based, patient-centered framework of the clinical consultation.(1–4)

Both Guides referenced previous work by Riccardi and Kurtz.(2, 5) The end product outlined the consultation as four sequential tasks:(2, 5)

* initiating the session
* gathering information
* explaining and planning
* closing the session.

Sandwiched in between 'gathering information' and 'explaining and planning' is the physical examination.(1, 3, 4)

Two additional tasks span all stages of the consultation:(1, 3, 4)

* building the relationship
* providing structure.

This model of the clinical consultation was adapted for use in veterinary medicine by Radford et al. in 2002.(6–8)

Note that each task requires the clinician to achieve specific objectives. The emphasis for this chapter is on the first task, initiating the session. Objectives for this task include:(4)

- preparation for the visit
- development of rapport with the patient
- identification of the presenting complaint.

19.1 Preparing for the Visit

Preparation for the visit is something that we are trained to do as veterinary students.

After graduation, when we acclimate to clinical practice and become more seasoned practitioners, we often downplay the importance of this step. Sometimes this is intentional: we may feel that we are adept at "winging it."

More often, this is less because of ego and more to do with case load. A busy day in the teaching hospital, for a student, involves tending to two or three patients, on average. Contrast that with a private practitioner, who may average three to four patients per hour, for 8 or more hours each day. She or he may visit with 24–32 patients a day, not including his or her responsibilities to those who are hospitalized.

In addition, veterinarians are often pressurized by time constraints and increasing demands – both self-imposed and by management – to "fit in" appointments to keep the customer, the veterinary client, happy. Additionally, veterinarians are faced with walk-in emergencies and/or overnight coverage. The result is that they often feel stretched thin.

Veterinarians may experience the same pressures that veterinary students do, only magnified. These pressures include:

- workload intensity
- content overload
- having to "cram" because there is too much to know and too little time.(9, 10)

All of the above contribute to anxiety, stress, fatigue, mental health concerns, fluctuations in weight, and/or altered sleeping patterns.(9, 11–14)

Compassion fatigue is a real phenomenon in clinical practice that occurs when providers become consumed with the pain of those in their care.(15–25) Repeated exposure to critically ill or otherwise injured patients may result in unchecked anxiety.(23, 26) Over time, the provider becomes numb as a means of self-protection.(23, 24)

If compassion fatigue is not addressed, it results in burnout.(22–25) A caregiver experiences burnout when s/he is unable to continue on in his/her current role due to mental, physical, and/or emotional exhaustion.(22–25) Environmental factors, such as time constraints and increased workload, accelerate the path to burnout.(25, 27)

To guard against mental health risks, we may be tempted to take shortcuts to trim the excess from our already overbooked days. We may feel that cutting out 5 minutes of prep work per case may, in the long run, be a time saver. We may feel that we no longer need to prepare for consultations because our experience and clinical acumen can carry us through.

In reality, preparation is essential.

19.1.1 Preparing Yourself for What Is to Come

First and foremost, preparation is a means of self-care. It allows you to tend to yourself and to consider your own needs. Ask yourself the following questions.

- What, if anything, do I need to do, for me, so that I am able to "turn off" the last task and focus all of my energy on the next?
- Do I need to take a breath?
- Do I need to stretch my back?
- Do I need a drink of water?
- Do I need to use the washroom?
- Do I need to jot down a few notes for myself about the last case so that my memory is jogged later?

This brief pause offers a moment of respite. At times, we have to "power through," but none of us can "power through" forever.

We all need that brief moment or two to gather our thoughts and to recharge. Only when we take that time can we fully invest in the next case. Only then can we truly get to know the client and patient as individuals, and serve them in the best way that we know how.

19.1.2 Preparing for the Next Case

After tending to yourself, take another moment to prepare for the case.

Preparation means something different to each and every practitioner. Sections 4.3 and 4.4 briefly touched upon the importance of being prepared for clinical practice. This section will afford greater detail.

When I engage in case prep, I take care to establish the following key pieces of information.

- The client's name:
  - Who will I be visiting with today?
  - Have I met this individual before?
- The patient's name and sex:

- ▪ Which dog or cat is presenting to me today?
- ▪ Is the patient a he or a she?

It matters to the client. Gender misidentification does not create a favorable first impression. Clients do not appreciate when you reference their beloved pet using the wrong pronoun.

- • The presenting or chief complaint (cc):
    - ▪ Why is the patient being examined today?
    - ▪ What is the purpose of the visit?
    - ▪ Is there more than one issue to resolve?

Recognize that the presenting complaint provides you with a starting point, but take it with a grain of salt.

The presenting complaint may have changed since the appointment was scheduled. Maybe the patient was exhibiting left pelvic limb lameness last week, when the client telephoned, but today the patient is exhibiting lameness of the right front limb. Maybe the complaint indicates that the patient is vomiting, however, the patient is now exhibiting diarrhea.

Maybe the presenting complaint is not at all helpful. In the United States, ill patients often present for ADR – "ain't doing right." Customer service representatives often list this in the appointment ledger, without additional details. All this tells you is that the patient is ill; it fails to elucidate how or why that may be so.

- • Past pertinent health history, if known:
    - ▪ Does the patient have pre-existing disease?
    - ▪ Is the pre-existing disease well managed?
    - ▪ What, if anything, is the patient taking by way of medication to manage this condition?
    - ▪ Could the patient's condition have worsened? If so, in what way? What might you on the lookout for?
- • Past pertinent diagnostic test results, if known:
    - ▪ Does the patient have abnormal values on bloodwork, urinalysis, fecal analysis, etc.?
    - ▪ Was the cause of the abnormal labwork ever identified?
    - ▪ Are the abnormalities expected to normalize?
    - ▪ Are the abnormalities expected to worsen?

Case preparation does not provide you with all the answers, nor is it intended to. Instead, case preparation helps you to anticipate who you are about to meet, and what you may be walking into when you enter the next consultation room.

Case preparation provides focus. Like blinders for horses, they help to narrow our attention to the case at hand and to minimize outside distractions.

As a student or new graduate, you may never feel 100% ready for the consultation. This is normal. However, the more you can commit to prep work, the less your jitters will get the best of you.

You will also enter into the consultation room with greater confidence. The practice of veterinary medicine is much like detective work, and preparation gives you your very first clues.

19.2 Developing Rapport

Relationship building begins from the very first moment you enter a consultation room. (28–31) Your entry and how you conduct yourself creates a lasting first impression. Your goal is to make your first impression a good one.

The importance of appropriate and effective nonverbal communication cannot be overstated. What we might consider to be inconsequential, our client may value immensely. Refer to Chapter 7 for a greater understanding of effective versus ineffective nonverbal cues.

Clients also appreciate the so-called "personal touches" of healthcare, and equate it with having a good "bedside manner".(32) Recall from Chapter 4 that greeting the client involves much more than just saying, "hi."

A proper greeting in western culture incorporates the following gestures:(4, 28, 30, 33–41)

- eye contact
- welcome statement
- handshake
- acknowledgement of the patient by name
- introduction of self and role
- acknowledgement of anyone else in the exam room
  - introduction of support staff and their role
  - recognition of the patient's support network, and understanding their relationship to the patient
- non-medical inquiries or "small talk."

Review Sections 4.5 and 4.6 to develop familiarity with patient/client preferences concerning the greeting stage of the clinical consultation.

19.3 Identifying the Presenting Complaint

Once you have made your introductions and properly greeted the veterinary client, it is essential for you to establish the reason for the consultation.(4)

To establish the presenting complaint, you can make use of any of the communication skills that you were introduced to in Part 2 of the text. However, I find the following three communication skills to be particularly helpful as you go about this task:

1. eliciting the client's perspective (for a summary of this skill, refer to Chapter 11)
2. open-ended questions (for a summary of this skill, refer to Chapter 8)
3. reflective listening (for a summary of this skill, refer to Chapter 5).

In addition, five further communication skills are nice add-ons. As such, I consider their use to be supplemental:

4. assessing the client's knowledge (for a summary of this skill, refer to Chapter 13)
5. checking in (for a summary of this skill, refer to Chapter 15)
6. asking for permission (for a summary of this skill, refer to Chapter 12)
7. signposting (for a summary of this skill, refer to Chapter 14)
8. partnership (for a summary of this skill, refer to Chapter 10).

19.3.1 Identifying the Presenting Complaint(s) in a Wellness Appointment

Let us see how these three skills might come together by exploring a clinical vignette in which an apparently health patient presents for examination. For the purpose of this example, assume that introductions between veterinarian and client have already been made.

Background

A new client, Mr. Engles, presents his recently purchased, 12-week-old, spayed female British shorthair kitten, "Bliss," to your clinic.

Clinical Conversation

Veterinarian: Now that I've met you both – Bliss is lovely, by the way – how can I be of service to you today? **eliciting the clients perspective / open-ended question**

Client: The contract that I signed with the breeder requires me to get her checked out within the first week of purchase. I brought her home with me last Saturday. I haven't noticed any signs of illness, but I do have a few questions about whether or not some of her behaviors are normal.

Veterinarian: Tell me more about that. **open-ended statement**

Client: For the most part, Bliss is quite gentle. She doesn't like to be picked up, but she will sit beside me while I'm typing at the keyboard and ever so softly tap my arm, with her paw, as if to tell me that I need to pay her attention. That part about her, I like very much. The problem is when I am getting up from the couch. She likes to hide under there. When I start to walk away, she has twice now come sprinting out from under the couch, wrapped her paws around my legs, and bitten down as hard as she could.

Its like she's out of her mind when she does this. I yelled ouch! but that doesn't seem to deter her!

Veterinarian: It sounds like she is settling in well other than these two episodes that have you concerned? **reflective listening**

Client: Yes, that's right. What could that be?

Veterinarian: It sounds to me like something we call play aggression. Have you heard of this before? **assessing the clients knowledge**

Client: [Shaking head to indicate no]

Veterinarian: This is very normal in kittens that are around her age. At her age, she is learning key lessons through play about hunting. She's figuring out her coordination, balance, and accuracy, all of which would be essential if she were going to be a mouser. Does that make sense? **check-in**

Client: Yes.

Veterinarian: Well, unfortunately, she thinks of you as a littermate, and littermates can play rough at times. As my Dad used to say with any type of play, sometimes laughing turns to crying. We need to teach Bliss that her teeth on your skin means no more play. Are you open to hearing more about what that might look like in your home environment? **asking for permission**

Client: Sure.

Veterinarian: Before we discuss ways to modify her behavior, is there anything else that you would like to discuss today? **eliciting the clients perspective**

Client: I am a bit confused about which vaccines she needs and when.

Veterinarian: Great, let's take a look at her schedule and come up with a plan that will work for all of us. **partnership**

Note that agenda-setting was successful: the clinician was able to establish the presenting complaints.(41–43)

Through an open-ended question that elicited the client's perspective, the veterinarian was able to establish that the kitten was here for a new patient check-up, as was required by the contract that he signed with the breeder. Because the clinician did not interrupt the client's opening statement, the client was able to share his concern about a behavioral issue at home.

Also, the clinician did not assume that the client had only a single concern. Instead, she took a moment to elicit the client's perspective for a second time, when she asked, "Is there anything else that you would like to discuss?" Because of this follow-up question, the client was also able to express interest in discussing vaccinations today.

Follow-up questions play an important role in agenda-setting because most patients have more than one concern to share.(42, 44–48)

19.3.2 Identifying the Presenting Complaint(s) at a Sick Visit

Let us now take a look at how these same communication skills might be of use when an ill patient presents for examination. In addition to the communication skills that were useful in wellness appointments, empathy is a valuable add-on skill when patients present to us with an illness. As was true of the last example, for the purpose of this vignette, please assume that introductions between veterinarian and client have already been made.

Background

A new client, Mr. Gregory, presents his 12-year-old, castrated male Miniature Poodle, "Wicket," to be evaluated for acute onset of unsteadiness.

Clinical Conversation

Veterinarian: I understand from what my technician has shared with me that Wicket suddenly seems to be losing his balance. `reflective listening`

Client: [affirmative head nod to indicate, yes]

Veterinarian: Can you tell me more about that? `open-ended question / eliciting the client's perspective`

Client: Two days ago, I came home from work to find Wicket splay-legged on the floor. When he saw me, he struggled to get up, but it was like he couldn't get his bearings. When I finally helped him up, he could stand, but he seemed to be leaning to one side and shaking. Maybe he was dizzy? He would take a few steps and stumble, take another few steps and stumble. He seemed aware of what was going on, but unable to regain his footwork.

Veterinarian: That must have been really scary for you to see. `empathy`

Client: At first I thought he was having a seizure, but then I realized that, no, that wasn't it. It's almost like he has vertigo.

Veterinarian: It's true that dogs can develop symptoms that look just like vertigo. In fact, what you're describing makes me think about a condition called vestibular syndrome, which we tend to see in older patients like Wicket. Have you ever heard of that condition? `assessing the client's knowledge`

Client: No, that sounds really complicated. ·

Veterinarian: Would it be alright for me to share a little bit about what that condition is, in dogs? `asking permission`

Client: Absolutely, especially if that's something you think he could have.

Veterinarian: Yes, it's a good possibility, based upon your description of what you saw. We don't fully understand what causes vestibular syndrome, but when it occurs in the form that I am most familiar with, patients become uncoordinated and severely

---

off-balance. Sometimes this causes them to fall over, like Wicket. Sometimes they lean to one side when they stand up. Other times they circle, or even roll to one side. Does that make sense? **check-in**

Client: [affirmative head nod, confirming yes]

Veterinarian: Many dogs have a head tilt. Have you noticed that with Wicket? **eliciting the client's perspective**

Client: Now that you mention it, yeah, he did seem to look at me funny, like his head was cocked to the right. In fact, sometimes I think he's still doing it.

Veterinarian: Yes, you're right. I also notice a right-sided head tilt as I stand here watching him.

[pause]

Veterinarian: Sometimes dogs with vestibular syndrome also get nauseous. Have you noticed any changes to his appetite or has he vomited at all? **eliciting the client's perspective**

Client: Now that you mention it, yes, he's a bit sluggish to eat. I almost have to coax him to, but he's kept it all down.

Veterinarian: That's very good to hear. I'm going to take a look at him shortly, but first I would like to ask one more question. **signposting**

Veterinarian: It sounds like you're very concerned about Wicket's balance. **reflective listening**

Veterinarian: Is there anything else, other than his coordination, that is weighing on your mind today? **eliciting the client's perspective**

Client: I really just don't want him to suffer. Is he in any pain?

Veterinarian: I don't believe he is, he's probably just more confused than anything else. But I will take a look just now and that will help me to answer you more definitively. **signposting**

Veterinarian: How does that sound? **check-in**

Client: That would make me feel a lot better, thank you.

Veterinarian: You're welcome, we are a team. **partnership**

When a patient presents with illness, particularly when the reason for illness is unknown, clients may experience any number of emotions. Emotions often run high and may include:

- stress
- confusion
- fear
- sadness
- worry

- frustration
- anger.

Although our primary purpose is to deliver high-quality medical care, we are reliant upon the client to agree to diagnostic and/or treatment recommendations. We also must rely heavily on the client for insight into the patient's presentation and the impact that it has on him or her.

We are not mind readers. We can speculate about a patient's history, but we do not know for sure what the client saw or what the client is presently experiencing.

If we are to effectively move forward with case management, then we need to start with an open-ended inquiry.

- "What brings you here today?"
- "How can I help?"

That inquiry is incomplete unless there is follow-up.

- "Is there anything else on your mind?"
- "Are there any other concerns that you have about …"
- "Is anything else going on with your dog at home that I should know about?"
- "Do you have any other concerns to share with me today?"

Sharing concerns between members of the veterinary team is a valuable part of relationship building and case management. When the client is given the freedom to share, she or he is more likely to focus on what we have to say. The efficiency of the consultation improves.(42)

The veterinarian is also able to consider a complete clinical picture. Now she or he can prioritize problems and address those that require immediate attention.(42)

References

1. Denness C. What are consultation models for? InnovAiT. 2013;6(9):592–9.
2. Kurtz SM, Silverman JD. The Calgary–Cambridge Referenced Observation Guides: an aid to defining the curriculum and organizing the teaching in communication training programmes. Med Educ. 1996;30(2):83–9.
3. Kurtz S. Teaching and learning communication in veterinary medicine. J Vet Med Educ. 2006;33(1):11–9.
4. Silverman J, Kurtz S, Draper J. Skills for communicating with patients. Oxford: Radcliffe Medical Press; 2008.
5. Riccardi VM, Kurtz SM. Communication and counselling in health care. Springfield, IL: Charles C. Thomas; 1983.
6. Englar RE, Williams M, Weingand K. Applicability of the Calgary–Cambridge Guide to dog and cat owners for teaching veterinary clinical communications. J Vet Med Educ. 2016;43(2):143–69.

7. Adams CL, Ladner LD. Implementing a simulated client program: bridging the gap between theory and practice. J Vet Med Educ. 2004;31(2):138–45.

8. Radford A, Stockley P, Silverman J, Taylor I, Turner R, Gray C. Development, teaching, and evaluation of a consultation structure model for use in veterinary education. J Vet Med Educ. 2006;33(1):38–44.

9. Pelzer JM, Hodgson JL, Werre SR. Veterinary students' perceptions of their learning environment as measured by the Dundee Ready Education Environment Measure. BMC Res Notes. 2014;7:170.

10. Sutton RC. Veterinary students and their reported academic and personal experiences during the first year of veterinary school. J Vet Med Educ. 2007;34(5):645–51.

11. Jackson EL, Armitage-Chan E. The challenges and issues of undergraduate student retention and attainment in UK veterinary medical education. J Vet Med Educ. 2017;44(2):247–59.

12. Ryan MT, Irwin JA, Bannon FJ, Mulholland CW, Baird AW. Observations of veterinary medicine students' approaches to study in pre-clinical years. J Vet Med Educ. 2004;31(3):242–54.

13. Hafen M, Jr., Reisbig AM, White MB, Rush BR. Predictors of depression and anxiety in first-year veterinary students: a preliminary report. J Vet Med Educ. 2006;33(3):432–40.

14. Kogan LR, McConnell SL, Schoenfeld-Tacher R. Veterinary students and non-academic stressors. J Vet Med Educ. 2005;32(2):193–200.

15. Manifold S. Minimizing the impact of euthanasia on veterinary teams. Veterinary Team Brief. 2017(April):49–52.

16. Sanders CR. Killing with kindness – veterinary euthanasia and the social construction of personhood. Sociol Forum. 1995;10(2):195–214.

17. Morris P. Blue juice: euthanasia in veterinary medicine. Philadelphia, PA: Temple University Press; 2012.

18. Yeates JW, Main DC. Veterinary opinions on refusing euthanasia: justifications and philosophical frameworks. Vet Rec. 2011;168(10):263.

19. Mitchener KL, Ogilvie GK. Understanding compassion fatigue: keys for the caring veterinary healthcare team. J Am Anim Hosp Assoc. 2002;38(4):307–10.

20. Rank MG, Zaparanick TL, Gentry JE. Nonhuman-animal care compassion fatigue: training as treatment. Best Pract Ment Health. 2009;38(4):307–10.

21. Shaw JR, Lagoni L. End-of-life communication in veterinary medicine: delivering bad news and euthanasia decision making. Vet Clin N Am - Small. 2007;37(1):95–108; abstract viii-ix.

22. McArthur M, Mansfield C, Matthew S, Zaki S, Brand C, Andrews J, et al. Resilience in veterinary students and the predictive role of mindfulness and self-compassion. J Vet Med Educ.44(1):106–15.

23. Lloyd C, Campion DP. Occupational stress and the importance of self-care and resilience: focus on veterinary nursing. Ir Vet J. 2017;70:30.

24. Hunsaker S, Chen HC, Maughan D, Heaston S. Factors that influence the development of compassion fatigue, burnout, and compassion satisfaction in emergency department nurses. J Nurs Scholarsh. 2015;47(2):186–94.

25. Wu S, Singh-Carlson S, Odell A, Reynolds G, Su Y. Compassion fatigue, burnout, and compassion satisfaction among oncology nurses in the United States and Canada. Oncol Nurs Forum. 2016;43(4):E161–9.

26. Figley CR. Compassion fatigue: psychotherapists' chronic lack of self care. J Clin Psychol. 2002;58(11):1433–41.

27. Perry B, Toffner G, Merrick T, Dalton J. An exploration of the experience of compassion fatigue in clinical oncology nurses. Can Oncol Nurs J. 2011;21(2):91–105.

28. Frankel RM, Stein T. Getting the most out of the clinical encounter: the four habits model. The Permanente Journal. 1999;3(3):79–88.
29. Manning P. Veterinary consultations: the value of reflection. In Practice. 2008;January:47–9.
30. Ranjan P. How can doctors improve their communication skills? JCDR. 2015;9(3):1–4.
31. Corsan JR, Mackay AR. The veterinary receptionist: essential skills for client care. China: Elsevier, Ltd; 2008.
32. Goldstein SA, Burkgren T. Client relations. IA State Univ Vet. 1993;55(2):75–7.
33. Makoul G, Zick A, Green M. An evidence-based perspective on greetings in medical encounters. Arch Intern Med. 2007;167(11):1172–6.
34. Thompson TL. The initial interaction between the patient and the health professional: communication for health professionals. Lanham, MD: Harper & Row Publishers, Inc.; 1986.
35. Zeldow PB, Makoul G. Communicating with patients. In: Wedding D, Stuber ML, editors. Behavior & medicine. Cambridge, MA: Hogrefe & Huber Publishers; 2006. pp. 201–18.
36. Lipkin M, Frankel RM. Performing the interview. In: Lipkin M, Putnam SM, Lazare A, editors. The medical interview: clinical care, education, and research. New York: Springer-Verlag NY Inc.; 1995. pp. 65–82.
37. Coulehan JL, Block MR. The medical interview: mastering skills for clinical practice. Philadelphia, PA: FA Davis Co Publishers; 1997.
38. Makoul G. The SEGUE Framework for teaching and assessing communication skills. Patient Educ Couns. 2001;45:23–34.
39. Billings JA, Stoeckle JD. The clinical encounter: a guide to the medical interview and case presentation. St. Louis, MO: Mosby Year Book Inc.; 1999.
40. Lloyd M, Bor R. Communication skills for medicine. New York: Churchill Livingstone, Inc.; 1996.
41. Smith RC. The patient's story: integrated patient–doctor interviewing. Boston, MA: Little Brown & Co. Inc.; 1996.
42. Marvel MK, Epstein RM, Flowers K, Beckman HB. Soliciting the patient's agenda: have we improved? JAMA. 1999;281(3):283–7.
43. Beckman HB, Frankel RM. The effect of physician behavior on the collection of data. Ann Intern Med. 1984;101(5):692–6.
44. Robinson JD, Tate A, Heritage J. Agenda-setting revisited: when and how do primary-care physicians solicit patients' additional concerns? Patient Educ Couns. 2016;99(5):718–23.
45. Braddock CH, 3rd, Edwards KA, Hasenberg NM, Laidley TL, Levinson W. Informed decision making in outpatient practice: time to get back to basics. JAMA. 1999;282(24):2313–20.
46. Heritage J, Robinson JD, Elliott MN, Beckett M, Wilkes M. Reducing patients' unmet concerns in primary care: the difference one word can make. J Gen Intern Med. 2007;22(10):1429–33.
47. Middleton JF, McKinley RK, Gillies CL. Effect of patient completed agenda forms and doctors' education about the agenda on the outcome of consultations: randomized controlled trial. BMJ. 2006;332(7552):1238–42.
48. Rost K, Frankel R. The introduction of the older patient's problems in the medical visit. J Aging Health. 1993;5(3):387–401.

Chapter 20

Using Communication Skills to Gather Data

History Taking

According to the Calgary–Cambridge model, a clinician must complete four sequential tasks during a consultation: (1–8)

* initiating the session
* gathering information
* explaining and planning
* closing the session.

The physical examination traditionally takes place between the second and third task.(1, 3, 4) However, as clinicians gain experience, they learn to multitask. That is, they may take a patient history during the physical examination to be efficient.

Recall that two additional tasks span all stages of the consultation:(1, 3, 4)

* building the relationship
* providing structure.

Chapter 19 outlined how communication skills can be utilized to successfully complete the first task, initiating the session. This chapter will continue where the last left off. After the clinician has established the reason(s) for the consultation, it is his or her responsibility to take a comprehensive patient history.

Recall from Chapter 8 that history taking serves many purposes, not the least of which is to paint a complete clinical picture. The history in and of itself is a valuable tool in the day-to-day detective work of clinical practice. It alone can lead to the correct diagnosis in 60–80% of cases in human healthcare.(9–14)

However, the history is also an opportunity for relationship building. When the clinician invites the client to share his or her experience with the veterinary team, the client feels respected and bonded to the team in partnership. The client is also able to share what is going on, in his or her own words, and why it is concerning.(15–19)

The client may not always know which information is relevant to case management or which information is most useful. The burden falls upon the clinician to ask the right questions in the right way. It is the clinician's role to navigate the patient profile and direct the flow of conversation in a way that is time efficient, yet relationship centered.

The clinician may redirect the flow, as necessary, but should refrain from interrupting the client. Interruptions may inhibit the client from answering subsequent questions thoroughly or honestly.(16) If clients truncate their answers, then the anamnesis is likely to be incomplete.

All new patient histories should be thorough, barring an emergency presentation, in which case patient stabilization takes precedence. Relevant topics for new patient histories include:(20–24)

- signalment
- patient acquisition history
- the client's expectations for the visit
- the client's expectations for the patient
- the patient's lifestyle
- activity level
- travel history
- serological status
- diet history
- current medications and supplements
- past pertinent history (PPHx)
- past pertinent diagnostic tests and test results
- past pertinent therapeutic trials and outcomes.

For more information, refer to Section 8.1.

Gathering this level of detail requires efficiency and finesse, as well as an appropriate balance of open- and closed-ended questions. Recall the difference between these two lines of questioning.(15)

- Closed-ended questions elicit an abbreviated response:(25)
  - confirmation: yes/no
  - numerical answer: 1, 2, 3, and so on.
- Open-ended questions and statements invite clients to share their story in greater detail:(6)
  - clients have the freedom to expand upon their answers
  - a two-way dialogue is encouraged.

Both types of questions have a place in the consultation, which can be structured to mirror the shape of a funnel.(4, 25, 26) Open-ended questions are good starting points because they allow clients to share what is on their minds (wide open mouth of the funnel). Follow-up questions are often closed-ended for the purpose of clarification or to provide key details (getting narrower to the stem). This means that we must consider how to phrase our questions so that we obtain the information we need without obstructing the flow of conversation and without alienating our clients.

To take an appropriate history, you can make use of any of the communication skills that you were introduced to in Part 2 of the text. However, in addition to open-ended questions, I find the following three communication skills to be particularly helpful as you go about this task:

1. eliciting the client's perspective (for a summary of this skill, refer to Chapter 11)
2. reflective listening (for a summary of this skill, refer to Chapter 5)
3. summarizing (for a summary of this skill, refer to Chapter 15).

In addition, six further communication skills may augment the flow of conversation:

4. asking for Permission (for a summary of this skill, refer to Chapter 12)
5. signposting (for a summary of this skill, refer to Chapter 14)
6. partnership (for a summary of this skill, refer to Chapter 10)
7. assessing the client's knowledge (for a summary of this skill, refer to Chapter 13)
8. replacing medical jargon with easy-to-understand language (for a summary of this skill, refer to Chapter 9)
9. chunking and checking in (for a summary of this skill, refer to Chapter 15).

20.1 Taking a Complete History at a Wellness Appointment

Let us see how these three skills might come together by exploring a clinical vignette in which an apparently health patient presents for examination. For the purpose of this example, please assume that introductions between the veterinarian and client have already been made, and the reason for the consultation (annual check-up, with or without vaccination boosters) has been established.

Background

A new client, Ms. Skye, presents her recently adopted 10-week-old, spayed female domestic longhaired (DLH) kitten, "Aura," to your clinic.

Clinical Conversation

Veterinarian: I am excited to hear all about your new arrival. Tell me how it was that Aura came to join your household. **open-ended statement**

Client: I didn't expect to fall in love with her. To be honest, I'm not exactly what you'd call a "cat person." I grew up with dogs underfoot. I haven't had a pet since I moved

---

away from home. Truthfully, she was an unexpected surprise.

Veterinarian: Cats have a way of doing that, don't they?

[Both share a laugh]

Veterinarian: Tell me more about where you found her. (open-ended statement)

Client: I am a junior high science teacher. We were visiting the shelter last week as part of outreach for our school. We try to get students involved with the community and to make connections for volunteer opportunities. I agreed to chaperone the trip to the shelter. During our tour of the facility, Aura kept on coming up to the cage front and extending a paw out to tap me. She made it very clear she wanted out. I made the mistake of opening the cage door. Once she jumped into my arms, she never left.

Veterinarian: It sounds like she knew exactly who to target. Smart girl! (reflective listening)

[Pause]

Veterinarian: Before I take a look at her today, I'd like to ask you some questions about her general health and her home environment. Would that be okay with you? (sign-posting / asking permission)

Client: Absolutely. It's been forever since I've owned a pet and I've never owned a cat before so I want to be sure that I'm not missing anything that I should be doing.

Veterinarian: You're in for a real treat, being a new cat owner. We can work together to get you up to speed so that you do not miss out on key aspects of kitten care. (reflective listening / partnership)

Client: Thank you so much.

Veterinarian: My pleasure.

[Pause]

Veterinarian: Let's start out by chatting about Aura's new life with you. Can you tell me a little bit about how she has settled into her new home? (open-ended question)

Client: She's been really easy. She came to me litter-trained, so I haven't had to worry about that. I found a clumpable litter that I really like that doesn't have any fragrances. I scoop it twice a day and so far, so good. She's been pooping and peeing normally. I haven't seen any diarrhea. She's also eating the same food that the shelter fed her – they gave me a small bag to get her started. I can't remember the name – but it's a yellow bag, with X and O shaped kibble. She eats whenever she wants. She doesn't overeat. She seems to snack throughout the day, so I just leave the bowl out. I've seen her drink some, but not a lot. She isn't really grooming herself, but maybe her mom never taught her how?

Veterinarian: Yes, it's possible that she was separated from her mom before she developed those life skills. Some cats also care a lot more about their appearance than others, just like people! We can talk about getting her used to grooming – brushing her and nail care – if that is something you are interested in. **reflective listening / eliciting the client's perspective**

Client: For sure, those nails are like needles! They are shark tooth sharp!

Veterinarian: I know exactly what you mean! She's practically climbing up my jacket now! In that case, I'll introduce you to our technician at the end of today's visit so that she can get you started on basic cat care. How does that sound to you? **signposting / eliciting the client's perspective**

Client: That would be great.

Veterinarian: You've given me a lot of great information about her eating and elimination habits. What about her lifestyle? Are you planning on keeping her indoors? **closed-ended question**

Client: Yes. I live by a busy intersection. I don't want to risk her getting hit by a car.

Veterinarian: I understand.

[pause]

Veterinarian: Did the shelter give you a record of her shots or any of her other health history? **closed-ended question**

Client: Thank you, yes, I knew I forgot something.

[Client fumbles in her purse before finding a folded-up piece of paper that she then hands over]

Client: Here it is. They said that it lists her shots and dewormer. Does that mean she had worms?

[Veterinarian reviews chart]

Veterinarian: It does look like she had roundworms, yes. **reflective listening**

Veterinarian: Have you heard of roundworms before? **assessing the client's knowledge**

Client: Uck, no! Is that something that I can catch?

Veterinarian: Yes, roundworms are something that we can catch. **reflective listening**

Veterinarian: But the good news is that they can be prevented, by washing your hands well after scooping her litter, and she has been given the proper medication by the shelter. Sometimes it takes a couple of doses to clear the infection entirely. I suggest that you bring in a stool sample so that we can make sure that the roundworms have cleared up. Is that something you would be interested in? **check-in / eliciting perspective**

Client: Yes, I don't like the idea of worms.

Veterinarian: Neither do I.

Veterinarian: Coming back to Aura's medical records, I see here that she tested negative for feline leukemia and for feline immunodeficiency virus! Did they share that with you? **eliciting perspective**

Client: Yes, that's a good thing, right?

Veterinarian: Yes, very good. Are you familiar with those two viruses? (assessing knowledge)

Client: I think both cause immune problems, right? And they are transmitted cat-to-cat?

Veterinarian: Yes, that's right. Because Aura tested negative, we do not have to worry that she has either disease.

Veterinarian: I also see here that when she was first brought to the shelter, Aura had a snotty nose and an eye infection. Both were treated with antibiotics. Have you noticed anything since? (closed-ended question)

Client: Nope, they warned me about it and said that a lot of kittens come to them already exposed to a virus – herpes, I think? If she has that, then she is prone to it coming back. But so far, no – no sneezing, no goopy eyes.

Veterinarian: You're absolutely right, many kittens have been exposed to and infected with herpesvirus. (reflective listening)

Veterinarian: If it's alright with you, may I share what to look out for? (asking permission)

Client: Yes, please.

Veterinarian: You'll want to look for green/yellow discharge from her nose or eyes, and let me know if ever she sounds congested. Sometimes the eye discharge makes them squint.

Client: Got it, thanks.

Veterinarian: No problem.

Veterinarian: Based upon Aura's medical records, it also looks like she's already on the right track in terms of her shots: she received her first vaccine for FVRCP two weeks ago. How familiar are you with the vaccines that kittens get? (assessing the client's knowledge)

Client: Not really, I just remember getting a parvo shot for my dogs way back when.

Veterinarian: That's great because kittens also get their own version of the parvo shot. Parvo in cats looks a little bit different than in dogs. Cats can still get diarrhea, just like dogs, but in addition, cat parvo causes something called panleukopenia. Would you like to know more about that? (eliciting the client's perspective?)

Client: Yes, please.

Veterinarian: Panleukopenia is a condition that makes cats, especially kittens, very sick. They become anemic – so they don't have as many red blood cells as they should. This makes them very weak. Their white blood cells are also suppressed, so that they cannot fight off infections properly. Does that make sense? (easy-to-understand language / check-in)

Client: I think so, yes.

Veterinarian: The FVRCP vaccine protects against this. It also protects against common viruses, like calicivirus, that can cause upper respiratory and eye infections. (chunk)

[Pause ← (silent check-in)]

Client: Oh, that makes sense.

Veterinarian: Aura received her first FVRCP vaccine two weeks ago, which means that it is too early to give her a booster. She is not due for another booster for another 1–2 weeks. She will then need a third booster about a month later to give her the best protection possible, ok? **check-in**

Client: [affirmative head nod]

Veterinarian: We'll also want to protect her against rabies when she's old enough, but that's something we can discuss next time, if that's alright with you? **signposting / check-in**

Client: Yep, that works.

Veterinarian: Okay, great! I think that covers all of the main points that I had hoped to before taking a look at Aura. To be sure that I am not missing anything, let me just recap for a moment. **chunk / signposting about summarizing**

Veterinarian: You adopted Aura last week. Other than a history of a cold and eye infection, both of which were medically managed before you met her, she's been the picture of perfect health. She's negative for feline leukemia and FIV. She's the only pet. She's going to remain indoor-only. And she is eating, drinking, and using the litterbox well? **summarizing / check-in**

Client: Yes, you've got it right.

Veterinarian: In that case, let's take a look at Miss Aura. Then we can chat more about what her healthcare needs are, moving forward. How does that sound to you? **signposting / check-in / eliciting perspective**

Client: Sounds great.

Consider the completeness of history taking in the example above. The following content areas were explored, with the assistance of a wide selection of communication skills:

- patient acquisition: where (shelter) and when (last week)
- client's past experience with pet ownership (some, but not recent)
- client's past experience with cat ownership (none)
- client's intentions (companion animal; single-pet household)
- client's interest in being educated concerning basic kitten care, including nail trims
- patient lifestyle (indoor-only)
- litter type (clumpable and fragrance-free) and use (no issues)
- litter maintenance (client scoops twice/day)
- bowel movements (normal consistency, no diarrhea)
- voiding history (urinating okay)
- dietary history (commercial dry food diet, fed ad libitum; brand unknown, but provided by shelter)
- thirst (drinking some water, but "not a lot")
- grooming history (kitten is not really attending to hygiene)
- serological status (negative for FeLV/FIV)
- vaccine history (needs additional FVRCP boosters and a rabies vaccination when she is of age)

- deworming history (history of roundworms; dewormed once; need to repeat fecal analysis)
- past pertinent medical history (previous upper respiratory infection and eye infection; resolved with antibiotic therapy)
- latency reactivation and recrudescence of herpesvirus, including which clinical signs to keep an eye out for.

By investing in about 5 minutes of conversation, the veterinarian gained a great deal of useful information. The client was able to share freely because open-ended questions were used to lead off the consultation. When additional details were required, the clinician asked specific closed-ended questions to gain clarification. Although there was, by necessity, a lot of talking on the part of the veterinarian, she or he did not dominate the conversation. The consultation was effectively broken up into segments by opportunity areas for the client to participate in dialogue. Ultimately, the client was able to weigh in on several important issues. The client also is left with a very clear understanding of what the veterinarian is hoping to achieve today, and in what order.

On paper, this dialogue may seem a bit stilted. It is true that it can be difficult to capture the nuances of clinical conversations in writing, when they are best explored by doing, and through observation.

However, recognize that as you begin to learn the communication skills and practice them, you will discover your own way of phrasing that makes the consultation uniquely yours. As you figure out which skills comes naturally and how to express them, you will feel increasingly comfortable navigating the flow of conversation. In that way, you will evolve into the doctor that you were meant to be.

Each and every one of us brings a great many strengths to the table. Each and every one of us carries our own weaknesses, too. Clinical communication is not about forcing everyone to sound like a carbon copy of each other. It is about finding your own way in a field that needs diversity in every sense of the word.

20.2 Taking a Complete History at a Sick Visit

Let us now take a look at how these same communication skills might be of use when you need to gather history about a patient that is unwell.

In addition to the communication skills that were useful during history taking in wellness appointments, empathy and unconditional positive regard are valuable supplemental skills when patients present to us with an illness.

As was true of the last example, for the purpose of this vignette, please assume that introductions between veterinarian and client have already been made, and the reason for the consultation (emesis) has been established.

Background

Ms. Cohen presents her 6-year-old, female spayed Burmese cat, Tigris, to you for acute onset of vomiting. Tigris belongs to a single-cat household; Ms. Cohen is the only person with whom she resides.

Ms. Cohen is a regular customer; you have known her and Tigris since Tigris was 12-weeks-old. You're very familiar with her lifestyle (indoor-only), her home environment, her biomedical data (FeLV/FIV negative), and her prescription history (topical Revolution® once/month).

Your history will primarily focus on a description of her presenting complaint as well as checking in to see if anything else at home has changed that might account for the vomiting.

Clinical Conversation

Veterinarian: It sounds like Tigris' recent bout of vomiting came about all of a sudden and it is unusual for her because she's never vomited once since the day you brought her home. Is that right? `reflective listening / check-in`

Client: Yes, that's right, she's never even thrown up a hairball. I am so worried. She's my baby, and seeing her so sick makes me feel so helpless.

Veterinarian: I can see how much you care about her. It's hard when one of our loved ones is feeling not at all like their usual self. `empathy`

[Pause]

Veterinarian: Let's work together to get to the bottom of this so that we can hopefully get her back to 100%. `partnership`

Client: Thank you. I really need this to turn out okay. She's my whole world.

Veterinarian: I can sense how important she is to you. `reflective listening / empathy`

Veterinarian: In order for me to help you help her, I need to ask some questions first. Then I will examine her. Is that okay with you? `signposting / asking permission / check-in`

Client: That works. Whatever I can do to help her, I will.

Veterinarian: I have no doubt, you always do. `unconditional positive regard`

Veterinarian: To start with, tell me what you've noticed in terms of Tigris vomiting ... `signposting`

Client: It started yesterday morning. I woke up to find a pile of kibble on the carpet next to the bed. It looked like it was fresh food – like it hadn't been digested – which was strange because her last meal was the night before. It should have been digested, don't you think?

Veterinarian: Yes, I agree, that doesn't sit well with me. Tell me more. `open-ended statement`

Client: I cleaned up the mess and went looking for her. She was underneath the coffee table. I think she felt bad for throwing up. Or maybe she just felt sick. Who feels good after they throw up anyway? So, I coaxed her out and told her that it wasn't her fault. I went to the kitchen to gather her breakfast. But you know what? She didn't even follow me. I had to bring the food to her. She took one sniff, licked her lips, then hightailed it back to the bedroom. She then vomited three more piles before laying on her side. It seemed to take a lot out of her. And she gave this awful cry.

Veterinarian: That must have been so awful for you to see. **empathy**

Client: [affirmative head nod] I really wanted to bring her in yesterday, but I couldn't. Work has been really chaotic lately. We've had a turnover in management and we're all on pins and needles waiting to hear who gets the axe. So, I didn't want to – I couldn't take off. I couldn't risk it.

Veterinarian: No, of course not, you did what you had to do. **unconditional positive regard**

Client: I also thought that when I got home, she would have perked up.

Veterinarian: Of course you would hope for the best. I would have, too, had I been in your shoes. **empathy / unconditional positive regard**

Client: By the time I got home last night, it was very late. I found six more piles of vomit. They were small, but thick and sticky, somewhat slimy, like mucus. They were also very yellow. The last one looked like it had a few specks of pink in it when I cleaned it up with a paper towel.

Veterinarian: Six more piles of vomit, on top of what she'd already produced, is definitely concerning. You were right to bring her in today. **reflective listening / regard**

Veterinarian: I know it may be hard right now, but tell me, have there been any changes at home that could have precipitated this event? **closed-ended question**

Client: Changes? No, not really. She's still indoor-only, and I haven't introduced any new pets or people to her.

Veterinarian: Okay, what about her diet? Has that changed at all? **closed-ended question**

Client: Nope. Same food, same amount. It's not even a new bag of food, so I know it's not as if I purchased a bag that was spoiled or something.

Veterinarian: Is there anything else, anything at all that she could have been exposed to? Something you didn't want her to eat, something you didn't think she would eat, but she maybe did?

[pause]

Client: Not that I can think of …

[pause]

Client: Well, actually, now that you mention it, I did receive some flowers the other day.

Veterinarian: Flowers? **reflective listening**

Client: A friend sent me a beautiful bouquet as a sort of pick-me-up. She knew how stressed I've been at work.

Veterinarian: How lovely! Can you think back and describe for me what kind of flowers were in the bouquet? **open-ended question / eliciting perspective**

Client: Pink carnations, some white roses, and – thinking – oh yes, Tiger lilies. My friend thought that'd be a nice touch in honor of Tigris.

Veterinarian: This information is really quite helpful. I'm afraid that I have some news that may be difficult to hear. **warning shot**

Veterinarian: That kind of lily is very toxic to cats. Is there any chance that she could have gotten into the lilies? **eliciting perspective**

Client: Oh no! I didn't mean to hurt her!

Veterinarian: No, of course you didn't, you would never do anything to hurt her. It was an accident. **regard / reflective listening**

Client: Tigris was up on the counter 2 days ago, dipping her paw in the water. I fussed at her to get down, which she did, but yes, there were bits and pieces of the flower scattered on the table. She may very well have eaten some.

Veterinarian: If she did eat them, then that would explain her symptoms. Lilies can hurt the kidneys. When the kidneys are injured, they do not filter out the toxins in the bloodstream. That can make a cat very sick. **appropriate, easy-to-understand language / chunk**

Veterinarian: What that means is we are going to need to do some bloodwork, after I complete my physical exam, to check her kidney function and to confirm our suspicion. Is that okay? **signposting / asking permission**

Client: Of course, anything we need to do, let's do it, if it means that she will get better.

Veterinarian: Lily poisoning can be a difficult road, I'm not going to lie, but we are certainly going to work hard to reverse kidney damage – if there is any – assuming that lilies caused her illness. The truth is, we don't know yet. **transparency**

Client: I have a bad feeling that you're right. I just can't believe this is all my fault. I should have come in sooner.

Veterinarian: What matters is that you are here now. Together, let's see how we can help Tigris. **regard / partnership**

[pause]

Veterinarian: Is there anything else that I should know before I get started on her physical exam? **eliciting perspective / check-in**

Client: No, let's just get her better.

Veterinarian: We will certainly do our best. **partnership**

Note that in this clinical scenario, history taking emphasized the presenting complaint.

When an ill patient presents for evaluation, patient stabilization takes a priority. All of the following aspects of background, pertinent to the chief complaint of emesis, were touched upon during data gathering:

- the onset of vomiting
- the frequency of vomiting
- the progression of vomiting
- the contents of the vomitus
- the color of the vomitus.

In addition, patient attitude and appetite were both addressed.

When the index of suspicion was raised that this presentation could indicate toxicosis, additional questions were raised.

- Could Tigris have gotten into something?
- Did she have access to the bouquet?
- What kind of flowers were in the vase?

Closed-ended questions were essential to flush out key details and to refresh the client's memory. Ultimately, the client recalled that Tigris was exposed to lilies and in fact may very well have ingested portions of them.

Note that the diagnosis is not definitive yet. The patient still requires a complete physical examination, and labwork is indicated for confirmation of acute kidney injury (AKI).

However, the history provided the driving force behind a targeted investigation. In this clinical scenario, the history held the clues to the patient's diagnosis. In order for the clinician to reach that discovery, she or he had to know which questions to ask and how to ask them.

I also want to point out that the patient's history was abbreviated in this clinical scenario. That may cause some of you to wonder why, particularly, when so much of this text has emphasized the importance of being thorough and taking a comprehensive anamnesis.

Just because the history was not fully outlined in the clinical scenario above does not mean that it is not important. It does not mean that there are times when a complete history is unnecessary. A comprehensive diagnosis plays an important part in diagnosis and case management.

So why did the clinician truncate the history in the case of Tigris?

When patients present with illness, particularly when patients are in a critical state, the primary goal is triage, followed by stabilization.

Accordingly, there are a number of topics that take a backseat in the moment.

- Is the patient sneezing?
- Is the patient coughing?
- Has the patient developed ocular discharge?
- Has the patient developed nasal discharge?

These content areas may need to be addressed later, but in the moment, they are not relevant to the presenting complaint. They do not help us get one step closer to solving the patient's problem.

Veterinary students may initially struggle with this because they do not always know what is or is not relevant. They are still learning to find links between health history and disease. They are still developing clinical acumen and discovering pattern recognition.

As you become more experienced in clinical practice, you start to appreciate which questions need to be asked now versus those that can be tabled for later.

In that sense, the doctor that you are today evolves into the doctor that you will become tomorrow.

Be patient with yourself.

Be patient with the process of history taking. There is an art to it. It takes time to master. Even then, you never stop learning how to improve the flow of conversation, the connectivity between you and your client, and the quest to glean sufficient data from your history to make the correct diagnosis.

References

1. Denness C. What are consultation models for? InnovAiT. 2013;6(9):592–9.
2. Kurtz SM, Silverman JD. The Calgary–Cambridge Referenced Observation Guides: an aid to defining the curriculum and organizing the teaching in communication training programmes. Med Educ. 1996;30(2):83–9.
3. Kurtz S. Teaching and learning communication in veterinary medicine. J Vet Med Educ. 2006;33(1):11–9.
4. Silverman J, Kurtz S, Draper J. Skills for communicating with patients. Oxford: Radcliffe Medical Press; 2008.
5. Riccardi VM, Kurtz SM. Communication and counselling in health care. Springfield, IL: Charles C. Thomas; 1983.
6. Englar RE, Williams M, Weingand K. Applicability of the Calgary–Cambridge Guide to dog and cat owners for teaching veterinary clinical communications. J Vet Med Educ. 2016;43(2):143–69.
7. Adams CL, Ladner LD. Implementing a simulated client program: bridging the gap between theory and practice. J Vet Med Educ. 2004;31(2):138–45.
8. Radford A, Stockley P, Silverman J, Taylor I, Turner R, Gray C. Development, teaching, and evaluation of a consultation structure model for use in veterinary education. J Vet Med Educ. 2006;33(1):38–44.
9. Lichstein PR. The Medical Interview. In: Walker HK, Hall WD, Hurst JW, editors. Clinical methods: the history, physical, and laboratory examinations. Boston, MA: Butterworths; 1990.
10. Takemura Y, Atsumi R, Tsuda T. Identifying medical interview behaviors that best elicit information from patients in clinical practice. Tohoku J Exp Med. 2007;213(2):121–7.
11. Hampton JR, Harrison MJ, Mitchell JR, Prichard JS, Seymour C. Relative contributions of history-taking, physical examination, and laboratory investigation to diagnosis and management of medical outpatients. Br Med J. 1975;2(5969):486–9.
12. Kassirer JP. Teaching clinical medicine by iterative hypothesis testing. Let's preach what we practice. N Engl J Med. 1983;309(15):921–3.
13. Peterson MC, Holbrook JH, Von Hales D, Smith NL, Staker LV. Contributions of the history, physical examination, and laboratory investigation in making medical diagnoses. West J Med.

1992;156(2):163–5.

14. Sandler G. The importance of the history in the medical clinic and the cost of unnecessary tests. Am Heart J. 1980;100(6 Pt 1):928–31.

15. Robinson JD, Heritage J. Physicians' opening questions and patients' satisfaction. Patient Educ Couns. 2006;60(3):279–85.

16. Beckman HB, Frankel RM. The effect of physician behavior on the collection of data. Ann Intern Med. 1984;101(5):692–6.

17. Robinson JD. Closing medical encounters: two physician practices and their implications for the expression of patients' unstated concerns. Soc Sci Med. 2001;53(5):639–56.

18. Robinson JD. An interactional structure of medical activities during acute visits and its implications for patients' participation. Health Commun. 2003;15(1):27–57.

19. Heritage J, Robinson JD. The structure of patients' presenting concerns: physicians' opening questions. Health Commun. 2006;19(2):89–102.

20. Cameron S, Turtle-song I. Learning to write case notes using the SOAP format. J Couns Dev. 2002;80(3):286–92.

21. Rockett J, Lattanzio C, Christensen C. The veterinary technician's guide to writing SOAPS: a workbook for critical thinking. Heyburn, ID: Rockett House Publishing LLC; 2013.

22. Borcherding S. Documentation manual for writing SOAP notes in occupational therapy. Second edn. Thorofare, NJ: SLACK Incorporated; 2005.

23. Kettenbach G, Kettenbach G. Writing patient/client notes: ensuring accuracy in documentation. 4th edn. Philadelphia, PA: F.A. Davis; 2004.

24. Kettenbach G. Writing SOAP notes: with patient/client management formats. 3rd edn. Philadelphia, PA: F.A. Davis Company; 2004.

25. Shaw JR. Four core communication skills of highly effective practitioners. Vet Clin North Am Small Anim Pract. 2006;36(2):385–96, vii.

26. Kurtz SM, Silverman JD, Draper J. Teaching and learning communication skills in medicine. Grand Rapids, MI: Radcliffe; 2004.

Chapter 21

Using Communication Skills to Gather Data

Explaining and Planning

Up to this point in the text, we have sufficiently explored the first two tasks that are associated with the Calgary–Cambridge model: initiating the session and gathering information.(1–8) At this point, the physical examination would commence.(1, 3, 4) The end of the physical examination marks the beginning of the third task, explaining and planning.(1–8)

As veterinarians, we are educators as much as we are healthcare providers. We spend much of our time in the examination room explaining to clients the following content areas:

- abnormal findings on the physical exam
- differential diagnoses
- presumptive diagnosis
- diagnostic data
  - labwork
  - imaging
  - histopathology
- definitive diagnosis
- the missing link: why disease "X" causes clinical sign "Y"
- options for medical management
- options for surgical management
- potential adverse effects of treatment
- pain management
- prognosis.

Educating our clients is an essential part of clinical practice because we alone are incapable of executing decisions for our patients. We know what we would do if the pet were ours. But it is not. It belongs to another person on the other end of the leash or holding the carrier.

We need the client to be on the same page as us so that she or he understands the patient's condition and what needs to happen in order to see improvement. This requires us to be a teacher, but not the "sage on the stage" variety, who dictates care and expects the client to follow through without hesitation.

We need to engage the client and encourage active participation. Much as didactic lectures have given way to interactive tools in the new age of digital classrooms, we, too, need to rethink, revise, and reconfigure how we present the case to the client.

We achieve nothing if all we do is educate. We need to effect action through education. That means involving the client in the process and actively inviting him or her to weigh in on the proposed plan.

Planning is a critical part of case management because it allows for the sharing of options (Plan A, Plan B, Plan C, and so on) and establishes realistic expectations for care. Planning may involve:

- discussing financial constraints
- providing an estimate for care that is needed in the future
- scheduling a diagnostic test
- scheduling a diagnostic procedure
- scheduling a surgical procedure
- hospitalizing
- referring to a specialist or a tertiary care facility
- anticipating patient needs relative to disease progression
- discussing the process of euthanasia and aftercare of the patient's body
- working through anticipatory grief that may precede euthanasia.

Both explaining and planning can be time intensive. Both tasks are associated with content-rich material to share, and both risk the potential of overwhelming the client.

Because of their inexperience, students often bombard the client with every fact about every diagnostic test or procedure. This is (usually) unintentional. Students are often very excited about what they have learned in the classroom, and have been trained – for better or worse – by most faculty to memorize facts and regurgitate them for testing.

It is tempting to recite pages of textbooks about disease "X" or medication "Y" in the consultation room because that is our comfort zone. But we are tasked to break it down for our client. Is it any wonder that we struggle?

We live and breathe in that circle of medical knowledge. We immerse ourselves with it. It envelops us. We feel at home with it. We may have difficulty paring it down for the client in a way that is complete, without overwhelming.

The purpose of this chapter is to provide you with examples of how you might more effectively navigate the processes of explaining and planning, by reaching for your communication toolbox.

To explain your findings in a client-friendly manner, you can make use of any of the communication skills that you were introduced to in Part 2 of the text. However, I find the following communication skills to be particularly helpful as you go about this task:

1. asking for permission (for a summary of this skill, refer to Chapter 12)
2. eliciting the client's perspective (for a summary of this skill, refer to Chapter 11)
3. assessing the client's knowledge (for a summary of this skill, refer to Chapter 13)
4. signposting (for a summary of this skill, refer to Chapter 14)
5. replacing medical jargon with easy-to-understand language (for a summary of this skill, refer to Chapter 9)
6. chunking, checking in, and summarizing (for a summary of these skills, refer to Chapter 15).

To engage in forward planning, you can make use of any of the communication skills that you were introduced to in Part 2 of the text. However, I find the following further communication skills to be particularly helpful as you go about this task:

7. signposting (for a summary of this skill, refer to Chapter 14)
8. contracting for next steps (for a summary of this skill, refer to Chapter 16)
9. partnership (for a summary of this skill, refer to Chapter 10)
10. assessing the client's knowledge (for a summary of this skill, refer to Chapter 13)
11. replacing medical jargon with easy-to-understand language (for a summary of this skill, refer to Chapter 9)
12. chunking, checking in, and summarizing (For a summary of these skills, refer to Chapter 15).

Let us see how these skills might come together by exploring two clinical vignettes.

21.1 Explaining Physical Examination Findings in an Apparently Healthy Patient

We will begin with the simplest clinical scenario, a consultation in which an apparently healthy patient presents for an annual wellness examination. For the purpose of this scenario, assume that you have already taken a complete patient history, and you have just now completed your physical examination. You are ready to share your physical exam findings with the client.

Background

A new client, Mr. Darcy, presents his recently purchased 14-week-old, castrated male Tonkinese kitten, "Mr. Bingley," to your clinic. The kitten was acquired 3 days ago from a local "cattery." According to the scant records that have been provided, the kitten has not yet received any vaccinations, dewormer, or medical attention. Mr. Darcy found the advertisement for the kitten online and shares with you that he was greatly displeased by the conditions in which he found the litter. The "breeder" is not registered, and he questions the kitten's lineage and breed. In spite of this inauspicious start, Mr. Darcy felt an instant connection to this kitten and did not want to leave him there. He is here today to have the kitten examined. He says that the kitten seems well. However, on physical examination you notice a few areas that you would like to address.

Clinical Conversation

Veterinarian: I can see why you bonded with Mr. Bingley, he's definitely a keeper! Thank you so much for bringing him in to let me take a look at him. He was such a good boy for his exam! If it's okay with you, I'd like to discuss a few of my findings with you before we chat about getting him up to date on his shots. (regard / asking permission / signposting)

Client: That sounds good to me.

Veterinarian: Have you noticed him shaking his head or pawing at his ears at home? (eliciting the client's perspective)

Client: Hmmm, well, now that you mention it, maybe a little? I guess I just thought that was normal.

Veterinarian: That makes sense, I can understand that. We all can get an itch now and again. (regard)

Veterinarian: Unfortunately, Mr. Bingley has more than just an itch. He has a fair amount of dark brown discharge in his ears, and when I took a closer look with my scope, I could actually see ear mites crawling around in there. Have you heard of ear mites? (chunk and check-in / easy-to-understand language / assessing the client's knowledge)

Client: No, I haven't. Is that a type of mange? Is it contagious?

Veterinarian: No, the good news is that it is not a type of mange, and thankfully, it's not contagious to you. (reflective listening)

Veterinarian: Ear mites are really common in young cats and they are very easy to treat! (easy to understand language / chunk)

Client: That's great news.

Veterinarian: Before we talk about treatment options, I'd also like to talk with you about another common issue that I found while examining Mr. Bingley. Is that okay? (chunk and check-in / signposting / asking permission)

Client: Yes, is it serious?

Veterinarian: Nope, not serious. (reflective listening)

[Pause]

Veterinarian: Just a nuisance. I'm afraid that Mr. Bingley has fleas.

Client: Oh no, I hate fleas!

Veterinarian: You and me both. May I ask, what has been your experience with fleas in the past? (partnership / eliciting perspective)

Client: Years ago, I rescued a cat off the street. I brought him into the house on a cold winter's night because I felt bad, it was snowing out. He was in my house for less than 24 hours. The very next morning, I took him to the vet's. By the time I got home, the whole house was infested! It took weeks to get that under control. I didn't realize at the time that a lot more is needed than just treating the cat. You really need to treat the whole house!

Veterinarian: You are absolutely right. Fleas require you to treat the house as well as the cat. If you only treat one, the problem doesn't go away. Do you recall what you did that worked for you to manage the problem? **reflective listening / eliciting the client's perspective**

Client: I remember that I vacuumed … A LOT! Other than that, no, it was a long time ago. I'd be interested in hearing what better ways have been developed since then.

Veterinarian: Indeed, flea control has come a long way. There are a lot of really great products out there on the market that we can discuss. But before we do, there's one last concern that I have regarding Mr. Bingley's physical exam. Can we discuss that? **reflective listening / chunk and check-in / signposting / asking permission**

Client: Poor Mr. Bingley. What now?

Veterinarian: I don't know if you've noticed, but he has a very round belly, even though he's underweight. **easy-to-understand language / chunk and check**

Client: I guess now that you mention it, yes, he does have a bit of a belly.

Veterinarian: Most of the time, that's because of internal parasites – worms. There are a lot of different types of them. We see roundworms the most. Are you familiar with them? **assessing the client's knowledge**

Client: Aren't those the ones that look like spaghetti when they are pooped out?

Veterinarian: Yes, you're absolutely right, adult roundworms that exit the body look very much like spaghetti. **reflective listening**

Client: But I'm not seeing any of those in his litter box, so how could he have worms?

Veterinarian: Kittens can carry different stages of the worm. Adult worms are just one part of the life cycle. Many times, kittens' intestines are packed full of eggs. We can't see those with the naked eye. Does that make sense? **easy-to-understand langauge / check-in**

Client: I think so.

Veterinarian: When kittens have worms, they may irritate the intestines. The intestines get a sort of doughy feel to them, and the affected kittens look bloated. That's the same kind of feeling I'm getting from Mr. Bingley.

[Pause] ← **silent check-in**

Client: So what do we do about them?

Veterinarian: The first thing we need to do is to examine a sample of his stool. That way, we know exactly what we are treating. He could have other worms, too, not just round ones. `signposting`

Veterinarian: Before we move on to planning next steps for Mr. Bingley, do you have any questions or concerns about his physical exam? `signposting / eliciting the client's perspective`

Client: No.

Veterinarian: We've covered a lot today. The good news is that Mr. Bingley is overall healthy on exam, he just has a few problem areas to address that almost every new kitten has that comes in to see me. He has three items that we can take care of today: ear mites, fleas, and probable roundworms. `summarizing / signposting`

Veterinarian: Shall we begin with treatment options for the ear mites? `asking permission`

You can appreciate from the clinical scenario above that there is no such thing as *just* a wellness examination. Even though this patient presented as being apparently healthy, the clinician identified specific areas on physical exam that needed to be addressed.

Mr. Bingley's problem areas centered on endo- and ectoparasites.

Other patients may require explanations about other problem areas. For kittens and puppies, common physical exam abnormalities include:

- abdominal wall defects
  - is there a hernia?
  - if so, how big is it?
  - is it reducible?
- coughing
- dentition
  - malocclusion
  - retained deciduous teeth
- reproductive organs
  - if the patient is a male, are both testicles descended?
  - if not, is the missing testicle palpable within the inguinal canal?
- heart murmurs
  - are they physiologic?
  - are they pathologic?
- nasal discharge
  - laterality
    - unilateral
    - bilateral
  - progression
  - color and consistency
- ocular discharge (especially kittens)
  - did the patient come from a cattery or shelter, or other region of densely populated cats?
  - is exposure to or infection with feline herpesvirus probable?

Older patients often involve discussions about weight, the emergence of or growth of lumps and bumps, and/or dental disease.

Regardless of topic, explanations about physical exam findings need to be simple and direct. Clients are not typically interested in a description that they can read out of an encyclopedia. They want the bottom line.

- What is the problem?
- What is the significance of the problem?
- Can the problem be managed and/or resolved?
- What will the impact be if the problem is not resolved?
- What are next steps in the management of the condition?

A successful explanation leads into a discussion involving forward planning:

- What needs to happen?
- Where do we go from here?

21.2 Explaining Physical Examination Findings in an Ill Patient

Sick patients also require their share of explanations so that clients can process what may be causing the illness in order to understand options for treatment.

In some cases, the link between symptoms and disease is obvious. For example, a snotty nose is easily associated with an upper respiratory infection (URI).

In other cases, the link between symptoms and disease is unclear. Consider, for instance, the classic cases involving endocrinopathy. As clinicians, we benefit from having studied the pathophysiology of disease. We understand how hormonal imbalances can contribute to organ and/or body system dysfunction. We can connect the dots, for instance, between poor wound healing and hyperadrenocorticism.

Most of our clients do not have that luxury. So, it is not apparent, without an explanation, why dogs with "ring-around-the-collar" or "rat tail" need to be tested for hypothyroidism.

Clients benefit from explanations that demystify medicine. They need to hear which next steps are indicated and why.

Let us consider how these explanations might work in companion animal practice for a more complicated consultation involving a clinically ill patient.

For the purpose of this scenario, assume that you have already taken a patient history, and you have just now completed your physical examination. You are ready to share your physical exam findings with the client.

Background

A new client, Mrs. Briar, presents her 9-year-old domestic medium haired (DMH) cat, "Lightweight," to your clinic. Lightweight is not so trim. Lightweight weighs 18.6

pounds today. The client claims that he weighed over 20 pounds last week.

Mrs. Briar and her husband, who is not present for today's consultation, took a 5-day business trip out of town last Thursday. They had hired a pet sitter to tend to Lightweight both morning and night; however, the pet sitter claims that he refused to eat anything for the second through fifth day.

When the clients returned home, Lightweight was unusually quiet. He didn't come to the door to greet them. At first, they thought he was just pouting. Then they noticed him laying underneath the dining room table, on his side, breathing hard.

They called out his name. It took several attempts to get him to look up.

When he did, his eyes seemed sunken in.

Mr. Briar had to head back into the office, so Mrs. Briar rushed him in to your clinic to be seen on emergency.

Lightweight's physical examination discloses a body condition score (BCS) of 8/9 and 8–10% dehydration. His peri-auricular skin is discolored yellow. His sclera are bilaterally icteric. He is also tender on abdominal palpation. He licks his lips and exhibits non-productive retching when deep pressure is applied to the cranial abdomen. You suspect hepatic lipidosis.

Clinical Conversation

Veterinarian: It is a good thing that you brought Lightweight in when you did. I share your concern that he is very sick. I am very worried by what I found on his examination. **transparency / warning shot**

[pause]

Client: What do you think is going on? Do you think that our pet sitter hurt him?

Veterinarian: No, I don't think it's anything like that, but I do think that something happened to him when you were away. I know that you have travelled before, on business. Tell me, how has his appetite been in the past when you've gone away? **open-ended question**

Client: It's never been great, he's a social eater – but he really prefers me or my husband to be around. The last time we went away, we were able to have one of Brandon's friends look after him. He needed to be coaxed to eat, but she got him to munch on a little something every day. Now that you mention it, I remember it took a lot of time and effort on her part. She wasn't available to pet sit this time, so we had to go with someone new. We had wanted him to meet Lightweight in advance of the trip, but our schedules just didn't line up. I trust that he came every day, but maybe he couldn't get him to eat? Why do you ask? What are you thinking?

Veterinarian: Cats are not like small dogs. Dogs can go a long time without eating. But cats can get very sick if they go on hunger strike. Especially heavy or overweight cats. **easy-to-understand language**

Client: He's not *that* fat, Doc. I just think he's big-boned.

Veterinarian: I know it's hard to think of him in that way, but he is significantly overweight. That can set the stage for some serious conditions involving his metabolism, particularly if he chooses not to eat. **(transparency)**

Client: Oh.

Veterinarian: When cats turn down food, their body needs to find an energy source to stay alive. Heavy cats break down their own body fat for fuel. Does that make sense? **(chunk and check / easy-to-understand language)**

Client: Yes.

Veterinarian: That sounds good. The problem is that the body can't make use of the fat fast enough, so it plugs up the liver. The result is a life-threatening condition called hepatic lipidosis. Have you ever heard of that term before? **(chunk / easy-to-understand language / assessing the client's knowledge)**

Client: No. What does that even mean?

Veterinarian: The build-up of fat in the liver can cause his liver to fail. I'm not going to lie to you, this is serious. **(chunk / easy-to-understand language / transparency)**

[pause] ← **(silent check-in)**

Veterinarian: Are you with me? **(check-in)**

Client: So this is all my fault?

[Client begins to cry]

Veterinarian: You had no idea that this would happen. You've gone away before without any issue. You did everything you could to make sure that he was well cared for. You got a pet sitter. You did everything right. **(regard)**

[pause]

Veterinarian: Unfortunately, Lightweight didn't read the textbook, he didn't know just how bad it could be for him if he didn't eat. Okay? **(check-in)**

Client: Yes, but I'll never forgive myself if something bad happens to him.

Veterinarian: It's normal to feel that way. But what I need you to do is focus all of your energy right now on getting Lightweight back to health. We need to put our heads together and come up with the best plan for him to help his liver recover. How does that sound? **(regard / empathy / signposting / partnership)**

Client: Yes, I'll do anything.

Veterinarian: Just remember, we are a team, we are in this together, we are going to work through this. **(partnership)**

[Client dries her eyes]

Veterinarian: Is there anything else that I can do for you to make this easier? **(eliciting the client's perspective)**

Client: No, just help him get better.

Veterinarian: Okay, that's precisely what we're going to do. Now let's get down to business and talk about what we need to do for Lightfoot … **(partnership / signposting)**

When patients present for illnesses, clients' emotions often run high. Guilt is a frequent undertone, particularly in discussions in which client action (or inaction) led to a less-than-ideal outcome for the patient.

Sometimes it is easy to accept a client's guilt. For example, it is easy to understand why a client might feel guilty if she or he administered a toxic drug or the wrong dose of a medication to the dog or cat. You might feel the same way were you in their shoes.

Other times, it is difficult to see how a client could possibly blame himself. In those situations, try to avoid saying the following.

- "Don't be silly."
- "Don't be ridiculous."
- "That's crazy thinking."
- "Why would you ever think that?"
- "How could you possibly feel that way?"

These statements are often said with good intent. They are an attempt on our part to relieve the client of a guilty conscience, particularly when we do not feel that the client is responsible for his or her pet's condition.

Similar statements are often heard in public, in conversations between friends.

As a society, we tend to negate each other's feelings with such comments.

- "Don't worry!"
- "That's not true!"
- "Don't feel that way!"
- "Don't give it a second thought!"

On the surface, these sound kind and comforting. They are our way of saying, "You didn't do anything wrong, so don't blame yourself."

Unfortunately, these statements are usually anything but helpful. Try as we might to relieve clients of guilt, clients feel what they are going to feel. Isn't that true for most of us? We do not feel what we feel because it is right. We just feel.

Clients need to be free to express themselves and how they are feeling in a safe and supportive environment. Clients need to know that what they are feeling is normal. The only way to move on from the emotion is to acknowledge it.

Review the case of Lightweight again. Consider how the veterinarian handled the client's expression of guilt. The veterinarian avoided telling the client how to feel. Instead, she or he reframed the situation: "It's normal to feel that way."

Other ways of reframing statements include.

- "I can see why you might feel that way."
- "I might feel the same way if I were in your shoes."
- "I might blame myself, too."

In the case of Lightweight, above, reframing also made use of an action statement to redirect the client's emotions into something positive.

- "What I need you to do is ..."
- "Focus all of your energy right now on ..."
- "We need to put our heads together ..."

Ultimately, it is patience and understanding, empathy and unconditional positive regard that move the consultation towards forward planning.

21.3 Forward Planning

Forward planning is essential to the consultation because it drives effective case management. Forward planning establishes expectations concerning the following.

- Tasks that the veterinarian agrees to do.
    - "As the primary care veterinarian, I will contact the board-certified ophthalmologist to inquire if there are any clinical trials for dogs that have glaucoma."
    - "As the specialist involved with surgical repair of Bristol's limb, I will reach out to your primary care veterinarian to discuss aftercare options for Gwen."
    - "I will formulate a home-cooked elimination diet for Bliss that is nutritionally complete."
    - "I will send the biopsy to the lab."
    - "I will contact you in 3–5 business days with the test results."
- Tasks that the veterinary support staff agree to do.
    - "I will text you with an update as soon as Katniss recovers from anesthesia."
    - "I will be taking care of Peeta in the ICU over the holiday weekend."
    - "I will borrow Cinna for a moment to draw some blood for his heartworm test."
    - "I will transfer your call to the front desk so that you can schedule an appointment for Rue to be rechecked."
    - "I will get that test started. It takes about ten minutes."
    - "I will teach you how to assess Finnick's blood sugar at home."
    - "I will express Cato's anal glands in the treatment area."
    - "I will trim Gale's nails."
- Tasks that the veterinary team asks the client to do.
    - "Please schedule an appointment for 3–5 days from now so that we can recheck Haymitch's eye."
    - "Please bring in a stool sample so that we can check Primrose for intestinal parasites."
    - "Please bring Seneca back to see us before he completes his two-week course of antibiotics so that we can recheck his urine for evidence of lingering infection."

- ▪ "Please email or fax Glimmer's proof of rabies vaccination to us before the end of the week."
- ▪ "Please telephone us with an update about how Foxface is adjusting to life as a new mom."
- ▪ "Please make a list of all the foods that Thresh has been exposed to so that we can formulate an elimination diet to rule out food allergies."

Forward planning also helps with goal setting.

- • "Let's recheck Marvel's red blood cell count before the end of the week to be certain that it is not continuing to drop."
- • "Let's recheck Clove's chemistry panel in two weeks to see how her kidney values are responding to treatment."
- • "Let's plan on getting Triumph's teeth cleaned within the next three months."

To be successful, forward planning relies heavily upon the following communication skills:

- • partnership (for a summary of this skill, refer to Chapter 10)
- • signposting (for a summary of this skill, refer to Chapter 14)
- • contracting for the next steps (for a summary of this skill, refer to Chapter 16)
- • asking for permission (for a summary of this skill, refer to Chapter 12)
- • eliciting the client's perspective (for a summary of this skill, refer to Chapter 11)
- • summarizing and checking in (for a summary of these skills, refer to Chapter 15).

Patient care requires teamwork and client "buy-in." If the client is onboard, then case management will be that much easier. If the client is not sold on the treatment plan, then rework the treatment plan. Otherwise, you are setting up the case for failure.

21.4 Planning Next Steps in an Apparently Healthy Patient

To appreciate forward planning, we will revisit the case of Mr. Darcy and his cat, Mr. Bingley. Recall from Section 21.1 that Mr. Bingley's physical exam disclosed the following three abnormalities:

- • ear mites
- • fleas
- • probable roundworms.

Each of these items were identified by you on physical exam and reported to Mr. Darcy. Now you must formulate a treatment plan and convince the client to take action. Let us consider how that clinical conversation might unfold.

Clinical Conversation

Veterinarian: To recap, Mr. Bingley has three problem areas that we need to address today: ear mites, fleas, and probable roundworms. (summarizing / signposting / partnership)

Veterinarian: If it's okay with you, I would like to start with a discussion about ear mites. (asking permission / signposting)

Client: Sure. I would like them to go away as soon as possible. That can't feel good, them crawling around in there.

Veterinarian: No, I can't imagine that they would feel good. It's got to be uncomfortable. (empathy / reflective listening)

Client: [shudders] Bugs give me the creeps.

Veterinarian: You and me both. (partnership)

Veterinarian: First, we need to clean out Mr. Bingley's ears. If it's alright with you, we can do that for you here. We use mineral oil, so it's going to make him a bit slick and greasy, but it's the best cleaner for this and it's non-irritating. Is that okay? (signposting / asking for permission / easy-to-use language)

Client: And you're sure that I can't catch these bugs?

Veterinarian: Absolutely sure. No, you can't catch them. (reflective listening)

Veterinarian: After we clean the ears out today, we need to start treatment right away. There are a couple of different ways we can do that. Would you be open to hearing about these? (signposting / eliciting perspective)

Client: Sure, but I'm really not good at pilling so I would much rather you give a shot of something.

Veterinarian: I understand: it can be really challenging to pill a cat. They can be the calmest of calm until there's a pill to be had and then suddenly they're Houdini! (empathy / regard)

Veterinarian: There are two options that I might suggest, given your situation. One option is to apply ear drops – something called Acarexx®. We can do that here for you – it's a suspension of ivermectin that will kill the mites. (signposting / easy-to-understand language / contracting for the next steps)

[pause] ← (silent check-in)

Client: [Affirmative head nod]

Veterinarian: If Mr. Bingley did not have fleas, I might suggest this approach because most of the time, one treatment is effective. (chunk)

[pause] ← (silent check-in)

Client: Okay.

Veterinarian: But Mr. Bingley also has fleas. Fleas can be a huge problem for the household, so we need to get on top of that right away. Right? (summarizing / check-in)

Client: Absolutely, I want to do whatever possible not to relive a flea infestation again.

That was a nightmare!

Veterinarian: I can only imagine! (empathy)

Veterinarian: The good news is this: we can apply one of our topical products, RevolutionPLUS®, to the skin at the base of Mr. Bingley's neck today. That product not only treats ear mites, it also treats fleas. (contracting for the next steps)

[pause] ← (silent check-in)

Veterinarian: It starts killing fleas in as few as 6 hours. It also interrupts the flea's life cycle by killing the adults before they can lay new eggs. We would still need to treat the environment – your home – but at least this kills two birds with one stone. Does that make sense? (chunk / easy-to-understand langage / check-in)

Client: Yes, I like the sound of that.

Veterinarian: The other great thing about RevolutionPLUS® is that it effectively treats roundworms and hookworms. So, in a way, you're getting three different treatments for three different problems for the price of one!

Client: That's great! I also like that it's not three different medications. One sounds like less for his little body to handle.

Veterinarian: I like the way you think. In my experience, RevolutionPLUS® is very gentle on the system and my other clients have had good success with it. I also have used it safely on my own pets so I can say that it truly works!

Client: That makes me feel a lot better. So then how do we treat the house for fleas so that they don't just re-infest Mr. Bingley?

Veterinarian: We can treat the house for fleas any number of ways. (reflective listening)

Veterinarian: Can you describe your home for me? Are there any carpets throughout the house? (open-ended question / eliciting the client's perspective)

Client: Yes, the whole second floor and the stairs leading up to it is all carpet.

Veterinarian: Okay, so we will need to treat the carpet. That means that you will need to vacuum – including carpet edges and room corners, under beds and other furniture. Flea eggs, larvae, and pupae love carpeting. This will help to break the cycle.

[pause] ← (silent check-in)

Client: Okay.

Veterinarian: You're going to need to vacuum every other day until the flea infestation is gone. It's a lot, but it will work. Does that sound reasonable to you? (eliciting the client's perspective / contracting for next steps)

Client: Yeah, it's going to be a pain, but if it will work, then it's worth it.

Veterinarian: It absolutely is. Do you have a vacuum cleaner with or without bags? (reflective listening / eliciting the client's perspective)

Client: It's an old model, it still has bags.

Veterinarian: That's okay, a vacuum with bags will still work well, as long as you throw out the bag each time you vacuum and replace it with a fresh one. This will prevent eggs from hatching in the vacuum bag and coming out when you vacuum. The goal is to reduce the flea population rather than contribute to it. (contracting for next steps / easy-to-understand language)

Client: Understood.

Veterinarian: I know that I've given you a lot of homework to consider. We've discussed Revolution to target Mr. Bingley's ear mites, fleas, and worms. (summarizing)

Veterinarian: Would you be open to hearing about other options for flea control at home? (eliciting perspective)

Client: Absolutely!

Veterinarian: Other things that we can do include washing all of Mr. Bingley's pet bedding and any small area rugs. (partnership / signposting)

Client: What about bombing the house or flea sprays that I see for sale at the market?

Veterinarian: I would prefer that you hold off on bombing the house or flea sprays unless you snap a photo of the ingredient label and send it my way. I could review it for you. Many flea bombs and sprays contain permethrin or pyrethrin, which have the potential to be toxic to cats. Does that make sense? (reflective listening / easy-to-understand language / contracting for next steps – what the veterinarian will do for the client / check-in)

Client: I understand. I don't want to do something that will hurt Mr. Bingley.

Veterinarian: No, of course not. (regard)

Veterinarian: Some of those products can be very scary. I've even had some cats pass away because of ones that were marketed as being safe for cats when they weren't. (transparency)

Client: I'll definitely double-check with you before I spray down the house with anything. Thanks for the heads-up.

Veterinarian: Certainly.

Veterinarian: We will also need to continue treating Mr. Bingley with RevolutionPLUS® once a month for at least three months because it takes that long to remove all of the life stages of the flea from your house. (contracting for next steps / partnership)

Client: Okay. Do I purchase that here?

Veterinarian: That would be my preference. We offer prescription products that are safest for Mr. Bingley and we know that they are effective. (transparency / contracting for next steps)

Client: Makes sense.

Veterinarian: Fleas can also carry tapeworms, so it is possible that Mr. Bingley is also infected with those. Have you had any experience with tapeworms in pets before? (assessing knowledge)

Client: Yes, I remember that my last cat had them as a kitten. I had noticed these little white flecks, they kind of looked like rice – crawling around her rear end. Sometimes I found them on the carpet where she'd been laying. Sometimes they made her really itchy and she would overgroom. I seem to recall though that it wasn't hard to treat – we needed to give her a medication that started with a "p."

Veterinarian: Praziquantal?

Client: Yes! That's it! It worked like a charm. Never had an issue with them again. But then again, I guess, if I'm understanding you right, they were probably because of the fleas. Once the fleas are treated, they shouldn't come back, right?

Veterinarian: Exactly!

Veterinarian: Do you have any additional questions about flea control before we move on to discuss Mr. Bingley's shots? `check-in`

Client: Nope.

Veterinarian: Great, in that case, let's talk about …

Forward planning requires transparency about expectations for case management. In the above example, the veterinarian expressed transparency about:

- resolving flea infestations: it takes time and can be a problem for the entire household
- the dangers of over-the-counter flea medications, particularly for cats.

Contracting for next steps was an effective way of identifying which veterinary team member was responsible for which arm of treatment. For example, contracting for next steps outlined that the veterinarian would take the lead in terms of:

- educating the client about different products that manage infestations
- cleaning both ears prior to onset of topical medication to manage ear mites.

Moreover, the veterinarian expressed willingness to research over-the-counter home and premise sprays. This agenda item is conditional upon the client forwarding a photograph of the ingredient label.

Contracting for next steps works both ways. Even though the client is the one seeking help from the veterinarian, the veterinarian is powerless to effectively create positive patient outcomes on his or her own.

More often than not, the client is required to assist with patient care. In the case of Mr. Bingley, the veterinarian will be relying upon the client to take charge of the following tasks:

- vacuuming every other day
- tossing out used vacuum bags, each and every time
- washing pet bedding
- washing area rugs.

Note that contracting for next steps is only effective when it is paired with partnership and eliciting the client's perspective. In other words, the veterinarian did not just prescribe one type of medication and assume that it would work well for the client. Instead, the veterinarian actively engaged the client to determine which aspects of patient care would be within reach. The veterinarian made certain to ask the client whether they:

- preferred a topical ear medication (Acarexx®) or a topical skin formulation (Revolution®PLUS)
- would be able to vacuum every other day
- would toss out the vacuum bags after each use
- were open to additional instructions concerning flea control within the home environment
- would hold off on applying premise sprays unless they were approved.

The veterinarian also asked for permission to:

- clean Mr. Bingley's ears
- initiate treatment for ear mites, fleas, and presumptive roundworms
- share additional details about at-home flea control
- move on to the next topic of vaccinations.

Contracting for next steps is effective only when it centers on dialogue, rather than dictation. Refer to Chapter 16 to review this communication skill in greater depth.

21.5 Planning Next Steps in an Ill Patient

Forward planning also takes place when managing patients that are ill. Let us revisit the case of Lightweight and Mrs. Briar from Section 21.2. Recall that Lightweight's anorexia has resulted in presumptive hepatic lipidosis. Physical examination disclosed that the patient was obese, with a history of weight loss, marked dehydration, and icterus. He was also tender on cranial abdominal palpation. The veterinarian expressed significant concern about the cat's present state. Transparency was key to the client understanding that this is not a minor event for Lightweight. Empathy and unconditional positive regard were essential components in navigating the client's guilt so that the client's attention could be focused on forward planning: what should be done now for Lightweight.

Let us see how that treatment plan is conveyed to the client and if it can convince the client to take action.

Clinical Conversation

Veterinarian: To review, Lightweight's yellow skin and eyes, in combination with his weight loss, dehydration, and abdominal pain, have me concerned. (summarizing / transparency)

Veterinarian: If it's okay with you, I would like to start by drawing some blood to con-

---

firm my suspicions. **asking permission / signposting**

Client: What would that involve, in terms of cost?

Veterinarian: The cost for a full CBC and chemistry panel – to evaluate his organ function and whole body health – would be about $150. I can have my receptionist draw up an exact estimate for you. Would that help? **reflective listening / transparency / contracting for next steps**

Client: Yes, but I'm sorry for all the extra work.

Veterinarian: It's quite alright. If I were in your shoes, I would want to know what I was looking at, too, in terms of pricing. **regard**

Veterinarian: I should also warn you, though, that's just the price of the bloodwork. If Lightweight does have hepatic lipidosis, then it is not easily managed at home. In fact, I really would suggest hospitalizing him today either way because his dehydration is serious. **transparency / contracting for the next steps**

Client: How long would he need to stay here for?

Veterinarian: How long he stays with us would really depend upon his starting point as well as how he responds to treatment. In my experience, it could take 3–5 days, easy, for him to get back on track. **reflective listening / chunk**

[Pause] ← **silent check-in**

Client: [Affirmative head nod]

Veterinarian: While in the hospital, we will hook him up to an IV to rehydrate him. We will also need to jumpstart his appetite. **chunk**

[pause] ← **silent check-in**

Client: [affirmative head nod]

Veterinarian: If we cannot get him to eat on his own, we may have to take a more aggressive approach to treatment. He may need a feeding tube. **chunk / transparency**

Client: I don't like the sound of that.

Veterinarian: I know that it sounds very scary. In truth, it's a simple procedure that can do a lot of good. Know that we might have to go down that route, but let's only cross that bridge if we have to. We're not quite there yet. **reflective listening / empathy / signposting**

Client: Phew, I'm okay with that. I'd much rather take a conservative approach. I don't want to do anything drastic.

Veterinarian: I hear you. You would like to take a step by step approach and only place a feeding tube if it is absolutely necessary. **reflective listening**

Client: Yes.

Veterinarian: That sounds like a perfectly reasonable plan to me. We also don't know for sure what we're up against until we run the bloodwork. At that point, we'll know more about Lightweight's needs. How does that sound to you? chunk / check-in

Client: Okay.

Veterinarian: In that case, let me get that estimate prepared for you – in fact, I will prepare two. contracting for next steps / signposting

[Pause]

Veterinarian: The first will cover the cost of hospitalization. The second will outline the cost of bloodwork and imaging. The truth is that we really need to see what is going on in there, and we have the ability to ultrasound his belly while the bloodwork is running.

[Pause]

Veterinarian: Is that okay with you? asking permission / eliciting perspective

Client: Will the ultrasound hurt him? I don't want to see him in any more pain.

Veterinarian: I know you don't, it is clear to me how much you care for him. He is very lucky to have you here with him today. regard / empathy

Veterinarian: The ultrasound in and of itself won't hurt, but he already has a painful belly. With your permission, I would like to give him some medication now to take the edge off. reflective listening / transparency / asking permission

Client: That would make me feel a lot better, too.

Veterinarian: Great! In fact, let me get started on that now so that we can make him feel at least a bit more comfortable while he waits. signposting / partnership / contracting for next steps

Veterinarian: Before I go grab his meds, is there anything else that you would like to discuss at this time? signposting / check-in

Client: No, let's get him feeling better first, then we can talk more.

Veterinarian: Sounds good. I'll be right back. signposting

Forward planning is a part of every consultation; however, it is even more critical in case management for patients that are ill and for whom care needs to be expedited. Sick patients need attention immediately, and the best way for us to initiate care is to be transparent and direct about patient care needs.

In this example, the veterinarian made it clear that Lightweight's condition is serious and that the cat not only needs bloodwork, he will also benefit from imaging and hospitalization.

The veterinarian also addresses the urgency of the situation, expressing that if Lightweight does not start eating again, then he will require a feeding tube. This allows for a brief discussion with the client about how she or he feels concerning a conservative versus aggressive approach to treatment. The veterinarian hears loud and clear that the client does not want to pursue a feeding tube unless it is absolutely essential. However, the veterinarian makes use of transparency to plant the seed that a feeding tube may be indicated, depending upon how Lightweight responds to treatment.

When case management involves a sick patient, contracting for next steps often involves discussions about finances.

- Which type of care is indicated?
- How much will that type of care cost?
- Is there a Plan B if Plan A is unaffordable?
- How are payments handled by the practice?
  - Is payment expected up front, in full?
  - Is a deposit required?
  - Does the practice accept third party payment?
  - Does the practice offer payment plans?

Finances are often one of the most frustrating topics for veterinarians to discuss with clients because we are trained to deliver high-quality healthcare. Unfortunately, healthcare is not free. There is always a cost associated with care, and that price is often not cheap.

Our client's budget may require the clinician to adjust his or her approach to case management. Sometimes a client's budget may prevent the clinician from providing care altogether. Contracting for next steps requires veterinarians to initiate discussions about care, anticipated cost, client expectations, and patient prognosis for recovery.(10, 14) Most pet owners in the United States and Canada do not subscribe to pet health insurance.(11, 14–16) Without transparency about the anticipated care needs of the patient, and both short-term and long-term costs, clients may be taken back when they receive an unexpectedly high bill. They may feel that they have been gouged.(10, 13, 17–20) They are also unlikely to understand the value of in-clinic services unless their value is specifically spelled out, in easy-to-understand terms.

Clients are often self-conscious about financial constraints, and veterinarians may react defensively when clients question cost of care.(10, 14) Both emotions detract from patient care.

Remember that the patient represents common ground. Also recognize that just because a client declines a treatment option does not mean that she or he does not care.

Use contracting for next steps to work with the client, not against the client, to establish what is within their means and how best to make use of finite resources. Stage diagnostic tests and treatment options, when necessary, but be sure to provide the complete clinical picture as part of your explanation.

This was demonstrated effectively in the example above. The clinician did not just say, "Let's start with bloodwork" period. Instead, the clinician made it clear that bloodwork was the starting point, and that hospitalization for 3–5 days, with IV fluid therapy, would be an essential part of care.

This was stated clearly, with transparency. This constitutes effective communication. There are no hidden costs or hidden agendas. Mrs. Briar knew what to expect and in what order. Mrs. Briar also felt safe and supported.

As a veterinarian, you cannot control what clients can and cannot afford or what clients will and will not agree to do as part of the patient care plan. All you can do is be upfront and maintain a judgment-free zone within the practice.

You may not be able to change the course of healthcare for that specific patient. For whatever reason, your hands may be tied.

But at least you can set the stage for open, frank discussion. Forward planning is all about honesty. You need to establish what can be done for the patient today, so that hopefully you are both set up for a better tomorrow.

References

1. Denness C. What are consultation models for? InnovAiT. 2013;6(9):592–9.
2. Kurtz SM, Silverman JD. The Calgary–Cambridge Referenced Observation Guides: an aid to defining the curriculum and organizing the teaching in communication training programmes. Med Educ. 1996;30(2):83–9.
3. Kurtz S. Teaching and learning communication in veterinary medicine. J Vet Med Educ. 2006;33(1):11–9.
4. Silverman J, Kurtz S, Draper J. Skills for communicating with patients. Oxford: Radcliffe Medical Press; 2008.
5. Riccardi VM, Kurtz SM. Communication and counselling in health care. Springfield, IL: Charles C. Thomas; 1983.
6. Englar RE, Williams M, Weingand K. Applicability of the Calgary–Cambridge Guide to dog and cat owners for teaching veterinary clinical communications. J Vet Med Educ. 2016;43(2):143–69.
7. Adams CL, Ladner LD. Implementing a simulated client program: bridging the gap between theory and practice. J Vet Med Educ. 2004;31(2):138–45.
8. Radford A, Stockley P, Silverman J, Taylor I, Turner R, Gray C. Development, teaching, and evaluation of a consultation structure model for use in veterinary education. J Vet Med Educ. 2006;33(1):38–44.
9. Is the gold standard the old standard? 2016 [Available from: http://veterinarymedicine. dvm360.com/gold-standard-old-standard].
10. Coe JB, Adams CL, Bonnett BN. A focus group study of veterinarians' and pet owners' perceptions of the monetary aspects of veterinary care. J Am Vet Med Assoc. 2007;231(10):1510–8.
11. Coe JB, Adams CL, Bonnett BN. Prevalence and nature of cost discussions during clinical appointments in companion animal practice. J Am Vet Med Assoc. 2009;234(11):1418–24.
12. Kipperman BS, Kass PH, Rishniw M. Factors that influence small animal veterinarians' opinions and actions regarding cost of care and effects of economic limitations on patient care and outcome and professional career satisfaction and burnout. J Am Vet Med Assoc. 2017;250(7):785–94.
13. Lue TW, Pantenburg DP, Crawford PA. Impact of the owner–pet and client–veterinarian bond on the care that pets receive. J Am Vet Med Assoc. 2008;232(4):531–40.
14. Brockman BK, Taylor VA, Brockman CM. The price of unconditional love: consumer decision making for high-dollar veterinary care. J Bus Res. 2008;61(5):397–405.
15. Brown JP, Silverman JD. The current and future market for veterinarians and veterinary medical services in the United States. J Am Vet Med Assoc. 1999;215(2):161–83.
16. Paws and claws: a syndicated study on Canadian pet ownership. Toronto: Ipsos Reid; 2001.
17. Volk JO, Felsted KE, Thomas JG, Siren CW. Executive summary of the Bayer veterinary care usage study. J Am Vet Med Assoc. 2011;238(10):1275–82.
18. Volk JO, Felsted KE, Thomas JG, Siren CW. Executive summary of phase 2 of the Bayer veterinary care usage study. J Am Vet Med Assoc. 2011;239(10):1311–6.

19. Volk JO, Thomas JG, Colleran EJ, Siren CW. Executive summary of phase 3 of the Bayer veterinary care usage study. J Am Vet Med Assoc. 2014;244(7):799–802.
20. DeHaven WR. Are we really doing enough to provide the best veterinary care for our pets? J Am Vet Med Assoc. 2014;244(9):1017–8.

Part IV

Testing Your Understanding of Oral Communication Skills in Veterinary Medicine

Chapter 22

End-of-Chapter Reading Comprehension Questions

At the conclusion of each chapter, you should be able to address the following learning objectives, which test your understanding of the material. Answers have *not* been provided. Learning objectives are intended to help you navigate your own personal growth as you strengthen your understanding of the role that oral communication skills play in the veterinary consultation.

Chapter 1 – What Do Our Clients Understand?

1. Compare and contrast the concepts of medical paternalism and relationship-centered care. Consider the advantages and limitations of each.
2. Explore the concept of patient autonomy as it relates to the modern-day practice of medicine: what are the patient's rights concerning healthcare?
3. Explain your understanding of health literacy and identify at least five patient-specific factors that influence it.
4. Identify the risks that are associated with overestimating your patient's/client's health literacy.
5. Expand upon the degree of health literacy that the average American citizen possesses.
6. Poor health literacy is associated with poor health outcomes. Provide at least five examples that demostrate your understanding of this link.
7. Explain how the use of medical jargon impacts health literacy.
8. Identify at least two factors that complicate oral health literacy, and explain why.
9. Consider additional barriers to physician–patient or veterinarian–client communication and expand upon them.
10. Explain why the veterinarian–client–patient relationship is unique as compared to the medical doctor–patient relationship.
11. Define compliance.
12. Explain three reasons for poor compliance.

Chapter 2 – How Can We Help Our Clients to Understand?

1. Define good bedside manner, and identify at least five character traits that are associated with a patient-centered clinician.
2. A growing body of literature has linked the attitudes and demeanor of healthcare professionals to patient outcomes. Identify at least five aspects of patient care that effective communication improves.
3. Summarize the Kalamazoo Consensus Statement and describe the impact that it had on the delivery of patient care.
4. Communication complaints are frequently filed with veterinary licensing boards. Provide at least five examples of the most prevalent communication-based complaints that the College of Veterinarians of Ontario has reported.
5. As the discipline of clinical communication transitioned from being seen as a soft and fluffy "nice-to-have" skill to a teachable one, veterinary curricula evolved. Describe the progression of communication training in curricular content of veterinary programs throughout the United States.
6. Describe the limitations that are associated with student–student role play.
7. Outline several advantages of student role play with trained actors to simulate clients in veterinary medical programs.
8. Outline arguments for and against the use of live animals in communication exercises, specifically within standardized client encounters.

Chapter 3 – How Can We Structure the Consultation?

1. Describe the Calgary–Cambridge model, including specific details as to how it structures the clinical consultation.
2. Expand upon what is meant by these two clinical tasks:
   - building the relationship
   - providing structure.
3. Consider the limitations of consultation models. Expand upon two of these.

Chapter 4 – First Impressions

1. First impressions are long lasting. Before we enter into a consultation room, what are some of the specific actions that we can take to prepare for the visit?
2. Describe at least two advantages of preparing for the consultation.
3. In traditional medical curricula, students are trained to complete several actions as part of a standard greeting. Identify at least five of these.
4. Consider that you are meeting a client for the first time and you are unsure how to pronounce the pet's name. Outline what you might say to clarify this with the client.

5. Consider that you are meeting a client for the first time and you are unsure of the patient's sex. Outline what you might say to clarify this with the client.
6. Explain why proper introduction of team members to clients is critical to the success of the consultation.
7. Strategize how you can attend to a client's comfort in the consultation room.
8. Strategize how you can attend to the patient's comfort in the consultation room.
9. Explain why patient anxiety at the veterinary clinic might be detrimental in the long term.
10. Define low-stress or fear-free practice.
11. Identify actions that we can take to reduce the likelihood that our greeting will be perceived as a threat by our canine and feline patients.

Chapter 5 – Reflective Listening

1. A clinical conversation implies that a dialogue between two people is occurring. Why should clinical conversations be two sided?
2. It has been said that listening humanizes medicine. Identify two other reasons why doctors should listen to their patients.
3. Explain why listening can be such a challenge for some doctors.
4. Define active or reflective listening.
5. Active or reflective listening requires preparation. Explain ways in which you can prepare yourself for active listening in the consultation room.
6. Explain why active or reflective listening is essential to the practice of veterinary medicine.
7. Provide at least three examples of statements that you might say to the client to demonstrate effective use of reflective listening.

Chapter 6 - Empathy

1. Compare and contrast cognitive versus emotional empathy.
2. Explain why there are missed opportunities for displays of empathy in healthcare.
3. Because of its ability to reinforce interpersonal connectivity, empathy is associated with several positive outcomes in human healthcare. Name at least three of these outcomes.
4. Differentiate empathy from sympathy.
5. Identify clinical scenarios that are more likely to trigger emotions in clients.
6. Identify the dangers of making assumptions about how a client feels or why she or he might feel that way.
7. In the process of trying to check in with our clients and clarify their perspective, we need to be cautious about how we phrase our questions. Explain why you might want to avoid asking clients questions that begin with "Why?"

8. Provide at least three examples of empathetic actions that a doctor might choose to display during a consultation.
9. Provide at least three examples of empathetic statements that a doctor might choose to make during a consultation.
10. Define compassion fatigue and consider how empathetic displays by the clinician might contribute to this state.
11. Strategize how to guard against compassion fatigue in clinical practice.

Chapter 7 – Nonverbal Cues

1. Consider the importance of nonverbal cues in clinical communication: how much of communication is nonverbal?
2. Outline four categories of nonverbal communication.
3. Define kinesics.
4. Identify at least five factors that are associated with body language.
5. When difficult conversations arise, clients may go into "fight or flight" mode. Identify body language that you might interpret in your client as being confrontational.
6. Differentiate good posture when standing from sitting.
7. Differentiate open versus closed body posture.
8. Explain what is meant by "mirroring the client's posture" and why it may be useful in the consultation.
9. Consider how a client might interpret finger tapping or toe tapping.
10. Explain how a client might interpret the clinician looking at his or her watch.
11. Consider how a client might interpret hand-wringing.
12. In western cultures, eye contact is established between the provider and the client during the initial stage of the visit, when an appropriate greeting is made. Explain how a client might interpret complete lack of eye contact.
13. Consider how a client might interpret a direct stare, that is, uninterrupted eye contact.
14. Explain how a client might interpret the clinician having a raised or furrowed brow.
15. Consider how a client might interpret the clinician having a clenched jaw.
16. Differentiate between procedural touch and expressive touch, and explain the purpose of each.
17. Several factors appear to influence how touch is used in clinical practice and by whom. Name at least two.
18. When touch is used in clinical practice, it is often restricted to safe zones. Identify these zones of the body.
19. Define proxemics.
20. Identify at least five physical barriers in the consultation room.
21. Consider the most effective way to position yourself relative to the client, when engaging in a clinical conversation.
22. Computer use by the veterinary team has increased in the consultation room. Identify at least three deleterious effects that computer use may have on clinical communication.

Chapter 8 – Open-Ended Questions and Statements

1. The diagnostic value of history taking cannot be understated. Identify the percentage of diagnoses in human healthcare that can be made based upon data obtained from history taking alone.
2. Define signalment.
3. In addition to signalment, outline at least eight broad categories of data that should be addressed when taking a clinical history.
4. Consider the potential implications that are associated with the clinician interrupting the client during history taking.
5. Describe what is meant by the question "funnel."
6. Compare and contrast open- versus closed-ended questions. Include an explanation as to when each line of questioning is of value.
7. Provide at least three examples of open-ended questions or statements.
8. Explain how you can soften an open-ended question or statement.
9. Provide at least three examples of closed-ended questions.
10. Consider the efficiency of asking open-ended questions or statements.

Chapter 9 – Reducing Medical Jargon

1. Define medical jargon and explain its purpose.
2. Outline several limitations to using medical jargon in the consultation. Consider the perspective of both the healthcare provider and the veterinary client.
3. Medical abbreviations are intended to simplify patient care instructions. Provide at least one example of how they can actually confuse and/or hinder patient care.
4. Explain how the changing face of healthcare has complicated our use and understanding of medical jargon.
5. Consider the following medical disciplines:
   - anatomy
   - oncology
   - anesthesia
   - surgery
   - internal medicine.

   Provide at least one example from each discipline to demonstrate how patient understanding in human healthcare can be compromised by the use of medical jargon.
6. Explain how physician recommendations may be misinterpreted by human medical patients.
7. Explain how symptom management may be compromised if caregivers (that is, veterinary clients) do not understand medical terminology (that is, drug names or drug functions).
8. Explain why the use of easy-to-understand language should not be considered "dumbing it down."

9. Explain why the use of easy-to-understand language should not include "baby talk."
10. Consider strategies for overcoming the use of medical jargon in the consultation.

Chapter 10 – Enhancing Relationship-Centered Care through Partnership

1. Consider how the human–animal bond has evolved over time and how the strength of this bond may impact the delivery of healthcare.
2. Define the communication skill of partnership, and explain how it enhances relationship-centered care.
3. Give at least two reasons why veterinary clients can be considered experts in their own right.
4. Provide at least three examples of phrases that effectively communicate partnership.
5. Consider how failure to incorporate partnership statements in the consultation may impact the consultation.

Chapter 11 – Eliciting the Client's Perspective

1. Explain why it is beneficial to elicit the client's perspective.
2. Provide at least three examples of phrases that effectively elicit the client's perspective.
3. Consider the clinical consequences that may result if clinicians do not elicit the client's perspective.

Chapter 12 – Asking Permission

1. Provide at least three examples of clinical scenarios in which it would be appropriate for the veterinarian to ask a client for permission in person.
2. Explain why it might be appropriate to ask a client for permission to share via telephone.
3. Consider how asking for permission might apply to the sharing of patient data with members outside of the veterinary team.
4. Indicate which words or phrases you might use to ask a client for permission. Be specific.

Chapter 13 – Assessing the Client's Knowledge

1. Provide at least three reasons why it might be beneficial to assess your client's knowledge.
2. Indicate which words or phrases you might use to assess your client's knowledge. Be specific.
3. Consider the potential consequences if you fail to assess your client's knowledge in clinical practice.

Chapter 14 – Mapping Out the Clinical Consultation: Signposting

1. Signposting is a term that is sometimes used to refer to the communication skill, "mapping out the consultation." Define this terminology.
2. Demonstrate how to map the consultation using ordinal numbers.
3. Demonstrate how to map the consultation using transitional words or phrases.
4. Explain how signposting may be used to effectively rein in a talkative client.
5. Explain why signposting is an important skill to use to preface actions, such as reviewing the medical record during the consultation, in the client's presence.
6. Define "warning shot."
7. Indicate which words or phrases you might use to deliver a warning shot. Be specific.
8. Consider why a warning shot is beneficial in the delivery of bad news.

Chapter 15 – Summarizing and Checking in with the Client

1. Explain how the communication skill of summarizing facilitates client comprehension and recall.
2. Differentiate internal summaries from end-of-consultation summaries.
3. Provide at least three examples of clinical scenarios for which internal summaries may be of assistance.
4. Consider how end-of-consultation summaries allow the clinician to double check accuracy in terms of the information that was gathered during history taking or the mutually agreeable plan that was decided upon.
5. Define "chunk" and "check-in," and explain the purpose of each.
6. Provide an example of a clinical scenario in which a pause may constitute a check-in.
7. Provide an example of a check-in statement.
8. Explain why it is possible to overuse check-in statements, and how doing so might make the client feel.

Chapter 16 – Contracting for Next Steps

1. In clinical practice, the patient is cared for by a veterinary team. Identify the members of this team.
2. Define the communication skill, "contracting for next steps."
3. Patient care can be thought of as a contract between caregivers.
4. Identify at least five actions that the veterinarian and/or veterinary support staff may take responsibility for delivering to the client and/or patient.
5. Identify at least five actions that the veterinarian and/or veterinary support staff may ask the client to take responsibility for.
6. Patient care responsibilities, for the client, may be basic, such as observing appetite or frequency of bowel movements. However, patient care responsibilities may also

be time or labor intensive. Provide at least three examples of how this might be so.

7. Indicate which words or phrases you might use, as a veterinarian, to contract for next steps, in order to convey that you will do something for the patient or the client. Be specific.

8. Indicate which words or phrases you might use, as a veterinarian, to contract for next steps, in order to ask the client to do something for you or the patient. Be specific.

9. Explain how contracting for next steps establishes your expectations for the client.

10. Explain how contracting for next steps reinforces our role in patient care.

11. Explain why you might choose to insert the word, "please," in front of a request that you have made of the client.

12. Strategize how you will handle a clinical scenario in which the client declines what you have asked him or her to do.

Chapter 17 – Agenda-Setting and the Final Check-In

1. Recognize that interruptions are common in the consultation room. How might clients interpret the clinician interrupting their opening statement?

2. Define "agenda-setting."

3. Explain the value of agenda-setting.

4. Agenda-setting often begins with an open-ended solicitation. Provide at least three examples of how this solicitation might be phrased.

5. Explain why follow-up questions play an important role in agenda-setting.

6. Although patient "X" may present for problem "Y," you need to consider the whole patient. Explain why it is important that you do not have tunnel vision during a clinical consultation.

7. Consider the purpose of the final check-in.

8. Provide an example that indicates your understanding of how the final check-in might be phrased.

9. Explain why it is important to pair the final check-in with appropriate nonverbal cues.

10. Provide an example of what might constitute inappropriate nonverbal cues for the clinician to display during the final check-in.

Chapter 18 – Compassionate Transparency and Unconditional Positive Regard

1. Jason Coe et al. (2008) conducted a focus group study to compare veterinarians' and pet owners' expectations concerning clinical communication. Several themes emerged. Identify at least five expectations that clients have of veterinarians concerning their ability to communicate.

2. Coe et al.'s 2008 study also asked veterinarians and pet owners to discuss breakdowns in communication. Identify at least three factors that clients singled out as contributing to communication failures.

3. Explain the concept of transparency in healthcare.
4. Identify several barriers to transparency in healthcare.
5. Provide several examples of how a clinician might demonstrate transparency through words.
6. Provide several examples of how a clinician might demonstrate transparency through his or her actions.
7. Explain the concept of unconditional positive regard in healthcare.
8. Explain how it is possible to demonstrate unconditional positive regard when you, the clinician, disagree with the client.
9. I conducted a focus group study in 2015 to evaluate dog and cat owner preferences concerning clinical communication. Describe how dog and cat owners differ in their desire for unconditional positive regard.
10. Provide at least three examples of clinical scenarios that might benefit from the use of unconditional positive regard.
11. Provide several examples of how a clinician might demonstrate unconditional positive regard through words.

Chapter 19 – Using Communication Skills to Initiate the Consultation

1. The Calgary–Cambridge Referenced Observation Guides were outlined by Kurtz and Silverman in 1996 as a skills-based, patient-centered framework of the clinical consultation. The resultant model breaks the consultation down into sequential tasks. Identify these tasks.
2. In addition to the tasks that you identified in Question 1, two tasks span all stages of the consultation. Which are these?
3. Consider why preparing for the next case is essential from the point of view of the clinician's health.
4. Identify strategies for building rapport with your client in the consultation room.
5. You can use any combination of communication skills to establish the presenting complaint. However, which three skills tend to be the most helpful?

Chapter 20 – Using Communication Skills to Gather Data: History-Taking

1. Refresh your understanding of key content areas that should be a part of every new patient history.
2. Recall that clinicians make use of two lines of questioning in the consultation: open ended and closed ended. Differentiate between these two types of questions.
3. Consider which supplemental communication skills may be beneficial when taking a case history for a patient that presents to us with an illness.

Chapter 21 – Using Communication Skills to Gather Data: Explaining and Planning

1. Explain why planning is a critical part of case management.
2. The consultation tasks of explaining and planning can be time intensive, and the clinician may inadvertently overwhelm the client with detail or jargon. Which communication skills might you rely upon to trim back the amount of information that you provide to the client at one sitting?
3. Consider why it is important not to assume that a patient that presents as being "healthy" is truly healthy.
4. When patients present for illnesses, clients' emotions often run high. Guilt is a frequent undertone, particularly in discussions in which client action (or inaction) led to a less-than-ideal outcome for the patient. Consider how you can acknowledge guilt without invalidating the client's emotions.
5. Why is it detrimental to the veterinarian–client relationship to negate how a pet owner feels?
6. How might you make use of reframing statements to acknowledge the client's emotions without necessarily agreeing with them?
7. Why is client buy-in essential to patient care and the success of case management?
8. Forward planning is a part of every consultation. It is even more critical in case management for patients that are ill and for whom care needs to be expedited. Explain why this is the case.
9. Strategize how to navigate clinical cases in which there are significant financial constraints.

Chapter 23

Workbook-Style Exercises

Aristotle once said that "We are what we repeatedly do. Excellence, then, is not an act, but a habit."

Practice does not make perfect, but it is a way to improve proficiency. The following exercises are intended to deepen your understanding of the communication skills that were covered in Chapters 1–21.

Exercise 23.1 – Defining Communication Skills I

Match each communication skill that is listed below in the left-hand column with the appropriate definition in the right-hand column.

A. Transparency
B. Open-ended question
C. Nonverbal cue
D. Empathy
E. Reflective listening
F. Regard

_____ 1. Asking the client something that cannot be answered with a simple one-word answer, such as "yes" or "no."

_____ 2. Restating back to the client what it is that s/he shared in order to let him/him know that s/he was heard.

_____ 3. Considering the client as a unique individual and making an effort to withhold judgment in order to improve connectivity and mutual understanding.

_____ 4. Being able to understand and share the feelings of another individual; putting yourself in his/her shoes and considering what it might be like to be him/her.

_____ 5. Being open and honest with the client about news that s/he may not want to hear, such as poor prognosis or terminal diagnosis.

_____ 6. That which is unspoken, yet communicates something to the client through body language or body positioning.

Exercise 23.2 – Defining Communication Skills II

Match each communication skill that is listed below in the left-hand column with the appropriate definition in the right-hand column.

A. Eliciting the client's perspective
B. Asking permission
C. Signposting
D. Easy-to-understand language
E. Chunk and check
F. Assessing client's knowledge
G. Offering partnership
H. Summarizing
I. Contracting for next steps
J. Final check-in

_____ 1. Using terms that are readily understood or relatable when describing or explaining medical conditions and treatment options.

_____ 2. Replacing "I" statements with "we" and being certain to ask the client to participate actively in discussions so as to honor his/her place as part of the veterinary team.

_____ 3. Breaking down big pieces of information into smaller bits to prevent information overload.

_____ 4. Reviewing what was discussed in brief as a way to check for accuracy and clarity of information-sharing.

_____ 5. Asking how the client feels about a particular situation or experience.

_____ 6. Taking a moment at the end of the appointment to make sure that the client is on the same page and to see if any information remains unclear.

_____ 7. Planning ahead by establishing what roles both the veterinarian and the client will play in the care of the patient.

_____ 8. Providing the client with an overview or 'road map' of where the conversation is going in order to structure the visit.

_____ 9. Establishing what the client already understands about a given disease process, test result, diagnosis, or treatment plan to determine what additional details are necessary to share.

_____ 10. Asking the client if it is okay to perform specific tests or procedures.

Exercise 23.3 – Examples of Communication Skills in Use I

Match each communication skill that is listed below in the left-hand column with an appropriate example in the right-hand column.

A. Transparency

B. Open-ended question

C. Nonverbal cue

D. Empathy

E. Reflective listening

F. Regard

_____ 1. "Of course you didn't mean for this to happen. You have always looked out for Turnip's health and have only ever done what you thought was best for him."

_____ 2. "My heart breaks for you. I don't know what I would do if I had to make the decision that you are being forced to make."

_____ 3. "Osteosarcoma is a very aggressive disease. Given that it has already spread through Priscilla's bloodstream into her lungs, I'm afraid that she doesn't have much time left."

_____ 4. Leaning forward into the conversation and maintaining eye contact.

_____ 5. "It sounds as though Jellyroll had a very difficult night because he experienced two seizures, each of which lasted for five minutes, and he hasn't been acting right since."

_____ 6. "How is Buttons fitting in to the household?"

Exercise 23.4 – Examples of Communication Skills in Use II

Match each communication skill that is listed below in the left-hand column with an appropriate example in the right-hand column.

A. Eliciting the client's perspective

B. Asking permission

C. Signposting

D. Easy-to-understand language

E. Chunk and check

F. Assessing client's knowledge

G. Offering partnership

H. Summarizing

I. Contracting for next steps

J. Final check-in

_____ 1. "Parvovirus is an infection that target's your dog's digestive tract. It causes a huge amount of water loss through diarrhea. Affected puppies get very dehydrated, very quickly. They can die. Does that make sense?"

_____ 2. "Would it be okay if I took Princeton to the treatment area to trim his nails? He tends to do better for us in the back."

_____ 3. "Have you ever heard that dogs and cats can get bladder stones?"

_____ 4. "First, I would like to discuss Fifi's bloodwork with you. Then I would like to consider the options that are available to you at this time."

_____ 5. "I need you to telephone with an update after the holiday weekend so that I can hear if the anti-anxiety medication helped to get Trolley through the fireworks."

_____ 6. "There is a plug of some sort that is blocking the exit of urine from his body. We need to remove the obstruction so that he is able to pee without straining."

_____ 7. "Is there anything else that I can do for you today?"

_____ 8. "How do you feel about having to administer subcutaneous fluids to Jenny?"

_____ 9. "To recap, Banjo's bloodwork showed mild anemia and high cholesterol. In combination with his hair loss around his collar and along his tail, this makes me suspect that he could be hypothyroid. The lab will do some follow-up tests that should clarify this for us in about three days."

_____ 10. "I would like for us to work together to find the best solution for Juniper."

Exercise 23.5 – Open- vs Closed-Ended Questions I

History taking requires you, the clinician, to obtain important details about patient health and lifestyle in order for you to conduct a thorough veterinary consultation. In order to take a comprehensive patient history, you need to ask a number of questions. Using the funnel approach and a mix of closed- and open-ended questions can be helpful.

The following statements and questions are items that you might choose to ask the client during history taking.

Identify whether each statement or question is closed- (C) or open (O)-ended in the blank provided.

_____ 1. Did Michael cough all night?

_____ 2. Show me what he looked like when you thought he was having trouble breathing.

_____ 3. Did he extend his head and neck like this when he was trying to breathe?

_____ 4. Did he cough anything up?

_____ 5. Describe the contents of what he produced when he retched.

_____ 6. Can you explain for me how he acted after he threw up?

_____ 7. What do you think is going on?

_____ 8. Tell me what concerns you most about Blitz.

_____ 9. Does Andy seem confused?

_____ 10. How would you describe your home environment?

Exercise 23.6 – Open- vs Closed-Ended Questions II

History taking requires you, the clinician, to obtain important details about patient health and lifestyle in order for you to conduct a thorough veterinary consultation. In order to take a comprehensive patient history, you need to ask a number of questions. Using the funnel approach and a mix of closed- and open-ended questions can be helpful.

The following statements and questions are items that you might choose to ask the client during history taking.

Identify whether each statement or question is closed (C) or open (O)-ended in the blank provided.

_____ 1. Tell me how you came to adopt Crys.

_____ 2. How are you and Lowell getting along?

_____ 3. Did Sage use the litterbox overnight?

_____ 4. What makes you say that?

_____ 5. How would you like us to proceed?

_____ 6. What is your goal for today's visit?

_____ 7. Can you deposit at least half of the estimate for today's care?

_____ 8. Does the estimate seem reasonable?

_____ 9. Is Christian an outdoor cat?

_____ 10. Tell me about Christopher's lifestyle.

Exercise 23.7 – Converting Closed-Ended Questions into Open-Ended Questions

History taking requires you, the clinician, to obtain important details about patient health and lifestyle in order for you to conduct a thorough veterinary consultation. In order to take a comprehensive patient history, you need to ask a number of questions. Using the funnel approach and a mix of closed- and open-ended questions can be helpful.

The following questions are closed-ended. Make each one open-ended.

1. "Is Tilly vomiting up blood?"

   _____

2. "Is Trill in labor?"

   _____

3. "Does Tidbit get along with Bruno?"

   _____

4. "Does Fishstick eat kibble or canned food?"

   _____

5. "Do you feed Merlot snacks?"

   _____

6. "Do you think that Champagne is overweight?"

   _____

7. "Does Pumpkin exercise?"

   _____

8. "Are you willing to take Pillsbury for walks?"

   _____

9. "Do you frequent the dog park?"

   _____

10. "Is it possible for you to medicate Dreamboat with a pill?"

    _____

Exercise 23.8 – Converting Open-Ended Questions into Closed-Ended Questions

History taking requires you, the clinician, to obtain important details about patient health and lifestyle in order for you to conduct a thorough veterinary consultation. In order to take a comprehensive patient history, you need to ask a number of questions. Using the funnel approach and a mix of closed- and open-ended questions can be helpful.

The following questions and statements are open-ended. Make each one closed-ended.

1. "How is housetraining coming along?"

   _____

2. "Describe Eggplant's appetite."

   _____

3. "How do you feel about giving insulin shots to Frenchie?"

   _____

4. "How would you cope if Sugar never went into remission and you had to manage her diabetes for life?"

   _____

5. "Paint a picture for me of what a typical day is in the life of Darcy."

   _____

6. "Describe what you see when you say that Lizzie has a seizure."

   _____

7. "Share what is going through your mind right now about Edna's diagnosis."

   _____

8. "Describe what is normal in terms of Fluffington's behavior?"

   _____

9. "Tell me what you're noticing at home that makes you worried Ghost is fainting."

   _____

10. "Tell me about the discharge that you've been noticing at the tip of Jack's penis."

    _____

Exercise 23.9 – Reflective Listening I

Reflective listening is an essential skill in veterinary practice. Because veterinary patients cannot speak our language to share their own story with us, we must rely heavily upon the client's perspective to gain insight into the patient's presenting complaint.

When clients share important details with us about their pets' healthcare, it is important that they feel heard.

Five statements below have been listed, from the client's perspective.

For each statement, create a response that you, the veterinarian, might say aloud to convey the communication skill of reflective listening.

1. Client's statement: "Tadpole hasn't kept anything down for the past 3 days. Not even water. He doesn't even have anything left in his stomach to bring up, so now he's dry-heaving."
    Your response: _____

    _____

2. Client's statement: "My greatest concern is making sure that Panda isn't in any pain. I don't want him to suffer. I would rather let him go, than force him to live in pain."
    Your response: _____

    _____

3. Client's statement: "Pickle is the only one in my life right now. If something happened to him, I would be lost. You have to fix him. He's all I have."
    Your response: _____

    _____

4. Client's statement: "Sampson loves playing Frisbee. When we were at the park yesterday, he chased the Frisbee for about two hours, on and off. At one point, he landed hard and yelped. Since then, he hasn't wanted to put weight on his back leg – the right one. I'm concerned that he broke something."
    Your response: _____

    _____

5. Client's statement: "I know you always say not to feed Pepper table scraps. But it was a holiday – and we were outside barbequing. And Pepper just looks at you with those wide eyes like he's starving. I give in. Every time. It seemed like a good idea until last night. He had explosive diarrhea. He asked to go outside ten or twenty times. I couldn't catch a break. Every time I went to bed, he had me up again."
    Your response: _____

    _____

Exercise 23.10 – Reflective Listening II

Reflective listening is an essential skill in veterinary practice. Because veterinary patients cannot speak our language to share their own story with us, we rely heavily upon the client's perspective to gain insight into the patient's presenting complaint.

When clients share important details with us about their pets' healthcare, it is important that they feel heard.

Five statements below have been listed, from the client's perspective.

For each statement, create a response that you, the veterinarian, might say aloud to convey the communication skill of reflective listening.

1. Client's statement: "I don't know what to do. On one hand, surgery could buy him an extra six months to a year of life. I wouldn't have to say goodbye. We could have another good year together. But is that selfish? How much am I asking him to go through on my behalf? Is that fair? Is that right? I am so confused. I don't know how to help him and I want to make the right choice for him, not because it's what's best for me."

   Your response: _____

   _____

   _____

2. Client's statement: "Cheeto has never been good in the car. From the first day we brought him home, he hasn't tolerated the ride. He gets motion sickness – and bad! It's to the point that I don't even want to bring him in to see you because it's just miserable – for him and me! And we're talking just short distances – ten minutes tops! Now we have to drive cross-country! How is that supposed to work?"

   Your response: _____

   _____

   _____

3. Client's statement: "Solo has always been a one-person dog. For 10 years, he's only known me. We've been together, just him and I. He never liked friends coming over, so we didn't force it. But now that I'm engaged, that's no longer an option. He's going to have to get used to sharing me with Derek. But every time Derek comes to visit, Solo growls at him and bares his teeth. I yell at him, but he snaps back. I don't see this transition working."

   Your response: _____

   _____

   _____

4. Client's statement: "Pivot started sneezing last week. At first, I thought it was allergies, so I let it go. It wasn't that frequent, so it really didn't bother me. But then it was paired with thick yellow snot. It got everywhere – all over me, the floor. It's getting worse. He wakes up sneezing. I can't get sleep because he's sneezing. And now his eyes are drippy, too. He was squinting his right eye yesterday as if it hurt, now both seem half-open. That seems a lot more serious than just allergies."

   Your response: _____

   _____

   _____

5. Client's statement: "When Trapper started to throw up on Saturday night, I tried what had worked for him in the past. I picked up his water bowl to give his belly a rest. I withheld his breakfast on Sunday. It seemed to work okay, until evening. He looked like he was up for eating, so I offered him dinner – just a half-portion. He took one bite, then started licking his lips. Then gagging. Then he upchucked – all over the floor. Clearly he's not getting better. That's why I called. We really could use your help."

   Your response: _____

   _____

   _____

Exercise 23.11 – Empathy I

The capacity to demonstrate empathy is an essential skill for the development and maintenance of interpersonal relationships.

1. There are two different types of empathy:
    - cognitive empathy
    - emotional empathy.

    How do these types of empathy differ?

    Your response: _____

    _____

    _____

    _____

2. Consider the following clinical vignette:

    You are an associate veterinarian at a companion animal practice. Your patient is a 10-year-old, castrated male Great Dane dog, Lion. You have just diagnosed the dog with proximal tibial osteosarcoma of the right pelvic leg. Three-view thoracic radiographs are negative for evidence of metastasis. You outline the treatment options, which include palliative care, right pelvic limb amputation, and chemotherapy.

    In response to treatment recommendations, your client makes the following statement:

    I'm not ready to let Lion go. He's been with me since my first semester in law school. He's seen me through the very worst of times – times when I didn't think there was a way out. I can't imagine life without him. But he's in a lot of pain. I'm worried about doing the wrong thing for the right reasons – keeping him alive to delay the inevitable.

    Give an example of a response that you might make that demonstrates <u>cognitive</u> empathy.

    Your response: _____

    _____

    _____

    _____

    _____

Give an example of a response that you might make that demonstrates <u>emotional</u> empathy.

Your response: _____

_____

_____

_____

_____

Exercise 23.12 – Empathy II

There are many missed opportunities for empathy in healthcare. Some clinical scenarios make us uncomfortable and we do not know how to respond. We may be unsure what constitutes an appropriate response. We may not even know where to begin, in terms of what to say or do. So rather than use it as an opportunity to connect to our client through empathy, we do something else. We offer advice. Maybe we change the subject or even terminate the conversation.

Consider the following clinical vignette.

You are an associate veterinarian at a companion animal practice. Your patient is an 11-year-old, spayed female Russian blue cat, Katerina, that presented for acute onset of vomiting and weight loss. Physical examination disclosed cranial abdominal pain and a mass effect within the cranial-to-mid-abdomen. Exploratory laparotomy confirmed the presence of a friable tumor that bridged two lobes of the liver. Partial liver lobectomies were performed, with tissue submitted for histopathology. The diagnosis is biliary cystadenocarcinoma. When you share this with the client, she begins to cry.

When she is able to compose herself, your client makes the following statement:

"There's no reason for me to live without Katerina."

This statement makes you very uncomfortable, so you say the first thing that comes to mind, even though it invalidates your client's emotions:

"Don't be silly. You have a lot going for you!"

Give an example of a response that would have more effectively demonstrated <u>cognitive</u> empathy.

Your response: _____

_____

_____

_____

Give an example of a response that would have more effectively demonstrated <u>emotional</u> empathy.

Your response: _____

_____

_____

_____

How might you effectively make use of a partnership statement to connect to your client?

Your response: _____

_____

_____

_____

You are concerned about the client's mental stability. Even though veterinarians are not licensed therapists, the client's statement has you worried that she might harm herself.

How might you elicit her perspective to gauge the likelihood that this will happen?

Your response: _____

_____

_____

_____

Your client catches your drift and clarifies:

"Oh, no, I didn't mean that! It's just a figure of speech. What I really mean is that I've had Katerina for half of my adult life. I just assumed she'd be with me forever. I never thought of what life would be like without her."

How might you effectively make use of reflective listening to let your client know that she has been heard?

Your response: _____

_____

_____

_____

Exercise 23.13 – Nonverbal Cues

Nonverbal cues are an essential part of interpersonal communication.

Four categories of nonverbal communication were introduced in Chapter 7.

Match each communication skill that is listed below in the left-hand column with the appropriate definition in the right-hand column.

A. Kinesics

B. Proxemics

C. Paralanguage

D. Autonomic shits

_____ 1. Volume, rate of speech, pausing, and tone

_____ 2. The study of gestures and body movements

_____ 3. Directed responses by nervous system that are outside of our control

_____ 4. The use of space: how space is configured to fit our needs

Exercise 23.14 – Barriers to Communication

In veterinary practice, a consideration of proxemics includes physical barriers that get in between the client and the veterinarian.

Name at least five NON-LIVING items in the examination room that could be considered physical barriers to communication.

1. _____

2. _____

3. _____

4. _____

5. _____

For each item that you have listed above, consider a potential strategy that you might use to get around it being a barrier:

1. _____

2. _____

3. _____

4. _____

5. _____

Exercise 23.15 – Reducing Barriers to Communication

In veterinary practice, communication is not limited to the veterinary team. Communication also takes place between veterinary patients. We must consider how these interactions may impact our patients. This includes a consideration of nonverbal cues, such as proxemics. Proxemics includes the spatial orientation of the waiting area.

It can be stressful for cats to encounter dogs in the waiting area. Identify at least three strategies to minimize this stress.

1. _____

2. _____

3. _____

Exercise 23.16 – Body Language and Communication I

Body language constitutes an important part of nonverbal communication.

Key components of body language have been listed below. Indicate how to make use of each item to FACILITATE clinical conversations with clients.

1. Body posture
   Your response: _____

   _____

2. Eye contact
   Your response: _____

   _____

3. Facial expressions
   Your response: _____

   _____

4. Gestures
   Your response: _____

   _____

5. Touch
   Your response: _____

   _____

Exercise 23.17 – Body Language and Communication II

Body language constitutes an important part of nonverbal communication.

Key components of body language have been listed below. Indicate one INAPPROPRIATE WAY of making use of each item below that will HINDER clinical conversations with clients.

1. Body posture
    Your response: _____

    _____

2. Eye contact
    Your response: _____

    _____

3. Facial expressions
    Your response: _____

    _____

4. Gestures
    Your response: _____

    _____

5. Touch
    Your response: _____

    _____

Exercise 23.18 – Medical Jargon I

Doctors-in-training, residents, and new graduates are likely to rely upon medical jargon to convey information to their patients. Medical terminology is frequently employed in conversations with patients about healthcare, yet such terms are often poorly understood by those without a medical background. An important clinical skill is the ability to replace medical jargon with easy-to-understand language. Note that during a consultation, you may still choose to make use of the medical term; however, when you incorporate jargon into your correspondence with clients, it is your responsibility to translate it.

For each procedural term below, please provide an appropriate translation that could be used with a client during a clinical consultation.

1. Orchiectomy
   Your response: _____

   _____

2. Ovariohysterectomy
   Your response: _____

   _____

3. Cystotomy
   Your response: _____

   _____

4. Thoracocentesis
   Your response: _____

   _____

5. Ovariectomy
   Your response: _____

   _____

Exercise 23.19 – Medical Jargon II

Doctors-in-training, residents, and new graduates are likely to rely upon medical jargon to convey information to their patients. Medical terminology is frequently employed in conversations with patients about healthcare, yet such terms are often poorly understood by those without a medical background. An important clinical skill is the ability to replace medical jargon with easy-to-understand language. Note that during a consultation, you may still choose to make use of the medical term; however, when you incorporate jargon into your correspondence with clients, it is your responsibility to translate it.

For each anatomical term below, please provide an appropriate translation that could be used with a client during a clinical consultation.

1. Inguinal
   Your response: _____

   _____

2. Umbilical
   Your response: _____

   _____

3. Perineal
   Your response: _____

   _____

4. Axillary
   Your response: _____

   _____

5. Pedal
   Your response: _____

   _____

Exercise 23.20 – Medical Jargon III

Doctors-in-training, residents, and new graduates are likely to rely upon medical jargon to convey information to their patients. Medical terminology is frequently employed in conversations with patients about healthcare, yet such terms are often poorly understood by those without a medical background. An important clinical skill is the ability to replace medical jargon with easy-to-understand language. Note that during a consultation, you may still choose to make use of the medical term; however, when you incorporate jargon into your correspondence with clients, it is your responsibility to translate it.

For each anatomical term below, please provide an appropriate translation that could be used with a client during a clinical consultation.

1. Cranial

    Your response: _____

    _____

2. Caudal

    Your response: _____

    _____

3. Lateral

    Your response: _____

    _____

4. Medial

    Your response: _____

    _____

5. Rostral

    Your response: _____

    _____

Exercise 23.21 – Medical Jargon IV

Doctors-in-training, residents, and new graduates are likely to rely upon medical jargon to convey information to their patients. Medical terminology is frequently employed in conversations with patients about healthcare, yet such terms are often poorly understood by those without a medical background. An important clinical skill is the ability to replace medical jargon with easy-to-understand language. Note that during a consultation, you may still choose to make use of the medical term; however, when you incorporate jargon into your correspondence with clients, it is your responsibility to translate it.

For each procedural term below, please provide an appropriate translation that could be used with a client during a clinical consultation.

1. Tarsorrhaphy
   Your response: _____

   _____

2. Laparotomy
   Your response: _____

   _____

3. Enucleation
   Your response: _____

   _____

4. Splenectomy
   Your response: _____

   _____

5. Lung lobectomy
   Your response: _____

   _____

Exercise 23.22 – Medical Jargon V

Doctors-in-training, residents, and new graduates are likely to rely upon medical jargon to convey information to their patients. Medical terminology is frequently employed in conversations with patients about healthcare, yet such terms are often poorly understood by those without a medical background. An important clinical skill is the ability to replace medical jargon with easy-to-understand language. Note that during a consultation, you may still choose to make use of the medical term; however, when you incorporate jargon into your correspondence with clients, it is your responsibility to translate it.

For each clinical pathology term below, please provide an appropriate translation that could be used with a client during a clinical consultation.

1. Anemia
    Your response: _____

    _____

2. Leukocytosis
    Your response: _____

    _____

3. Thrombocytopenia
    Your response: _____

    _____

4. Azotemia
    Your response: _____

    _____

5. Hypercholesterolemia
    Your response: _____

    _____

Exercise 23.23 – Medical Jargon VI

Doctors-in-training, residents, and new graduates are likely to rely upon medical jargon to convey information to their patients. Medical terminology is frequently employed in conversations with patients about healthcare, yet such terms are often poorly understood by those without a medical background. An important clinical skill is the ability to replace medical jargon with easy-to-understand language. Note that during a consultation, you may still choose to make use of the medical term; however, when you incorporate jargon into your correspondence with clients, it is your responsibility to translate it.

For each imaging term below, please provide an appropriate translation that could be used with a client during a clinical consultation.

1. Radiograph
   Your response: _____

   _____

   _____

2. Echocardiogram
   Your response: _____

   _____

   _____

3. Electrocardiogram (ECG)
   Your response: _____

   _____

   _____

4. Contrast urography
   Your response: _____

   _____

   _____

5. Barium study of the GI tract
   Your response: _____

   _____

   _____

Exercise 23.24 – Partnership

Today's veterinary client desires to be an active participant in decision-making for the pet. Healthcare is therefore seen as an opportunity for partnership, in which the veterinarian and client come together as one team for the benefit of common ground, the patient.

Sentences have been listed below that might be stated by the clinician to the client in general practice. These sentences LACK partnership.

Transform each sentence below into a statement that CONVEYS partnership. You may consider statements that BLEND partnership and eliciting the client's perspective, because quite often these will overlap.

1. I am prescribing an ophthalmic medication that comes in two formulations.
    Your response: _____

    _____

    _____

2. I have determined the best way to manage Harrison's anxiety.
    Your response: _____

    _____

    _____

3. I am telling you that the best way to proceed is with hind limb amputation.
    Your response: _____

    _____

    _____

4. My plan is to run bloodwork first, then consider hospitalization if Julip's kidney values are off the charts.
    Your response: _____

    _____

    _____

5. I have decided that the adrenocorticotropin hormone (ACTH) stim test is much better than the Low-Dose Dexamethasone Suppression (LDDS) test.
    Your response: _____

    _____

    _____

Exercise 23.25 – Eliciting the Client's Perspective

Eliciting the client's perspective is an important communication skill because it invites the client to share. The client that is allowed to share is more likely to feel heard by the clinician. Clients want to be heard. They value two-way conversation with healthcare providers because they see it as a sign of respect.

Sentences have been listed below that might be stated by the clinician to the client in general practice. These sentences would benefit from follow-up statements that elicit the client's perspective.

Add a sentence to each statement below that appropriately elicits the client's perspective.

1. Chronic kidney disease (CKD) can be challenging for cat owners.
   Your response: _____

   _____

   _____

2. I know that it comes as quite a surprise for you that Marshmallow is diabetic.
   Your response: _____

   _____

   _____

3. We need to keep a close watch on Ginny because eye ulcers can progress very fast. I'd also suggest that she wear an Elizabethan collar at all times. That should prevent her from creating more damage to herself.
   Your response: _____

   _____

   _____

4. I know we've covered a lot of material today, in terms of Teddy Bear's vaccine schedule.
   Your response: _____

   _____

   _____

5. Pilling a cat is never as easy as it looks, but it is essential that Wilson get his medication.
   Your response: _____

   _____

   _____

Exercise 23.26 – Assessing the Client's Knowledge

Assessing the client's knowledge is an important communication tool that helps you to explore what your client knows about a disease, disease process, diagnostic or treatment plan, medication, therapy, or prognosis.

When you invite your client to share their knowledge with you, you are accepting them as contributors to the conversation and to patient care. This demonstrates respect. The client feels welcome to share his or her knowledge base. The client may also feel less reluctant to share that he or she does not know something.

Sentences have been listed below that might be stated by the clinician to the client in general practice. These sentences would benefit from follow-up statements that assess the client's knowledge.

Add a sentence to each statement below that appropriately assesses the client's knowledge.

1. At-home blood sugar monitoring for diabetics can be challenging for cat owners.
   Your response: _____

   _____

   _____

2. Based upon Tilly's work-up, she has chronic kidney disease (CKD).
   Your response: _____

   _____

   _____

3. Pike would benefit from a 10-day course of metronidazole.
   Your response: _____

   _____

   _____

4. Skipper needs to receive a tapering dose of prednisone.
   Your response: _____

   _____

   _____

5. The ultrasound report shows that Trolley has a kidney stone.
   Your response: _____

   _____

   _____

Exercise 23.27 – Signposting I

Mapping out the consultation, or signposting, is a way to provide structure to the consultation. We acknowledge openly where the conversation is headed and what we are choosing to discuss now versus that which we will discuss later.

We can signpost using ordinal numbers. List at least five of these below:

1. _____

2. _____

3. _____

4. _____

5. _____

Exercise 23.28 – Signposting II

We can also signpost using transitions. List at least five transitional words or phrases that can be used for signposting:

1. _____

2. _____

3. _____

4. _____

5. _____

Exercise 23.29 – Signposting and Transparency

Consider the following clinical vignette.

> Your patient is a 6-year-old, spayed female domestic short hair (DSH) cat, Rose, that ingested lilies 48-hours ago. She presents with a 12-hour history of vomiting and anorexia. While the bloodwork is pending, you discuss the need for hospitalization and her guarded prognosis. Your client does not appreciate the severity of the situation, and asks for you to trim her nails.

How might you signpost to convey that you will be happy to trim her nails after she has been stabilized?

Your response: _____

_____

_____

How might you make use of transparency to convey that this situation is life-threatening?

Your response: _____

_____

_____

In response to your use of transparency above, the client begins to cry. It is difficult to make out her words, but you definitely hear her say, "This is all my fault."

How might you respond to the client using unconditional positive regard?

Your response: _____

_____

_____

Exercise 23.30 – Putting It All Together

Consider the following clinical vignette.

> Your patient is a 3-year-old, intact male Akita dog, Bitzie, who presents on emergency after being hit by an automobile. He sustains an open right femoral fracture, which the client is prepared to have you operate on; however, you advise that he be admitted first for observation and stabilization instead of going straight to surgery. Distal to the site of the fracture, the remainder of the limb appears mangled. He is non-weight-bearing and has no deep pain in the right pelvic leg. He is tachypneic, but not yet dyspneic. Thoracic radiographs are unremarkable. You are concerned that they will worsen over time.

> How might you use a warning shot to indicate that hit-by-car (HBC) patients often decompensate?

> Your response: _____

> _____

> _____

> How might you make use of signposting to indicate that it is best to postpone Bitzie's surgery?

> Your response: _____

> _____

> _____

> Your client picks up on your reluctance to go to surgery right this minute, and questions you for the delay: "Isn't it better to repair fractures as soon as they occur, to improve healing?"

> How might you make use of reflective listening to indicate that your client's concerns have been heard?

> Your response: _____

> _____

> _____

How might you make use of asking for permission in this clinical scenario?

Your response: _____

_____

_____

You are concerned about lung contusions. How might you assess the client's knowledge about this condition?

Your response: _____

_____

_____

Your client says that she agrees with your decision to hold off on surgery, but you can see that she is not convinced. How might you elicit her perspective?

Your response: _____

_____

_____

Chapter 24

Answer Key to Workbook-Style Exercises

Exercise 23.1 – Defining Communication Skills I

B   1. Asking the client something that cannot be answered with a simple one-word answer, such as "yes" or "no."

E   2. Restating back to the client what it is that s/he shared in order to let him/him know that s/he was heard.

F   3. Considering the client as a unique individual and making an effort to withhold all judgment in order to improve connectivity and mutual understanding.

D   4. Being able to understand and share the feelings of another individual; putting yourself in his/her shoes and considering what it might be like to be him/her.

A   5. Being open and honest with the client about news that s/he may not want to hear, such as poor prognosis or terminal diagnosis.

C   6. That which is unspoken, yet communicates something to the client through body language or body positioning.

Exercise 23.2 – Defining Communication Skills II

D   1. Using terms that are readily understood or relatable when describing or explaining medical conditions and treatment options.

G   2. Replacing "I" statements with "we" and being certain to ask the client to participate actively in discussions so as to honor his/her place as part of the veterinary team.

E   3. Breaking down big pieces of information into smaller bits to prevent information overload.

H   4. Reviewing what was discussed in brief as a way to check for accuracy and clarity of information-sharing.

A   5. Asking how the client feels about a particular situation or experience.

J   6. Taking a moment at the end of the appointment to make sure that the client is on the same page and to see if any information remains unclear.

I   7. Planning ahead by establishing what roles both the veterinarian and the client will play in the care of the patient.

C   8. Providing the client with an overview or 'road map' of where the conversation is going in order to structure the visit.

F   9. Establishing what the client already understands about a given disease process, test result, diagnosis, or treatment plan to determine what additional details are necessary to share.

B   10. Asking the client if it is okay to perform specific tests or procedures.

Exercise 23.3 – Examples of Communication Skills in Use I

F   1. "Of course you didn't mean for this to happen. You have always looked out for Turnip's health and have only ever done what you thought was best for him."

D   2. "My heart breaks for you. I don't know what I would do if I had to make the decision that you are being forced to make."

A   3. "Osteosarcoma is a very aggressive disease. Given that it has already spread through Priscilla's bloodstream into her lungs, I'm afraid that she doesn't have much time left."

C   4. Leaning forward into the conversation and maintaining eye contact.

E   5. "It sounds as though Jellyroll had a very difficult night because he experienced two seizures, each of which lasted for five minutes, and he hasn't been acting right since."

B   6. "How is Buttons fitting in to the household?"

Exercise 23.4 – Examples of Communication Skills in Use II

E   1. "Parvovirus is an infection that targets your dog's digestive tract. It causes a huge amount of water loss through diarrhea. Affected puppies get very dehydrated, very quickly. They can die. Does that make sense?"

B   2. "Would it be okay if I took Princeton to the treatment area to trim his nails? He tends to do better for us in the back."

F   3. "Have you ever heard that dogs and cats can get bladder stones?"

C   4. "First, I would like to discuss Fifi's bloodwork with you. Then I would like to consider the options that are available to you at this time."

I   5. "I need you to telephone with an update after the holiday weekend so that I can hear if the anti-anxiety medication helped to get Trolley through the fireworks."

D   6. "There is a plug of some sort that is blocking the exit of urine from his body. We need to remove the obstruction so that he is able to pee without straining."

J   7. "Is there anything else that I can do for you today?"

A   8. "How do you feel about having to administer subcutaneous fluids to Jenny?"

H   9. "To recap, Banjo's bloodwork showed a mild anemia and elevations in cholesterol. In combination with his hair loss around his collar and along his tail, this makes me suspect that he could be hypothyroid. The lab will do some follow-up tests that should clarify this for us in about three days."

G   10. "I would like for us to work together to find the best solution for Juniper."

Exercise 23.5 – Open- vs Closed-Ended Questions I

C   1. Did Michael cough all night?
O   2. Show me what he looked like when you thought he was having trouble breathing.
C   3. Did he extend his head and neck like this when he was trying to breathe?
C   4. Did he cough anything up?
O   5. Describe the contents of what he produced when he retched.
O   6. Can you explain for me how he acted after he threw up?
O   7. What do you think is going on?
O   8. Tell me what concerns you most about Blitz.
C   9. Does Andy seem confused?
O   10. How would you describe your home environment?

Exercise 23.6 – Open- vs Closed-Ended Questions II

O   1. Tell me how you came to adopt Crys?
O   2. How are you and Lowell getting along?
C   3. Did Sage use the litterbox overnight?
O   4. What makes you say that?
O   5. How would you like us to proceed?
O   6. What is your goal for today's visit?
C   7. Can you deposit at least half of the estimate for today's care?
C   8. Does the estimate seem reasonable?
C   9. Is Christian an outdoor cat?
O   10. Tell me about Christopher's lifestyle.

Exercise 23.7 – Converting Closed-Ended Questions into Open-Ended Questions

1. "Is Tilly vomiting up blood?"
   - "Tell me about Tilly's vomit."
   - "Describe the content of Tilly's vomit."
2. "Is Trill in labor?"
   - "Tell me what Trill is doing that suggests she is in labor."
   - "Tell me what you are noticing that makes you think that Trill is in labor."
3. "Does Tidbit get along with Bruno?"
   - "Share with me how Bruno and Tidbit are getting along."
   - "Can you describe the relationship between Bruno and Tidbit?"
4. "Does Fishstick eat kibble or canned food?"
   - "Tell me about Fishstick's diet."
   - "Can you tell me what you feed Fishstick?"

5. "Do you feed Merlot snacks?"
   - "How does Merlot snack?"
   - "Tell me about Merlot's snacking habits."
6. "Do you think that Champagne is overweight?"
   - "How do you feel about Champagne's weight?"
7. "Does Pumpkin exercise?"
   - "Tell me about Pumpkin's exercise habits."
8. "Are you willing to take Pillsbury for walks?"
   - "Tell me about your schedule as it relates to the exercise that Pillsbury has been getting."
   - "How would you feel about taking Pillsbury for walks?"
9. "Do you frequent the dog park?"
   - "How would you feel about visiting the dog park?"
10. "Is it possible for you to medicate Dreamboat with a pill?"
    - "Tell me about the possibilities of you medicating Dreamboat."
    - "Share with me your thoughts about pilling Dreamboat."

Note that this exercise does not have one right answer per question. There are multiple right answers for each question. If your phrasing is not listed above, then that does not necessarily mean that you are incorrect. Double-check with your instructor if there is any question or concern.

Exercise 23.8 – Converting Open-Ended Questions into Closed-Ended Questions

1. "How is housetraining coming along?"
   - "Is housetraining going well?"
   - "Is he using the pee pads?"
   - "Is he wetting inside of the house?"
   - "Is he having accidents?"
2. "Describe Eggplant's appetite."
   - "Is Eggplant eating well for you?"
   - "Is Eggplant a picky eater?"
   - "Does Eggplant eat what you feed him?"
   - "Is Eggplant a good eater?"
3. "How do you feel about giving insulin shots to Frenchie?"
   - "Are you willing to give insulin shots to Frenchie?"
   - "Are you able to administer insulin to Frenchie?"
   - "Do insulin shots sound possible for you to do to manage Frenchie's diabetes?"
4. "How would you cope if Sugar never went into remission and you had to manage her diabetes for life?"
   - "It is not always possible for cats to go into remission from their diabetes. If that were the case for Sugar, would you be able to give insulin shots to her for life?"

5. "Paint a picture for me of what a typical day is in the life of Darcy."
   - "Is Darcy active during the day?"
   - "Does Darcy go out during the day?"
   - "Does Darcy visit the park?"
   - "Does Darcy go to daycare?"
   - "Does Darcy visit with other dogs?"
   - "Does Darcy visit other homes to meet other people?"
6. "Describe what you see when you say that Lizzie has a seizure."
   - "When Lizzie has a seizure, does she fall on her side and paddle her feet?"
   - "When Lizzie has a seizure, does she lose control of her bladder and bowels?"
   - "When Lizzie has a seizure, does she vocalize?"
   - "When Lizzie has a seizure, does she lose consciousness?"
   - "Does she seem aware of her surroundings?"
7. "Share what is going through your mind right now about Edna's diagnosis."
   - "Does Edna's diagnosis worry you?"
   - "Does Edna's diagnosis make you question our decision to go to surgery?"
8. "Describe what is normal in terms of Fluffington's behavior?"
   - "Is Fluffington behaving well for you at home?"
   - "Is this normal behavior for Fluffington?"
9. "Tell me what you're noticing at home that makes you worried Ghost is fainting."
   - "When you say that Ghost is fainting, does she lose consciousness?"
   - "When you say that Ghost is fainting, does she seem weak immediately beforehand?"
   - "Is she stiff and rigid during the event?"
   - "Does the event last minutes?"
   - "Does the event last hours?"
   - "Does she act normal after she faints?"
10. "Tell me about the discharge that you've been noticing at the tip of Jack's penis."
   - "Is the discharge from Jack's penis bloody?"
   - "Is the discharge from Jack's penis green?"
   - "Is the discharge from Jack's penis cloudy?"
   - "Is there more discharge than normal?"
   - "Does the discharge look different today?"

Note that this exercise does not have one right answer per question. There are multiple right answers for each question. If your phrasing is not listed above, then that does not necessarily mean that you are incorrect. Double-check with your instructor if there is any question or concern.

Exercise 23.9 – Reflective Listening I

1. Client's statement: "Tadpole hasn't kept anything down for the past three days. Not even water. He doesn't even have anything left in his stomach to bring up, so now he's dry-heaving."

    Your response: "It sounds like Tadpole hasn't been able to keep down food or water for the past three days and he's still heaving, even though his stomach is empty, is that right?"

2. Client's statement: "My greatest concern is making sure that Panda isn't in any pain. I don't want him to suffer. I would rather let him go, than force him to live in pain."

    Your response: "So pain management at this point is what we need to focus on, and if ever there comes a time when we cannot manage his pain appropriately, then we will need to consider euthanasia?"

3. Client's statement: "Pickle is the only one in my life right now. If something happened to him, I would be lost. You have to fix him. He's all I have."

    Your response: "What I'm hearing you say is just how important Pickle is to you and that you depend upon him for survival."

4. Client's statement: "Sampson loves playing Frisbee. When we were at the park yesterday, he chased the Frisbee for about two hours, on and off. At one point, he landed hard and yelped. Since then, he hasn't wanted to put weight on his back leg – the right one. I'm concerned that he broke something."

    Your response: "So Sampson might have overdone it at the park? He landed hard yesterday and hasn't wanted to bear weight on his right hind limb. You're worried he has fractured his leg. Is that right?"

5. Client's statement: "I know you always say not to feed Pepper table scraps. But it was a holiday – and we were outside barbequing. And Pepper just looks at you with those wide eyes like he's starving. I give in. Every time. It seemed like a good idea until last night. He had explosive diarrhea. He asked to go outside ten or twenty times. I couldn't catch a break. Every time I went to bed, he had me up again."

    Your response: "It sounds like Pepper's decision to indulge caught up with him and he's had diarrhea 10–20 times overnight. It's keeping you both up, it's that bad."

Exercise 23.10 – Reflective Listening II

1. Client's statement: "I don't know what to do. On one hand, surgery could buy him an extra six months to a year of life. I wouldn't have to say goodbye. We could have another good year together. But is that selfish? How much am I asking him to go through on my behalf? Is that fair? Is that right? I am so confused. I don't know how to help him and I want to make the right choice for him, not because it's what's best for me."

    Your response: "It sounds like you're conflicted. You're trying to make the right decision for Twister: you would like to go to surgery to prolong life, but only if that's best for him."

2. Client's statement: "Cheeto has never been good in the car. From the first day we brought him home, he hasn't tolerated the ride. He gets motion sickness – and bad! It's to the point that I don't even want to bring him in to see you because it's just miserable – for him and me! And we're talking just short distances – ten minutes tops! Now we have to drive cross-country! How is that supposed to work?"

    Your response: "What I'm hearing you say is that Cheeto's motion sickness is a long-standing problem, but now it's about to become a big issue for you because you have to drive cross-country with him. Is that right?"

3. Client's statement: "Solo has always been a one-person dog. For ten years, he's only known me. We've been together, just him and I. He never liked friends coming over, so we didn't force it. But now that I'm engaged, that's no longer an option. He's going to have to get used to sharing me with Derek. But every time Derek comes to visit, Solo growls at him and bares his teeth. I yell at him, but he snaps back. I don't see this transition working."

    Your response: "It sounds like you need help figuring out how to integrate Derek into your household because Solo isn't fond of sharing you with anyone."

4. Client's statement: "Pivot started sneezing last week. At first, I thought it was allergies, so I let it go. It wasn't that frequent, so it really didn't bother me. But then it was paired with thick yellow snot. It got everywhere – all over me, the floor. It's getting worse. He wakes up sneezing. I can't get sleep because he's sneezing. And now his eyes are drippy, too. He was squinting his right eye yesterday as if it hurt, now both seem half-open. That seems a lot more serious than just allergies."

    Your response: "So Pivot's sneezing has progressed for the past week to the point that it's waking you up and the discharge has become thick and yellow. Now his eyes seem bothered as well. Did I get that right?"

5. Client's statement: "When Trapper started to throw up on Saturday night, I tried what had worked for him in the past. I picked up his water bowl to give his belly a rest. I withheld his breakfast on Sunday. It seemed to work okay, until evening. He looked like he was up for eating, so I offered him dinner – just a half-portion. He took one bite, then started licking his lips. Then gagging. Then he upchucked – all over the

floor. Clearly he's not getting better. That's why I called. We really could use your help."

Your response: "It sounds like you tried to rest Trapper's belly by withholding food and water for 24 hours. But things didn't go well when you re-introduced food and now he's throwing up again?"

Exercise 23.11 – Empathy I

1. There are two different types of empathy:
    - cognitive empathy
    - emotional empathy.
    How do these types of empathy differ?

    Being empathetic at a *cognitive* level simply means that you can identify with the individual with whom you are engaging. You may or may not agree with this person's perspective or insight, but you can appreciate his or her thought process. You get why s/he thinks the way s/he does about certain scenarios or events. This form of empathy is purely cerebral.

    Emotional empathy takes it a step further. Emotional empathy is the capacity to feel as another, instead of just feeling sorry for him or her. This figure of speech implies that, through empathy, we can become one with another person. We can connect to that individual through emotion. We can feel what they feel.

2. Consider the following clinical vignette:

    You are an associate veterinarian at a companion animal practice. Your patient is a 10-year-old, castrated male Great Dane dog, Lion. You have just diagnosed the dog with proximal tibial osteosarcoma of the right pelvic leg. Three-view thoracic radiographs are negative for evidence of metastasis. You outline the treatment options, which include palliative care, right pelvic limb amputation, and chemotherapy.

    In response to treatment recommendations, your client makes the following statement:

    I'm not ready to let Lion go. He's been with me since my first semester in law school. He's seen me through the very worst of times – times when I didn't think there was a way out. I can't imagine life without him. But he's in a lot of pain. I'm worried about doing the wrong thing for the right reasons – keeping him alive to delay the inevitable.

    Give an example of a response that you might make that demonstrates <u>cognitive</u> empathy.

    Your response: I can see that Lion holds a very important place in your heart. Because of this, I can appreciate why you want to be sure that the treatment you select for him is in his best interest, rather than your own.

Give an example of a response that you might make that demonstrates <u>emotional</u> empathy.

Your response: I can't begin to imagine how difficult this must be for you, knowing that Lion has been with you all along, through some really major milestones. I feel your pain in having to make a difficult choice, one that may have to put his needs before your own. That has got to be so hard.

Exercise 23.12 – Empathy II

Give an example of a response that would have more effectively demonstrated <u>cognitive</u> empathy.

Your response: I can understand that you feel like there's nothing left for you without Katerina.

Give an example of a response that would have more effectively demonstrated <u>emotional</u> empathy.

Your response: I have never loved anyone the way that you love Katerina, and I can see just how much the thought of losing her is tearing you apart.

How might you effectively make use of a partnership statement to connect to your client?

Your response: I know that I'm a poor substitute for Katerina right now, but we are in this together: you are not alone through these tough decisions; help me help you to make the best decision for her. We are not likely to cure her, but we can work together to make her comfortable.

You are concerned about the client's mental stability. Even though veterinarians are not licensed therapists, the client's statement has you worried that she might harm herself. How might you elicit her perspective to gauge the likelihood that this will happen?

Your response: I know this is a lot to take in right now and it may seem very overwhelming. Something that you said concerned me. When you say that there's no reason for you to live, what do you mean by that? Are you thinking of hurting yourself?

How might you effectively make use of reflective listening to let your client know that she has been heard?

Your response: I get that. Half of your adult life is a long time to be with someone. You've never before had to think about something like this until now.

Exercise 23.13 – Nonverbal Cues

C   1. Volume, rate of speech, pausing, and tone
A   2. The study of gestures and body movements
D   3. Directed responses by nervous system that are outside of our control
B   4. The use of space: how space is configured to fit our needs

Exercise 23.14 – Barriers to Communication

Name at least five NON-LIVING items in the examination room that could be considered physical barriers to communication:

1. medical record
2. computer
3. exam room table
4. patient's crate or carrier
5. patient's leash

Note that this exercise does not just have five right answers. If your answer is not listed above, then that does not necessarily mean you are incorrect. Double-check with your instructor if there is any question or concern.

For each item that you have listed above, consider a potential strategy that you might use to get around it being a barrier:

1. Acknowledge that the medical record is a barrier between you and the client: make use of signposting to acknowledge to the client when you need a moment to review the chart so that the client knows you're not intentionally ignoring him/her.

2. Acknowledge that the computer is a barrier between you and the client: make use of signposting to acknowledge to the client when you need a moment to turn your back on him/her in order to type something into the electronic medical record.

3. Rather than sit across from your client, with the exam room table in between, create an "L" shape by sitting at the end of the table and facing your client. This reinforces partnership.

4. Keep the crate or carrier outside of your line of vision so that it is not seated in between you and the client. It is best if placed off to the side.

5. The leash twisting around legs does not facilitate conversations, particularly if the content of the conversation is sensitive. If appropriate, you can ask the client to let go of the leash so that the dog is free to walk around the exam room; or perhaps have one of your team members hold onto the leash so as to allow the client to focus on your words.

Exercise 23.15 – Reducing Barriers to Communication

It can be stressful for cats to encounter dogs in the waiting area. Identify at least three strategies to minimize this stress:

1. Maintain separate waiting rooms – one for dogs and one for cats.
2. Encourage cat-owners to place a towel over the top of their cat carriers to decrease visual stimulation. They may still smell dogs, but at least they won't see them.
3. Do not force cat-owners to sit in the waiting room with dogs. Instead, direct cat-owners immediately into the exam room.

Note that this exercise does not just have three right answers. If your answer is not listed above, then that does not necessarily mean you are incorrect. Double-check with your instructor if there is any question or concern.

Exercise 23.16 – Body Language and Communication I

Key components of body language have been listed below. Indicate how to make use of each item to FACILITATE clinical conversations with clients:

1. Body posture
   Your response: Stand tall and straight, and keep your shoulders back. Allow your arms to hang naturally at your sides. Face your client.

2. Eye contact
   Your response: Maintain appropriate intermittent eye contact to demonstrate respect for the client. When eye contact is effective, it conveys that you are listening.

3. Facial expressions
   Your response: Be aware of your brow, eyebrows, facial muscles, mouth, and jaw tone. Clients can read your facial cues, even those that you don't think are apparent. Greet clients with a warm smile.

4. Gestures
   Your response: Offer a hand shake when meeting a client for the first time.

5. Touch
   Your response: Appropriate use of direct touch (body contact) in safe zones (hands or forearms).

Exercise 23.17 – Body Language and Communication II

Key components of body language have been listed below. Indicate one INAPPROPRIATE WAY of making use of each item below that will HINDER clinical conversations with clients:

1. Body posture
    Your response: Appear slouched and hunched over. Face away from your client. Turn your back on the client.

2. Eye contact
    Your response: Avoid eye contact altogether: look at the floor or ceiling. Look past the client instead of meeting the client's gaze. Alternatively, stare at the client at all times.

3. Facial expressions
    Your response: Frown and/or grimace when a client asks you to do something extra, for example, "Can you also trim Ginger's nails when she's in the back for her blood draw?" Doing so may convey annoyance or irritation.

4. Gestures
    Your response: Look at your watch, click your pen, and/or tap your foot against the floor when a client is longwinded with his/her requests. This implies that you are short on time and you are becoming impatient because you have somewhere else to be.

5. Touch
    Your response: Touch the client in non-safe zones – i.e. places other than the hands, forearms, upper arms, or shoulders – without their permission. For instance, if you were to touch your client on the thigh, this might be seen as an inappropriate advance. Touching clients out of context – i.e. during social situations that do not call for touch – would also be out of line.

Exercise 23.18 – Medical Jargon I

For each medical term below, please provide an appropriate translation that could be used with a client during a clinical consultation:

1. Orchiectomy
    Your response: castration or neuter; surgically removing both testicles to sterilize a patient.

2. Ovariohysterectomy
    Your response: spay or neuter; surgically removing the ovaries and uterus to sterilize a patient.

3. Cystotomy

    Your response: bladder surgery – that is, cutting into the bladder, typically to remove bladder stones.

4. Thoracocentesis

    Your response: tapping the chest – that is, inserting a needle into the space between the ribs and vital organs to remove air or fluid that shouldn't be there.

5. Ovariectomy

    Your response: surgically removing just the ovaries to sterilize a patient.

Exercise 23.19 – Medical Jargon II

For each procedural term below, please provide an appropriate translation that could be used with a client during a clinical consultation:

1. Inguinal

    Your response: at or near the groin

2. Umbilical

    Your response: at or near the belly button

3. Perineal

    Your response: at or near the rear

4. Axillary

    Your response: at or near the arm pit

5. Pedal

    Your response: pertaining to the foot

Exercise 23.20 – Medical Jargon III

For each anatomical term below, please provide an appropriate translation that could be used with a client during a clinical consultation:

1. Cranial

    Your response: nearer to the head

2. Caudal

    Your response: closer to the tail

3. Lateral
   Your response: to the outside

4. Medial
   Your response: to the inside

5. Rostral
   Your response: closer to the nose

Exercise 23.21 – Medical Jargon IV

For each procedural term below, please provide an appropriate translation that could be used with a client during a clinical consultation:

1. Tarsorrhaphy
   Your response: surgery to (temporarily) sew the eyelids together to narrow the eyelid opening.

2. Laparotomy
   Your response: cutting into the abdomen, usually for the purpose of an exploratory surgery.

3. Enucleation
   Your response: surgical removal of the eye.

4. Splenectomy
   Your response: surgical removal of the spleen.

5. Lung lobectomy
   Your response: surgical removal of one part of the left or right lung.

Exercise 23.22 – Medical Jargon V

For each clinical pathology term below, please provide an appropriate translation that could be used with a client during a clinical consultation:

1. Anemia
   Your response: low red blood cell count / too few red blood cells.

2. Leukocytosis
   Your response: high white blood cell count / too many white blood cells.

3. Thrombocytopenia
   Your response: low platelet count / too few platelets.

4. Azotemia

Your response: elevation in two blood parameters, BUN and creatinine, which may suggest dehydration or kidney issues; elevation in kidney values, which suggests that the kidney is having difficulty filtering the toxins out of the bloodstream.

5. Hypercholesterolemia

Your response: cholesterol level is too high.

Exercise 23.23 – Medical Jargon VI

For each imaging term below, please provide an appropriate translation that could be used with a client during a clinical consultation:

1. Radiograph

    Your response: x-ray.

2. Echocardiogram

    Your response: ultrasound of the heart.

3. Electrocardiogram (ECG)

    Your response: test that measures the electrical activity of the heart; this will tell us how the heart is working; this will tell us about the heart's rhythm.

4. Contrast urography

    Your response: using imaging and contrast material to evaluate for abnormalities in the urinary tract, such as blood in the urine, kidney or bladder stones, and/or masses within the urinary tract.

5. Barium study of the GI tract

    Your response: using imaging and contrast material to evaluate for abnormalities in the digestive tract, such as dilated esophageal (that may indicate megaesophagus) or an unusual intestinal pattern that may indicate an obstruction.

Exercise 23.24 – Partnership

Transform each sentence below into a statement that CONVEYS partnership. You may consider statements that BLEND partnership and eliciting the client's perspective, because quite often these will overlap.

1. I am prescribing an ophthalmic medication that comes in two formulations.

    Your response: We need to decide upon the best plan to treat Joey's eye ulcer. There are two options: an ointment that requires administration every eight hours – so 3x/day – or an eye drop that requires administration every four hours – so 6x/day. Which would you prefer?

2. I have determined the best way to manage Harrison's anxiety.

    Your response: Thank you for sharing your concerns about Harrison's anxiety. Based upon what you have shared with me, perhaps we could talk about behavior modification exercises that you could do with him at home?

3. I am telling you that the best way to proceed is with hind limb amputation.

    Your response: You and I both agree that a hind limb amputation is the best step to improve Triton's quality of life. Would you be open to hearing more about that procedure and what it would mean for you and Triton both if we were to proceed?

4. My plan is to run bloodwork first, then consider hospitalization if Julip's kidney values are off the charts.

    Your response: How would you feel about running bloodwork first and then considering hospitalization if Julip's kidney values are off the charts? I know that we are both concerned about how dehydrated he is and how poorly that is making him feel.

5. I have decided that the adrenocorticotropin hormone (ACTH) stim test is much better than the Low-Dose Dexamethasone Suppression (LDDS) test.

    Your response: Based upon my experience, we can run either the ACTH test or the LDDS test. Would you be open to hearing why I prefer the ACTH stim test?

Exercise 23.25 – Eliciting the Client's Perspective

Add a sentence to each statement below that appropriately elicits the client's perspective.

1. Chronic kidney disease can be challenging for cat owners.

    Your response: How do you feel about having to manage your cat's kidney disease at home?

2. I know that it comes as quite a surprise for you that Marshmallow is diabetic.

    Your response: What are your thoughts about having to administer insulin shots at home?

3. We need to keep a close watch on Ginny because eye ulcers can progress very fast. I'd also suggest that she wear an Elizabethan collar at all times. That should prevent her from creating more damage to herself."

    Your response: What is your opinion about how well Ginny might tolerate an E collar?

4. I know we've covered a lot of material today, in terms of Teddy Bear's vaccine schedule.

    Your response: What concerns might you have about getting Teddy Bear up-to-date on vaccinations?

5. Pilling a cat is never as easy as it looks, but it is essential that Wilson get his medication.
   Your response: How do you feel about having to medicate him at home?

Exercise 23.26 – Assessing the Client's Knowledge

Add a sentence to each statement below that appropriately assesses the client's knowledge.

1. At-home blood sugar monitoring for diabetics can be challenging for cat owners.
   Your response: What do you know about at-home equipment for monitoring blood sugar in cats?

2. Based upon Tilly's work-up, she has chronic kidney disease (CKD).
   Your response: Have you ever heard of CKD in cats before?

3. Pike would benefit from a ten-day course of metronidazole.
   Your response: Are you familiar with metronidazole?

4. Skipper needs to receive a tapering dose of prednisone.
   Your response: What is your understanding of tapering prednisone?

5. The ultrasound report shows that Trolley has a kidney stone.
   Your response: Did you know that dogs could get kidney stones?

Exercise 23.27 – Signposting I

We can signpost using ordinal numbers. List at least five of these below:

1. First
2. Second
3. Third
4. Fourth
5. Fifth

Exercise 23.28 – Signposting II

We can also signpost using transitions. List at least five transitional words or phrases that can be used for signposting:

1. In the beginning / initially
2. After / afterward

3. Then
4. Before
5. At the end / at the conclusion

Exercise 23.29 – Signposting and Transparency

How might you signpost to convey that you will be happy to trim her nails after she has been stabilized?

Your response: I would be more than happy to trim Rose's nails after we stabilize her; however, first what she really needs to have us do is to place an IV catheter.

How might you make use of transparency to convey that this situation is life-threatening?

Your response: I know that this has happened very fast, so it still may seem like a shock to you, but Rose is very sick. Not every cat that ingests lilies survives. We are going to do everything we can to help her and to help you, but I need you to prepare yourself. This is serious.

In response to your use of transparency above, the client begins to cry. It is difficult to make out her words, but you definitely hear her say, "This is all my fault."

How might you respond to the client using unconditional positive regard?

Your response: You brought Rose in as soon as you could, and are here, now, to do all you can to make her better. How could you have known that lilies were so toxic to cats? You did the best you could.

Exercise 23.30 – Putting It All Together

How might you use a warning shot to indicate that hit-by-car (HBC) patients often decompensate?

Your response: I know that this may be difficult to hear, but the femoral fracture may not be the worst of the damage that the car accident caused. Bitzie may have also sustained significant trauma to his internal organs. This could potentially be life-threatening.

How might you make use of signposting to indicate that it is best to postpone Bitzie's surgery?

Your response: Although surgery is necessary to repair Bitzie's femoral fracture, our first priority is to be sure that Bitzie can survive surgery.

Your client picks up on your reluctance to go to surgery right this minute, and questions you for the delay: "Isn't it better to repair fractures as soon as they occur, to improve healing?

How might you make use of reflective listening to indicate that your client's concerns have been heard?

Your response: Yes, you are right, it is important to repair fractures as soon as possible. However, in this case…

How might you make use of asking for permission in this clinical scenario?

Your response: May I share with you why, in this case, stabilization must take a priority to fracture repair?

You are concerned about lung contusions. How might you assess the client's knowledge about this condition?

Your response: Are you familiar with lung contusions?

After a lengthy discussion, the client says that she agrees with your decision to hold off on surgery, but you can see that she is not convinced. How might you elicit her perspective?

Your response: Please forgive me, but I can see that you still have a lot weighing on your mind. May I ask what concerns you most about delaying surgery?

Chapter 25

Clinical Vignettes for Role Play

The following scenarios have been scripted for use by doctors-in-training and veterinary educators to practice clinical communication in a safe, supportive learning environment. Role play is one type of experiential learning that offers several benefits, allowing the learner to:

- practice through repetition, trial and error, without fear of distressing a real client during emotionally charged encounters, by saying the wrong thing
- recognize that there is rarely one correct approach and one incorrect approach to clinical communication
- test out different word choices and phrases to find options that feel most natural to him or her
- receive immediate feedback.

Scripted scenarios can be test-piloted as part of in-class instruction and break-out sessions, or informally, as extracurricular practice.

One student can play the part of the veterinarian. Another can play the part of the client. The student who is playing the part of the client may ad lib details as necessary to make the case seem plausible.

Note that a full script has not been provided – only a brief background and a list of tasks that the veterinarian has been prompted to complete.

The student who is playing the role of the veterinarian is encouraged to identify at least one learning objective prior to the start of the encounter. This learning objective is intended to provide structure as she or he progresses through the exercise. The learning objective also serves as a tangible way for the student to self-reflect and assess his or her performance at its conclusion.

Note that these scripts can be completed in any order. However, I have ordered them from most simple to most complex.

Answers have intentionally *not* been provided so that students have an opportunity to develop their own strategies for managing casework from the standpoint of clinical communication. Double-check with your instructor if there are any questions or concerns.

Scenario 25.1: Greeting the Client at a Wellness Visit I

You are an associate veterinarian in clinical practice. Ms. Rebecca Mills is presenting her 3-month-old, intact female Ragdoll kitten, Biscuit, for wellness examination and her 1st FVRCP (feline viral rhinotracheitis – calicivirus – panleukopenia) vaccination.

Ms. Mills is new to the practice. This is her first experience meeting you.

Your task

To establish rapport through greeting the client.

Helpful hints

- What constitutes a proper greeting?
- What do you need to share about yourself (and your role) with the client?
- How should you address a client whom you have never met before?

Scenario 25.2: Greeting the Client at a Wellness Visit II

You are an associate veterinarian in clinical practice. Mr. Bruce Billows is presenting his 3-month-old, intact male Boston terrier, Cinnabar, for wellness examination and his 1st DA2PP (canine distemper – adenovirus – parvovirus – parainfluenza) vaccine.

Mr. Billows is new to the practice. This is his first experience meeting you.

Your task

To establish rapport through greeting the client.

Helpful hints

- What constitutes a proper greeting?
- What do you need to share about yourself (and your role) with the client?
- How should you address a client whom you have never met before?

Scenario 25.3: Greeting the Returning Client I

You are an associate veterinarian in clinical practice. Ms. Rebecca Mills is presenting her now 4-month-old, intact female Ragdoll kitten, Biscuit, for her 2nd and final FVRCP booster.

You met Ms. Mills for the first time 4 weeks ago.

Your task

To greet the client appropriately, given that she is a returning client and is right on schedule for Biscuit's last "feline distemper" vaccine.

Helpful hint

• What constitutes a proper greeting when you are visiting with a returning client?

Scenario 25.4: Greeting the Returning Client II

You are an associate veterinarian in clinical practice. Mr. Bruce Billows is presenting his now 5-month-old, intact male Boston terrier, Cinnabar, for his 2nd and final DA2PP booster. He is overdue for his vaccination by 4 weeks.

Your task is to greet the client appropriately, given that he is a returning client. He is unaware that his dog is overdue for vaccination and will now have to restart his series.

Helpful hint

• What constitutes a proper greeting when you are visiting with a returning client?

Scenario 25.5: Taking a Clinical History at the Wellness Visit – Feline

You are an associate veterinarian in clinical practice, and your next appointment has arrived.

Ms. Jennifer Bradley recently moved to the area from out-of-state with her 5-year-old, female spayed Abyssinian cat, Charlie.

Charlie is not, to Ms. Bradley's knowledge, due for any vaccinations. Ms. Bradley is simply hoping to establish a professional relationship with your practice to manage Charlie's healthcare, as she intends for them both to reside in this area for the long term.

Before you enter the consultation room, you are told that Charlie is an indoor-only cat and that she is petrified to be here today. The technician says that she is hiding underneath a towel in the examination room sink.

Your tasks

To:
• establish rapport with the client
• take a comprehensive patient health history.

Helpful hints

- What constitutes a proper greeting for a new client?
- What do you need to share about yourself (and your role) with the client?
- What do you need to know about addressing the client?
- Which content areas should be explored during anamnesis (history taking) for any new patient?
- Which style of questioning (open or closed) should you use to initiate history taking?
- Which style of questioning (open or closed) is preferred for follow-up, to flush out case details?

Scenario 25.6: Taking a Clinical History at the Wellness Visit – Canine

You are an associate veterinarian in clinical practice, and your next appointment has arrived.

Mr. Alan Finch recently adopted a 9-year-old, castrated male Vizla dog, Butters. Butters used to be owned by Mr. Finch's father, from whom Mr. Finch had been estranged until the past 3 months. Mr. Finch's father, Paul, had been admitted to hospice for pancreatic cancer. It was Paul's dying wish that he and his son would be reunited. Mr. Finch honored his father's wish, and agreed to take in Butters after his father passed.

Butters has only been living with Mr. Finch for the past 3 days. He's not really a "dog person," and he and Butters are still figuring each other out, but Mr. Finch is doing what he can to fulfill his promise.

Butters is not, to Mr. Finch's knowledge, due for any vaccinations. Mr. Finch is simply hoping to establish a professional relationship with your practice to manage Butters' healthcare.

Before you enter the consultation room, you are told that Butters is a happy-go-lucky dog, and seems to be excited to meet everyone! The technician says to be careful as you enter the room, or you may trip over the dog, he loves to be the center of attention and up in everyone's space.

Your tasks

To:
- establish rapport with the client
- take a comprehensive patient health history.

Helpful hints

- What constitutes a proper greeting for a new client?
- What do you need to share about yourself (and your role) with the client?
- What do you need to know about addressing the client?

- Which content areas should be explored during anamnesis (history taking) for any new patient?
- Which style of questioning (open or closed) should you use to initiate history taking?
- Which style of questioning (open or closed) is preferred for follow-up, to flush out case details?

Scenario 25.7: Taking a Clinical History at a Sick Visit – Feline I

You are an associate veterinarian in clinical practice, and your next appointment has arrived. Ms. Betty Swarthmore is presenting her 8-year-old, castrated male, Siamese cat, Sweet Pea, for evaluation of unusual episodes of "breathing trouble."

Sweet Pea is an indoor-only cat in a single-pet household. The only recent change to the house has been construction: one of the walk-in closets is being ripped out to create an additional toilet off the foyer. There has been a lot of construction dust.

Since the construction started, Ms. Swarthmore is concerned that Sweet Pea is wheezing. He stands with his head and neck extended, as if trying to draw in air. She used to think that he was trying to hack something up, like a hairball, based upon his posture, but now she truly believes it is his airway.

The patient is presently stable. The last episode took place on Friday night. It lasted for about 10 minutes.

Your tasks

To:
- establish rapport through greeting the client
- take a comprehensive patient health history, with emphasis on the presenting complaint
- elicit the client's perspective to discover Ms. Swarthmore's views on the presenting complaint: what it is and what may have triggered it.

Helpful hints

- How do you establish rapport with a client at a sick visit? What is the appropriate tone that you will set for the occasion?
- Which content areas should be emphasized during history taking, given the patient's presenting complaint?
- Which style of questioning (open or closed) should you use to initiate history taking?
- Which style of questioning (open or closed) is preferred for follow-up, to flush out case details?
- What do you need to know about the presenting complaint? Which details are essential?
- How will you elicit the client's perspective? What words will you use, specifically, to get Ms. Swarthmore to share her story with you?

Scenario 25.8: Taking a Clinical History at a Sick Visit – Feline II

You are an associate veterinarian in clinical practice, and your next appointment has arrived. Mr. Jon Swift is presenting his 6-year-old, castrated male, Maine Coon cat, Norton, for evaluation of acute onset of "being down" in his hind end.

Norton is an indoor-only cat in a single-pet household. He was fine last night. However, Mr. Swift awoke to a guttural cry. He found Norton at the base of his bed, unable to move either hind limb. When Mr. Swift tried to get him to rise, the best that Norton could do was to drag both pelvic legs.

Mr. Swift tried to touch Norton's toes, but Norton growled and tried to bite. Mr. Swift is concerned that he is in pain because Norton has never before lashed out at him.

After establishing contact with the client, you observe that Norton's pelvic limb paw pads are cyanotic. You prioritize a differential diagnosis of aortic thromboembolism (ATE). To confirm your suspicions, you reach out to touch each distal hind limb. They are both cold to the touch. You agree that Norton is in distress, and you cannot palpate either femoral pulse.

Your tasks

To:

- establish rapport with the client
- recognize that this patient's condition is far more serious than, for example, clinical scenario 25.7; as a result, you will take a more abbreviated patient health history at this time, with emphasis on the presenting complaint
- acknowledge and validate Mr. Swift's concern that his cat is in pain and could benefit from analgesia
- acknowledge how you plan to address Norton's pain.

Helpful hints

- How do you establish rapport with a client at a sick visit? What is the appropriate tone that you will set for the occasion?
- Which content areas should be emphasized during history taking, given the patient's presenting complaint?
- Which style of questioning (open or closed) should you use to initiate history taking?
- Which style of questioning (open or closed) is preferred for follow-up, to flush out case details?
- What do you need to know about the presenting complaint? Which details are essential?
- How will you let Mr. Swift know that his concern about Norton's pain level has been heard? Which communication skill(s) will assist you with this task?
- How will you let Mr. Swift know that you will address Norton's pain level? Which communication skill(s) will assist you with this task?

Helpful relevant medical notes

- ATE is a condition in which a thrombus (blood clot) forms within the vasculature, enters the aorta, and occludes arterial vasculature.
- The distal aorta is the most common site of obstruction in cats. Obstructions at this location result in a so-called "saddle thrombus."
- Cats with primary cardiomyopathy, particularly hypertrophic cardiomyopathy (HCM), are at increased risk for ATE. Maine coon cats appear to be predisposed to HCM.
- Affected patients present acutely with pelvic limb paresis or paralysis.
- Bilateral involvement is most common.
- Owners may witness the cat dragging the affected limb(s).
- The affected limb(s) often lack(s) a femoral pulse.
- Without blood flow, the affected limb(s) become(s) cold.
- Affected patients are acutely painful and often vocal.

Refer to Chapter 39 (Palpably Cool or Cyanotic Extremities) in my reference text, *Common Clinical Presentations in Dogs and Cats*, for additional information about pathophysiology of ATE.

Scenario 25.9: Taking a Clinical History at a Sick Visit – Canine I

You are an associate veterinarian in clinical practice, and your next appointment has arrived. Mr. Nick Tremaine is presenting his 2-year-old, spayed female, Miniature Schnauzer, Taffy, for evaluation of "passing out" yesterday on her morning walk.

Just prior to the episode, Taffy saw a squirrel and chased after it, barking loudly. Taffy seemed "fine one minute" and then not. "Out of the blue," she "fell over" onto her side.

At first, Mr. Tremaine thought that she'd had a seizure – he once owned a Doberman pinscher with epilepsy. However, he noticed that Taffy was not paddling her limbs as had his previous dog. Instead, she laid there, quietly.

Taffy got up after what seemed like "forever." She seemed unfazed, but this episode concerned Mr. Tremaine greatly.

Your tasks

To:

- establish rapport with the client
- recognize that all of the client's focus is on the presenting complaint; although you will ultimately need to take a comprehensive patient history, you must abbreviate some of the content for now in order to acknowledge and address the presenting complaint
- acknowledge and validate Mr. Tremaine's concern that his dog passing out is not normal and could be indicative of underlying cardiomyopathy.

Helpful hints

- How do you establish rapport with a client at a sick visit? What is the appropriate tone that you will set for the occasion?
- Which content areas should be emphasized during history taking, given the patient's presenting complaint?
- Which style of questioning (open or closed) should you use to initiate history taking?
- Which style of questioning (open or closed) is preferred for follow-up, to flush out case details?
- What do you need to know about the presenting complaint? Which details are essential?
- How will you let Mr. Tremaine know that his concern about Taffy's episode has been heard? Which communication skill(s) will assist you with this task?
- How will you let Mr. Tremaine know that, although syncope is a primary focus, you must also take a comprehensive patient history? This means that you may need to cover content area that seems entirely unrelated to the presenting complaint.

Helpful relevant medical notes

Taffy has presumptive sick sinus syndrome. This diagnosis can be confirmed on electro-cardiogram (ECG).

- Sick sinus syndrome is the condition by which the sinoatrial (SA) node of the heart fails to discharge as often as it should. This results in long pauses between heartbeats.
- If the pause is long enough, another part of the heart may fire off an escape rhythm.
- If the patient does not generate an escape rhythm, then s/he experiences true asystole. This results in a syncopal episode.
- Clients may note that weakness and incoordination often precede the episode.
- Miniature schnauzers are predisposed to this condition.
- Symptomatic patients may respond to positive chronotropic drugs, but most affected patients benefit from the implantation of a pacemaker.

Refer to Chapter 40 (Collapse) in my reference text, *Common Clinical Presentations in Dogs and Cats*, for additional information about pathophysiology and diagnosis of sick sinus syndrome.

Scenario 25.10: Taking a Clinical History at a Sick Visit – Canine II

You are an associate veterinarian in clinical practice, and your next appointment has arrived. Mrs. Dottie Paulson is presenting her 7-year-old, spayed female, German shepherd dog, Peanut, for evaluation of a one-time episode of epistaxis that took place yesterday afternoon.

Mrs. Paulson has racked her brain, but cannot think of any precipitating factors. She knows that she, personally, often gets nose bleeds when she is stressed, but she never knew that dogs could develop the same issue.

While hanging out in the waiting area, Mrs. Paulson has done some research on Google and is very concerned that her dog may have a nasal tumor. She read online that German shepherd dogs are predisposed.

Mrs. Paulson is adamant that you take skull radiographs today. "If it's cancer, then I want to know about it, and I want to know now."

Your tasks

To:

- establish rapport with the client
- recognize that all of the client's focus is on the presenting complaint; although you will ultimately need to take a comprehensive patient history, you must abbreviate some of the content for now in order to acknowledge and address the presenting complaint
- acknowledge and commend Mrs. Paulson for due diligence and researching her pet's condition
- acknowledge and validate Mrs. Paulson's concern that nose bleeds in dogs are not normal and could be indicative of underlying neoplasia
- acknowledge that other pathological states can also cause epistaxis in dogs, such as fungal infections of the nasal cavity and/or systemic bleeding disorders
- acknowledge that an investigation, with imaging studies, is essential; however, more advanced screening with computer tomography (CT) or magnetic resonance imaging (MRI) is of value because both modalities provide enhanced detail.

Helpful hints

- How do you establish rapport with a client at a sick visit? What is the appropriate tone that you will set for the occasion?
- Which content areas should be emphasized during history taking, given the patient's presenting complaint?
- Which style of questioning (open or closed) should you use to initiate history taking?
- Which style of questioning (open or closed) is preferred for follow-up, to flush out case details?
- What do you need to know about the presenting complaint? Which details are essential?
- How will you let Mrs. Paulson know that her concern about Peanut has been heard? Which communication skill(s) will assist you with this task?
- How will you let Mrs. Paulson know that a diagnosis of neoplasia is possible? Which communication skill(s) will assist you with this task?

- How will you explain that additional diagnoses are also possible? Which communication skill(s) will assist you with this task?
- How will you acknowledge Mrs. Paulson's desire to obtain a definitive answer as soon as possible? Which communication skill(s) will assist you with this task?
- How will you inform Mrs. Paulson that obtaining a definitive diagnosis may require a biopsy? Which communication skill(s) will assist you with this task?

Helpful relevant medical notes

In actuality, Peanut has sinorhinitis, caused by *Aspergillus fumigatus,* the causative agent of aspergillosis.

- Affected patients develop chronic nasal discharge that may be hemorrhagic.
- Affected patients may also develop depigmentation of the nasal planum or alar folds.
- Dogs become infected either through nasal trauma, or when they inhale spores, which are ubiquitous in the environment.
- Infection causes destruction of the patient's nasal turbinates.
- As the disease progresses, the cribiform plate, nasal bones, and orbit may be damaged. This may cause gross facial asymmetry and the visual appearance of a distorted face.
- Advanced imaging will demonstrate lytic changes. CT scans are particularly helpful.
- Rhinoscopy may disclose fungal granulomas and allow for sample collection for definitive diagnosis.
- German Shepherds are overrepresented.

Refer to Chapter 33 (Nasal Discharge) in my reference text, *Common Clinical Presentations in Dogs and Cats*, for additional information about pathophysiology of this infectious disease.

Scenario 25.11: Explaining Physical Examination Findings – Feline I

You are an associate veterinarian in clinical practice, and your next appointment has arrived.

Ms. Steph Timber is presenting her estimated 10–12-week-old, intact male, Siamese × domestic shorthaired (DSH) kitten, Captain, for evaluation of alopecia, an open wound, and a history of pawing at his left eye. Timber is one of a litter of five kittens that was born in her barn to a semi-feral queen. Ms. Timber has been attempting to socialize the kittens since they were approximately two weeks old, when their eyes first opened. At this time, the kittens live exclusively outdoors, so it is unclear what happened to Captain. Ms. Timber says that he disappeared for 24 hours only to return with the lesions evident in Figure 25.1.

Ms. Timber is squeamish and has not taken a close look at the wound. She is not aware that, given its location, damage could have been sustained to the left cornea. You note that Captain is exhibiting blepharospasm associated with the left globe. Closer

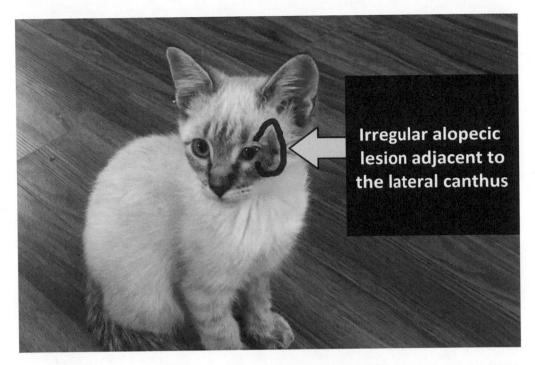

Irregular alopecic lesion adjacent to the lateral canthus

Figure 25.1 Courtesy of Rachel Sahrbeck, DVM Candidate, Kansas State University, Class of 2021

inspection reveals left ocular chemosis and corneal haze.

The remainder of Captain's physical examination discloses the following important, but unrelated findings:

- unilateral cryptorchidism
- low-grade (grade 1/6) parasternal systolic murmur
- doughy abdomen on palpation with diffusely thickened small intestines.

For the purpose of this case, please assume that you have already taken a complete patient history.

Your task

Summarize key physical exam findings. Which communication skill(s) will assist you with this task?

Scenario 25.12: Explaining Physical Examination Findings – Feline II

You are an associate veterinarian in clinical practice, and your next appointment has arrived.

Mr. Robert Wolfe found a kitten of unknown age curled up in a ball along the side of the road this morning. The kitten's coat was so dirty that Mr. Wolfe did not appreciate that this coat color contained white until after he had cleaned him up a bit with a warm washcloth and some gentle detergent.

Mr. Wolfe ultimately brought the kitten in to see you because the kitten appeared to be weak and minimally responsive.

On presentation, the kitten is an underweight intact male, estimated to be 8 weeks old. His appearance is captured in the photograph below:

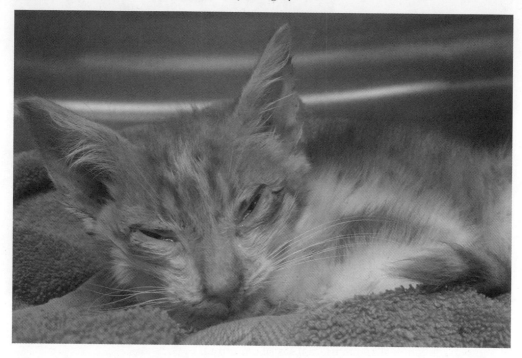

Figure 25.2 Courtesy of Genevieve LaFerriere, DVM

Physical examination discloses the following important findings:

- febrile: 103.5°F/39.7°C
- estimated to be 8–10% dehydrated
- ectoparasite infestation with the cat flea, *Ctenocephalides felis*
- diffuse pallor associated with the mucous membranes and conjunctiva
- bilateral conjunctivitis with serous-to-mucoid ocular discharge bilaterally and dried peri-ocular crusts
- audible upper airway congestion
- abdominal effort associated with respiration
- productive sneezing, with yellow discharge from both nostrils
- black-brown coffee-grounds-like aural debris bilaterally
- doughy abdomen on palpation with diffusely thickened small intestines.

For the purpose of this case, please assume that you have already taken a complete patient history.

Your task

Summarize key physical exam findings. Which communication skill(s) will assist you with this task?

Scenario 25.13: Explaining Physical Examination Findings – Canine I

You are an associate veterinarian in clinical practice, and your next appointment has arrived.

Mr. Ivan Newton is presenting his 4-month-old, intact male mixed breed dog, Gus, for wellness examination. He received the dog as a birthday gift from his wife. His wife found the dog advertised online. The dog is reportedly the progeny of "very skilled" bird dogs. She is hopeful that Gus can be Mr. Newton's new bird dog. Now that Mr. Newton is retired, he enjoys the outdoors and hunting fowl.

Physical examination discloses a reducible umbilical hernia. See photograph below: a close-up of the patient's ventral abdomen.

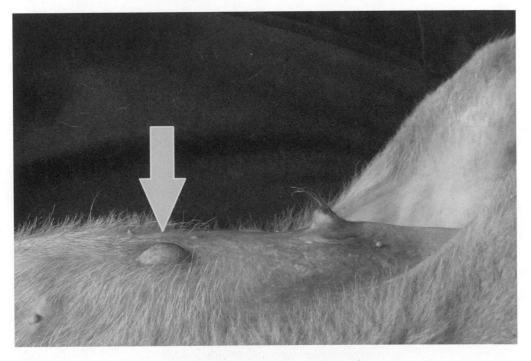

Figure 25.3 Courtesy of Rachel Sahrbeck, DVM Candidate, Kansas State University, Class of 2021

In addition, Gus' exam identifies these key findings:

* ectoparasite infestation with the cat flea, *Ctenocephalides felis*
* doughy abdomen on palpation with diffusely thickened small intestines.

For the purpose of this case, please assume that you have already taken a complete patient history.

Your task

Summarize key physical exam findings. Which communication skill(s) will assist you with this task?

Scenario 25.14: Explaining Physical Examination Findings – Canine II

You are an associate veterinarian in clinical practice, and your next appointment has arrived.

Ms. Jessica Filbert is presenting her 5-year-old, castrated male, Labrador retriever dog, Dobby, for evaluation of left pelvic limb lameness that began a little over a week ago and has gotten progressively worse.

Ms. Filbert reports that initially there were no obvious external wounds. However, over the past 24 hours, the area has become exceptionally raw, moist, and red. Dobby is intent on licking at it. Scolding him does little to take his mind off of the region. It seems to Ms. Filbert that he is intent on "eating his own foot!"

The following photograph depicts what you see on physical examination:

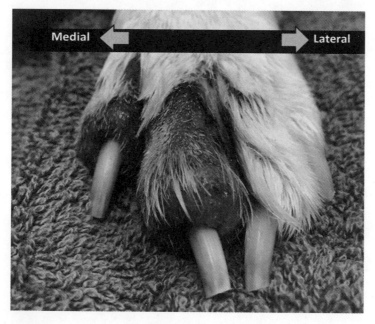

Figure 25.4 Courtesy of Alexis Siler, DVM

In addition, Dobby's exam discloses the following key findings:

- accumulation of thick, waxy, dark brown exudate at most nail beds associated with his other three feet
- greasy "feel" to his coat
- whole body pruritus.

For the purpose of this case, please assume that you have already taken a complete patient history.

Your task

To summarize key physical exam findings. Which communication skill(s) will assist you with this task?

Scenario 25.15: Explaining Radiographs I

You are an associate veterinarian in clinical practice, and your next appointment has arrived.

Mr. Stephen Finn is presenting his 2-year-old, intact female, domestic short haired (DSH) cat, Francesca, for evaluation of vulvar discharge that began three days ago and has gotten progressively worse. The discharge is whitish-green and thick. There is an odor to it.

Mr. Finn reports that Francesca is indoor-only and the only pet at home; however, she escaped twice from the house during the past month. On each occasion, she was missing for 3–4 days before she returned home of her own accord.

For the past 2 days, Francesca has been less interested in eating. Her thirst may also be increased.

On physical examination, you confirm the presence of vulvar discharge. You also palpate a tubular structure in the caudal abdomen. You recommend that two-view abdominal radiographs be taken to confirm your suspicion that Francesca has pyometra. The left lateral view has been made available to you in Figure 25.5.

For the purpose of this case, please assume that you have already taken a complete patient history and performed a complete physical examination. There were no additional remarkable findings.

Your tasks

To:

- summarize key physical exam findings.
- summarize key radiographic findings.

- establish what Mr. Finn knows about pyometra in cats.
- explain the diagnosis of pyometra to Mr. Finn.
- explain treatment options for pyometra: recommend that Francesca undergo ovari-ohysterectomy (OVH), both to manage the current condition and to prevent its recurrence.

Which communication skills will assist you with these tasks?

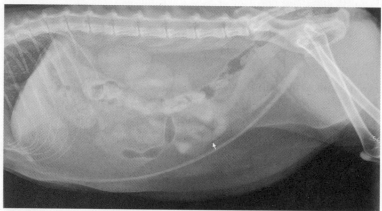

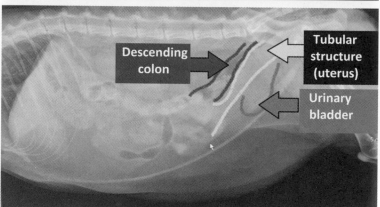

Figure 25.5a-b Courtesy of Dylan Dewitt and "Luci"

Scenario 25.16: Explaining Radiographs II

You are an associate veterinarian in clinical practice, and your next appointment has arrived.

Ms. Karen Olathe is presenting her 3-year-old, male castrated, Great Dane dog, Beanie, on emergency for acute onset of non-productive retching and an increasingly distended abdominal silhouette. You suspect gastric dilatation-volvulus (GDV) based upon the history and triage of the patient, and recommend that the patient submit to a right lateral abdominal radiograph to confirm the diagnosis. A cropped version of the image has been provided for you to review. Refer to Figure 25.6.

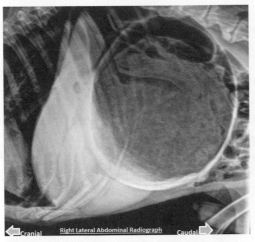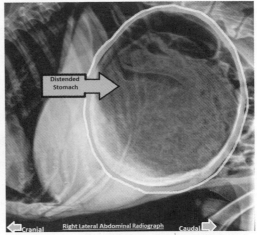

Figure 25.6a-b Courtesy of Pamela Mueller, DVM

Your tasks

To:

- summarize key radiographic findings.
- establish what Ms. Olathe knows about GDV in dogs.
- explain the diagnosis of GDV to Ms. Olathe.
- explain treatment options for GDV: recommend that Beanie undergo emergency surgery to fully explore the abdomen, de-rotate the stomach, and tack the stomach to a normal position to reduce the chance of recurrence.

Which communication skills will assist you with these tasks?

Scenario 25.17: Explaining Radiographs III

You are an associate veterinarian in clinical practice, and your next appointment has arrived.

Ms. Tina Stark is presenting her 4-year-old, castrated male, mixed-breed dog, Hoover, for evaluation of a three-day history of vomiting. The patient has a history of pica; however, in the past, his foreign bodies have always been able to pass through his digestive tract without incident. This time, Ms. Stark is afraid that something is "stuck."

Hoover is vomiting 7–10 times a day. Initially, the vomitus was food. Now, it appears to be just yellow bile and mucus, since he has not eaten for the past 24 hours.

Physical examination discloses that Hoover is an estimated 6–8% dehydrated, with reproducible splinting on superficial and deep cranial abdominal palpation that is suggestive of pain.

You recommend that the patient submit to two-view abdominal radiographs to evaluate his gut for potential foreign body obstruction. The left lateral view has been made available for you to review below.

Although you do not see an obvious foreign body, you are displeased by the accumulation of gas within the stomach and by the dilation of several loops of small bowel. This pattern is suggestive of an intestinal obstruction.

You recommend that you take Hoover to surgery for exploratory laparotomy.

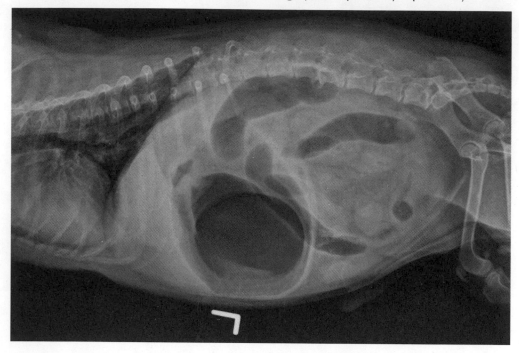

Figure 25.7 Courtesy of Daniel Foy, MS, DVM, DACVIM, DACVECC

Your tasks

To:

- summarize key radiographic findings.
- establish what Ms. Stark knows about abdominal surgery in dogs, including the potential need to cut into one or more parts of the digestive tract (that is, gastrotomy, enterotomy).
- explain that if a foreign body is identified at one or more bowel segments, then it will be surgically excised. This may require intestinal resection and anastomosis. Explore Ms. Stark's understanding of these procedures as well as potential complications.

Which communication skills will assist you with these tasks?

Scenario 25.18: Explaining Radiographs IV

You are an associate veterinarian in clinical practice, and your next appointment has arrived.

Ms. Helen Potter is a Good Samaritan who just arrived at your practice and is hoping that you can help. When she was tending to her horses in the pasture this morning, she heard a faint mew and stumbled across the path of a stray kitten that appeared to be alone wandering the field.

The kitten was non-weight-bearing on the right thoracic limb, which appeared to be edematous.

Your physical examination findings corroborate the client's observations, and you suspect that the limb is broken. You recommend that analgesia and sedation be administered to the kitten so that you can examine him. He appears to be 5–6 weeks old and a domestic short haired (DSH) kitten.

The client agrees to cover the cost of your diagnostic plan, as it is her intention to adopt him into her home if he is reparable.

Two-view radiographs of the right forelimb are taken, with comparison films of the left forelimb.

A cropped version of the lateral radiograph of the patient's right thoracic limb has been provided for your review.

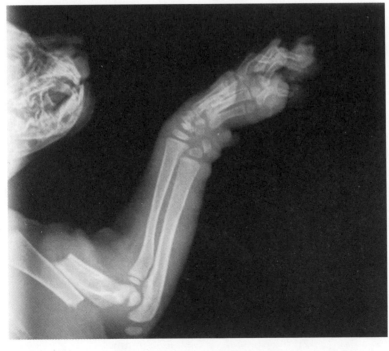

Figure 25.8 Courtesy of Genevieve LaFerriere, DVM

Your tasks

To:

- summarize key radiographic findings.
- establish what Ms. Potter knows about long bone fractures in one so young?
- explain to the client which bone is fractured and how that fracture impacts the patient's quality of life.
- consider the kitten's age and the fracture type (closed, transverse), and how these factors might impact your recommendations for how to manage this diagnosis.
- explain your recommendations for managing this fracture.

Which communication skills will assist you with these tasks?

Scenario 25.19: Explaining Bloodwork I

You are an associate veterinarian in clinical practice, and your next appointment has arrived.

Mr. John Snyder is a returning client. He is presenting his 9-year-old, castrated male, Burmese cat, Hal, for evaluation of a month-long history of increased clumps of urine in the litter box. You have known Hal for the past 4 years.

Hal lives with two other indoor-only cats, so it took Mr. Snyder a while to figure out who was eliminating, how much, and how often. Eventually, he caught Hal in the act. Although he is pleased that Hal is still using the litter box, he is concerned about the amount and frequency of his urination. Incidentally, Hal also seems to be drinking more water.

On physical examination, you note that Hal has lost 2.3 lb (1.05 kg) of body weight since his last visit four months ago. He also appears to have more pronounced, bilaterally symmetrical muscle atrophy over the hips and caudal thighs.

There is no palpable thyroid slip. The remainder of his exam is unremarkable other than mild focal gingivitis associated with the maxillary molars.

At your recommendation, Mr. Snyder agrees to proceed with baseline labwork, which includes a complete blood count (CBC), chemistry panel, and urinalysis. Hal isn't thrilled about submitting to venipuncture, and lets you and your team know of his dissatisfaction with a pulsatile tail swish.

You send the samples to an outside lab for analysis, but you do a spot-check for blood glucose and obtain the following preliminary results:

	Traditional units	SI
Sample: Serum		
Test: Blood glucose	320 mg/dL	17.76 mmol/L

Your tasks

To:

- consider the results of Hal's blood glucose spot-check in light of his attitude at today's visit: what could his resting hyperglycemia indicate?
- explain the results of Hal's blood glucose spot-check (and their significance) to the client. Which communication skill(s) will assist you with this task?
- consider if you need to change your treatment plan based upon this test result.
- consider any additional add-on tests that might be important. If so, how might you explain their necessity to the client, who has just paid a large sum of money for the initial round of diagnostic testing.

Which communication skill(s) will assist you with this task?

Scenario 25.20: Explaining Bloodwork II

You are an associate veterinarian in clinical practice.

This morning, you admitted a long-term patient into the hospital for day boarding. His name is Sunny D. Sunny D is a 7-year-old, castrated male, Sphynx cat that you diagnosed with diabetes mellitus 1 month ago.

You are still in the process of regulating his diabetes. He currently receives 1.0 unit (U) of twice daily, subcutaneous glargine insulin therapy.

At your recommendation, his "dad", Mr. Scott Shipley, dropped him off for a 12-hour blood glucose curve.

Mr. Shipley has just arrived to pick up Sunny D and to discuss the results of his blood glucose curve with you. The results are shown below:

Sample:	Serum	**Traditional units**	SI
Reading 1:	8AM	Blood glucose 480 mg/dL	26.64 mmol/L
Reading 2:	11AM	Blood glucose 373 mg/dL	20.70 mmol/L
Reading 3:	1PM	Blood glucose 391 mg/dL	21.70 mmol/L
Reading 4:	4PM	Blood glucose 246 mg/dL	13.65 mmol/L
Reading 5:	6PM	Blood glucose 320 mg/dL	17.76 mmol/L
Reading 6:	8PM	Blood glucose 456 mg/dL	25.31 mmol/L

Your tasks

To:

- consider the results of Sunny D's blood glucose curve:
  - is the insulin effective?
  - what is the duration of insulin effectiveness?
  - what is the glucose nadir?
- explain the results of Sunny D's blood glucose curve (and their significance) to the client.
- consider whether you need to change your treatment plan following these results. Do you? Why or why not? How will you explain your recommendations to the client?

Which communication skills will assist you with these tasks?

Index

abbreviations 171–2
access to information 9–11, 17
Accreditation Council for Graduate
    Medical Education (ACGME), on
    communication skills 33
active listening *see* reflective listening
active participation
    in treatment 9
    see also compliance with treatment
advice
    generic 14
    see also doctor-patient relationship;
        health literacy; veterinarian-cli-
        ent-patient relationship
agenda-setting 271–5
American Academy of Orthopedic
    Surgeons (AAOS), on communica-
    tion skills 11
American Animal Hospital Association
    (AAHA), on compliance with
    treatment 18
American Medical Association (AMA),
    ethical codes of practice 8
animal welfare
    and stress 80–2
    see also pets: patient care
anxiety 80–2
Aristotle 360
assumptions
    about clients 106, 124–5, 173–5
    about clinician 154–5
    about pets 70
autonomic responses 122, 140–1

bad news 19, 238–42
Balint model 52
barriers
    to communication 12–14, 239–40
    physical 136
    to transparency 286–7
bedside manner 28–9
biopsychosocial approach 28
blame 334–5
body language 121, 125–6
    see also nonverbal communication

Calgary–Cambridge model 52–61, 164,
    283, 299–300
Canadian Medical Association (CMA), on
    teaching communication skills 31
care
    lack of 34
    plan 265–6
cat owners, preferences of 221–2
chunk and check 257–9
clients
    access to information 17
    as advocates 15–16, 50
    assumptions about 106, 124–5, 173–5
    chatty 237–8, 278–9
    checking understanding 245–59
    comfort of 78–9
    compliance with treatment 16–19,
        153, 261–70
    dissatisfaction of 34
    educating 16–17
    and emotions 19, 106–7, 334–5
    expectations of 283–5

as experts 192–3
greeting 71–8
grief 191
guilt 334–5
information overload 233–4
medical knowledge 173–6, 184,
    224–30
perspective of 67–9, 105–6, 111, 127,
    154–5, 202–9
as 'pet parents' 105–6, 190–1
see also consultation; litigation;
    patients (human)
clinical conversations see consultation
closed-ended questions 156–9
Coe, J.B. 283–5
cognitive empathy 98–103
comfort, of client 78–9
communication
    barriers to 12–14, 239–40
    and bedside manner 29
    breakdown in 18–19
    chunk and check 257–9
    delivering bad news 19, 238–42
    distractions to 19
    effective 11, 19–20, 29–30
    failures of 34–5
    interpersonal skills 34
    and litigation 20, 30, 34
    mixed messages 142–3
    nonverbal 121–43, 238–9, 276–7
    and partnership 191–8
    poor 20
    practicing 40–2
    reflective listening 89–95
    as 'soft skill' 30, 42
    summarizing 247–57
    as teachable skill 36–9
    telephone 218–20
    training 30–43
    and understanding 14
    see also relationship-centered care
companion animals 50, 190
compassion fatigue 111–13

compliance with treatment 16–18,
    261–70
computers 136–8, 239–40
concern 28–9
connectivity 28
    see also relationship-centered care
consent 5
    see also permission
consultation
    agenda-setting 271–5
    data gathering 325–32
    empathy 98–114
    end-of-consultation summaries 252–7
    final check-in 276–9
    first impressions 67–82, 85–6
    forward planning 335–45
    greeting clients 71–8
    history taking 149–53, 311–23
    identifying presenting
        complaint 305–8
    models 50–1
    preparing for 70–1, 90, 300–3
    questions 108, 149–65
    rapport building 67–82, 303–4
    signposting 232–42
    see also Calgary–Cambridge model
Crossing the Quality Chasm: A New
    Health System for the 21st Century
    (2001) 286

death and dying 5, 241, 285–6
    see also grief
diagnosis
    and communication 15–16
    unexpected 241
    see also consultation; examination
doctor-patient relationship
    active participation 9
    bedside manner 28–9
    'doctor knows best' approach 4–6,
        211
    informed consent 5
    medical paternalism 4–7

origins of 3
patient autonomy 5–8
relationship-centered care 7–10,
    27–32, 50–2
withholding information 4–5
see also patients; veterinarian-cli-
    ent-patient relationship
dog owners, preferences of 221–2
Draper, J. 53

effective communication 11, 19–20,
    29–30
emotional empathy 103
emotions
    of clients 106–7, 334–5
    impact on compliance 19
empathy 28–9, 98–114
    compassion fatigue 111–13
    dangers of 111–12
    decline of 113–14
    human-animal bond 105
    showing 109–11
    versus sympathy 104–5
Engel, G. 28, 123
ethical codes of practice 8
ethics 9
examination 327–32
eye contact 130–1

facial expressions 131–2
false hope 5
feedback 37
feline anxiety 81
Fetzer Institute 31
final check-in 276–9
first impressions 67–82, 85–6
following-up 34
forward planning 335–45

gender
    and judgment making 124
    misidentification of 302
    and touch 134

gender-neutral names 70
generic advice 14
gestures 132–3
Great Gatsby, The 132
greeting clients 71–8
Gregory, J. 6–7
grief 191
guilt 334–5

handshakes 132–3
head shaking 130
health literacy 10–12, 15–16
height, differences in 135
Hippocrates 3
Hippocratic Oath 3–4, 211
history taking 149–53, 311–23
    see also consultation
human-animal bond 105
humanistic approach 28, 89

information
    access to 9–11, 17
    accuracy of 17
    cramming 19
    overload 233–4
    sensitive 220–1
    withholding 4–5
informed consent 5
Institute of Medicine, on
    patient-centeredness 28–9
internet, as source of information 17
interpersonal skills 34
    see also bedside manner;
        communication

jargon 12, 169–86

Kalamazoo Consensus Statement 31–2
Kedrowicz, A.A. 73
kinesics 125–6
Kurtz, S.M. 53

laughing 132

leaflets 12
    see also health literacy
LeBlanc, T.W. 40–1
listening 87–95, 153–4
    reflective listening 89–95
litigation 20, 30, 34
    prevalent complaints 34

Maguire, P. 30–1
Makoul, G. 72
malpractice claims 20, 30
Marvel, M.K. 154
medical documents 185–6
medical error 241
medical jargon *see* jargon
medical paternalism 4–7, 27, 49–50, 86, 211
medical records 238–40
medicine
    and relationship-centered care 8–10
    teaching and training 32
mirroring 129
mixed messages 142–3

negligence claims 34
    see also litigation
neoplasia 4
noncompliance 153
nonverbal communication 121–43, 238–9, 276–7
North American Veterinary Medical Education Consortium (NAVMEC), on communication training 36
numeracy skills 14

O'Donnell, R. 105
Oken, D. 4
oncology 176
open-ended questions 155–65
oral literacy 11, 13
Osler, W. 49–50
Ospina, N.S. 154
owners *see* clients

paralanguage 121, 138–9
partnership 191–8, 212–13
    see also relationship-centered care
paternalism *see* medical paternalism
patient-centeredness 28–9
patients (human)
    access to information 9–11
    autonomy of 5–8, 31–2
    families and support networks 31
    health literacy 10–12
    medical history 28
    medical knowledge 173–6
    perspective of 31–2, 67–8
    self-efficacy 12
    see also communication; pets
Pearce, C. 138
pediatric medicine 15–16
permission 213–14
'pet parents' 16, 105–6, 190–1
pets
    advocacy for 15–16, 50
    assumptions about 70
    care plan 265–6
    as companion animals 50, 190
    compliance with treatment 16–19
    death of 241
    diagnosis 16
    history taking 149–53, 311–23
    patient care 263–5
    stress during consultation 80–2
physical barriers 136
posture 128
    see also body language
print literacy 10–11, 12
privacy 79
professionalism, lack of 34
proxemics 135

questions 108
    closed-ended 156–9
    open-ended 155–65

rapport building 67, 303–4
reflective listening 89–95
regard 28–9
relationship-centered care 7–10, 27–32, 50–2, 67, 190–8
    as partnership 202–9, 211–22
    teamwork 261–3
RENO mnemonic 86
Rogers, C. 89, 290
role-play 37–8

self-efficacy 12
sensitivity 28–9
sharing information 220–1
signposting 232–42
Silverman, J.D. 53
sincerity 28–9
smiling 132
speech 139–40
    see also communication
stress 80–2
summarizing 247–57
sympathy 104–5
    see also empathy
symptom management 177–8

teamwork 261–3
telemedicine 60
terminal diagnosis
    disclosing 4–5
    see also death and dying
To Err is Human (1999) 285–6
touch 133–5
training
    in communication skills 30–43
    feedback 37
    role-play 37–8
transparency 285–9
    lack of 34
treatment, compliance with 16–18, 261–70
triage 13
tripartite relationship 51

see also veterinarian-client-patient relationship

unconditional positive regard 19, 290–4
United States Medical Licensing Examination (USMLE), on communication skills 33

veterinarian-client-patient relationship 51, 57, 86
    compliance with treatment 16–19
    damage to 35
    delivering bad news 19
    empathy 98–114
    and health literacy 15–16
    rapport building 67–82
    reflective listening 91–5
    relationship building 51
    see also communication; consultation
veterinarians
    as 'expert in charge' 211–12
    as 'pet parents' 16
veterinary education, and communication skills 33
Volk, J.O. 81

warmth 28–9
'warning shots' 238–42
Wible, P. 88
withholding information 4–5